KV-577-293

Acknowledgements

The authors would like to thank Gary Vaux, Margaret Richards and Luke Clements for their contributions to the checking of this new *Handbook*.

Special thanks are due to Sue Ramsden, without whose efforts in checking the law and practice relating to Scotland, which was beyond the knowledge and experience of the authors, this *Handbook* would not have been possible. Acknowledgements are also due for the assistance she received from Mark Brough of The Action Group, and from Money Advice Scotland and the Scottish Refugee Council.

Special thanks are also owed to Deborah Lyttelton at CPAG for her remarkably supportive and tolerant role in the editorial process which steered the *Handbook* past many icebergs, and to Peter Ridpath, Ela Sedzik and Chris Bullivant at CPAG for their roles in the production process. Thanks also to Paula McDiarmid for copy editing the book and Pam Scott for devising the index.

Geoff Tait is especially grateful (and hopeful they will never have cause to read a word of the final product) to Lorraine for her tireless support and inspiration and cups of tea during lost weekends, to Ben, Max and Gemma, and to Dr Steven Earnshaw for his postmodernist contributions.

Pauline Thompson would like to thank all the people she contacted while writing this book who gave invaluable information about community care practice. She is also grateful to the staff at the National Assembly for Wales for their patient checking of Welsh circulars, and explanations of where there are differences between Wales and England. Above all, she would like to thank Michael Mandelstam whose book *Community Care Law and Practice* and many phone conversations with him proved to be an invaluable starting point for finding the numerous pieces of legislation needed for this *Handbook*.

Helen Winfield is especially grateful to Jimmy for his encouragement and support, to Ciara who is too young to understand but did her bit by sleeping through the nights, and to mom and dad for their support and babysitting skills.

The authors have made their best endeavours to try to ensure that the law covered in this *Handbook* was correct as at 30th November 1999.

Contents

Part 6:   Future trends

Preface

The purpose and scope of this Handbook

Since the community care reforms came into force in 1993, there has been a revolution in social services law and practice as it applies to older people, people with physical disabilities, learning difficulties, long-term illnesses, mental health problems or addictions, and their carers. The current social security scheme is also the result of many revolutions, and remains massive in scope. Although it will affect nearly all individuals at some time in the course of their lives, it has a particular effect on vulnerable adults which, in turn also impacts on carers and the responsibilities of social services departments. It has become increasingly questionable whether the social security and community care schemes have kept up with the pace of change or the emerging policy directions of each other.

This *Handbook* aims to draw together the effects of the laws relating to social security and community care and consider how they work in practice and how they may be made to work better within the limitations which exist. It aims to provide a guide for adults in need of care and support, their carers and relatives, and professionals involved in administering or advising on the effects of each scheme.

It is clear that some people are fortunate enough not to require any financial assistance from social services or health authorities or the DSS to meet their needs even if they have significant personal care needs due to old age, health problems or disabilities. More commonly, however, many will need at least some assistance, whether by way of care, or by cash, or in kind. This applies whether they are able to live at home in the community, or whether they need to live in a care home. The costs of a care home in particular, however, are such that the majority of people will sooner or later need some financial assistance, usually from social services or the DSS, and commonly nowadays from both. There will often, however, be a significant price to be paid by those who need assistance with the costs of a care home, and this needs to be understood if proper consideration is to be given (not only by individuals in need of care and their relatives and carers, but also by social services and health authorities responsible for assisting them in meeting their needs) to alternative means available for supporting those who may otherwise be able to continue to live independently at home in the community instead.

The different responsibilities of government agencies for assisting those with insufficient means of their own to meet the costs of their care home have now largely replaced those which were previously the primary responsibility of the Department of Social Security. The Department of Social Security has retained the primary responsibility in the case of those with 'preserved rights' from the time before the community care reforms took effect in 1993. For those with 'preserved rights', the arrangements for claiming assistance are undoubtedly rather more straightforward than for those entering care homes since then, but such arrangements are not without their own problems.

For many of those who have entered a care home since 1993, it is undoubtedly the case that the new arrangements are adequately achieving their objectives, and the different responsibilities of social services and the Department of Social Security will often cause few problems. Whatever their own means, residents in care homes are likely to be left with a small personal allowance at least, which may suffice to meet their needs, and social services will often take on responsibility for sorting out any claims for benefits which may assist with the resident's costs (and thereby reduce their own expenditure).

For others, however, the way in which assistance is calculated may have a significant bearing on how much money they will be left with. Those who have been able to achieve significant incomes from independent sources (such as private pension schemes) will often find themselves no better off than those of more modest means. Others may be able to supplement their incomes from savings which are ignored by the means tests, but for those with capital assets, particularly the value of their own homes, the slightly different means tests applied by social services and the DSS will have a crucial bearing on whether or not it may be better (for them or their relatives who may otherwise stand to gain from the proceeds of the sale of a home) to arrange to pay for their care home without any contractual involvement by social services.

Part 1 sets out an overview of the community care and social security schemes, and covers the background, history and policy intention behind them. It also explains the different responsibilities and roles of the Department of Health, Department of Social Security, social services departments and health authorities in providing for the care and support needs of adults.

Part Two covers the range of services and assistance available to adults living at home in the community. It explains the range of community care services – and charges which may be paid for them (Chapter 2) – and social security benefits (Chapter 3) – on which charges for community care services (and the ability to pay them) also often depend – and other sources of financial assistance (Chapter 4) which may be available for independent living. It also explains the range of supported housing for which housing benefit may often be available to enable people to continue to live independently in the community as an alternative to residential or nursing care (Chapter 5).

Part 3 deals with the general provisions which relate to many of the social security benefits for people living at home in the community and which generally also apply if they need to live in care homes. It provides details of the means test which applies to certain benefits (Chapters 6-7) and the responsibilities of the liable relatives of those who claim them (Chapter 8). It also deals with how social security benefits are administered (Chapter 10), the special rules which apply to particular groups of claimant (Chapter 9) and common problems which arise (Chapter 11).

Part 4 deals with the general provisions which apply to social services departments and health authorities when a person needs residential or nursing care. It covers the duties of social services and health authorities in arranging for accommodation in care homes (Chapter 12); the means test in relation to income which social services must apply when assisting someone with the costs of a care home (Chapter 13) and, often more importantly, capital (Chapter 14); the amounts of any personal allowance which most people will be left with to meet their own expenses for any needs not provided in the home (Chapter 15); the responsibilities of their liable relatives (Chapter 17), and the responsibilities of other individuals to pay for care home charges (Chapter 16). It also deals with how social services departments may go about recovering any charges owing to them (Chapter 19); how social services assistance is administered (Chapter 20); and the special rules which apply to particular groups (Chapter 18).

Part 5 explains the effect of going into a care home on claims for benefits (Chapters 21 and 22); how social services calculate the charges people must contribute to the costs of their care home if help is being provided (Chapter 23); and common problems which arise (Chapter 24).

Finally *Part 6*, acknowledging that social security and community care provision is in a continuing state of evolution, looks towards the future to consider the impact of changes which may be more or less likely to occur in due course.

For reasons of space, there are a number of areas which are beyond the scope of this book. In particular, this *Handbook* does not attempt to cover in any significant detail the very different responsibilities of welfare agencies which may apply in respect of young people (under the age of 18) and children in need. Nor does this book cover the different private financial or insurance arrangements which individuals may have the opportunity to make so that they do not require state assistance for their care needs (although some of these are briefly referred to in Chapter 1). Where appropriate, however, references are made in the text to other sources of information on particular aspects which may be of interest but which are not covered in the *Handbook*.

How to use this *Handbook*

This *Handbook* aims to provide all the information you will need about claiming practical and financial assistance in meeting your care needs from social services, health authorities and the Department of Social Security. It aims to give practical help in the areas where disputes are likely to arise between those who need assistance and those who are responsible for administering and providing it. If you not satisfied with the help you are being offered, the *Handbook* aims to guide you in challenging decisions made about you.

The organisation of the **contents** is explained at the beginning of this preface. The main subjects in each chapter are also summarised in the contents page at the front of the *Handbook*. The main subject heads and page numbers are repeated at the beginning of each chapter.

It is often helpful to refer to the sources from which the information in the text is drawn, which is the relevant law and official guidance, as well as caselaw which often clarifies what the law and guidance should mean in practice. **References** to these are given in the notes found at the end of each chapter and are numbered in the order in which they appear in the text. The references are usually to Acts or Regulations, but sometimes they are to formal guidance issued by the Departments of Health or Social Security, and sometimes to caselaw. In order to save space, the notes are in abbreviated form, but the abbreviations used are explained in Appendix 6.

Abbreviations are often also used in the text to save space, but an abbreviation is always given in full the first time it is used in a chapter or section (followed by the abbreviation in brackets).

The **index**, like the contents, will also help you to find the information you are looking for. Entries in bold type direct you to the general information on the subject, or where the subject is covered more fully. Sub-entries under the bold headings are listed alphabetically and direct you to specific aspects of the subject.

There are many **cross-references** in the text which are also designed to assist you in finding other relevant information about a particular topic. They give either the chapter or page number(s), as appropriate.

Whereas many of the sources of information about social security benefits will be familiar to readers of other CPAG Handbooks (and these are set out in Appendix 4), the main **sources** of legislative powers and duties of social services departments may be less familiar, and for ease of reference these are set out in full in Appendix 1 (followed by a list of key guidance circulars in Appendix 2).

The contents of this *Handbook* are intended to set out the authors' understanding of the relevant law as it stood at the end of November 1999 (although every attempt has also been made to also include details of any changes anticipated to take effect by the time of publication). Further changes due to take effect by April 2000 are also referred to in the main text. Changes planned for the longer term are considered in Part 6. The *Handbook* covers the law and practice which applies in England and Wales (and includes references to some differences in sources of guidance and terminology). The different provisions which apply to Scotland, but which more often than not are of similar effect, have also been covered. Although much of the law relating to social security is similar in effect in Northern Ireland, the very different arrangements for health and social welfare generally (although also sometimes similar in effect) are such that it has not been possible to cover them in this *Handbook*.

Because the areas of policy, practice, law, caselaw and guidance covered in this *Handbook* are notoriously the subject of constant change, readers are urged to use the *Handbook* in conjunction with other sources which may provide regular updates or may provide more extensive detail on particular aspects which are beyond the scope of this *Handbook* (such as those sources referred to in Appendix 5). It is, however intended that this *Handbook* will be revised annually so that each new edition will aim to provide a guide which will be up-to-date at the time of publication and which will highlight particular areas which will be likely to change in the near future.

This *Handbook* has, moreover, been produced in a very short timescale to very tight deadlines and the authors readily acknowledge that some errors or omissions may become apparent, which the authors would wish to rectify in future editions. Any comments from any readers which may be considered to improve the contents of the text or the structure or the general usefulness of the *Handbook* in future editions would be gratefully received (and should be sent c/o CPAG).

Geoff Tait
Pauline Thompson
Helen Winfield
David Simmons
November 1999

Abbreviations used in the text

AA	Attendance allowance
AM	Assembly Member
AMA	Adjudicating medical authority
AO	Adjudication officer
BAMS	Benefits Agency Medical Service
CCG	Community care grant
CTB	Council tax benefit
DAT	Disability appeal tribunal
DLA mobility	Disability living allowance – mobility component
DLA care	Disability living allowance – care component
DPTC	Disabled person's tax credit
DSS	Department of Social Security
EC	European Community
ECJ	European Court of Justice
EEC	European Economic Community
EMO	Examining medical officer
EU	European Union
GP	General practitioner
HB	Housing benefit
IB	Incapacity benefit
ICA	Invalid care allowance
IS	Income support
MAT	Medical appeal tribunal
MP	Member of Parliament
MSP	Member of Scottish Parliament
PAYE	Pay-As-You-Earn
REA	Reduced earnings allowance
SDA	Severe disablement allowance
SERPS	State Earnings-Related Pension Scheme
SF	Social fund
SFI	Social fund inspector
SFO	Social fund officer
SHCU	Severe hardship claims unit
SHP	Severe hardship payment
SSAT	Social security appeal tribunal
SSP	Statutory sick pay
WFTC	Working families' tax credit

Benefit rates

April 1999 to April 2000

Income support (and income-based jobseeker's allowance)

Personal allowances
1999/00, 2000/01

Single

Under 18 years (usual rate)	£30.95
Under 18 years (higher rate)	£40.70
18 to 24 years	£40.70
25 years and over	£51.40

Lone parent

Under 18 years (usual rate)	£30.95
Under 18 years (higher rate)	£40.70
18 to 24 years	£51.40

Couple

Both under 18 years (higher rate)	£61.35
Both over 18 years	£80.65

Children

Under 16 years	£25.90
16 years and over	£30.95

Premiums

Family	Ordinary rate	£13.90
	Lone parent rate*	£15.75
Disability	Single	£21.90
	Couple	£31.25
Pensioner (60 to 74 years)	Single	£23.60
	Couple	£35.95
Enhanced pensioner (75 to 79 years)	Single	£25.95
	Couple	£39.20
Higher Pensioner	Single	£30.85
	Couple	£44.65
Severe disability	per qualifying person	£39.75
Disabled child	each child	£21.90
Carers		£13.95

Housing and council tax benefit

Personal allowances
Single

16 to 24 years	£40.70
25 years and over	£51.40

Lone parent

Under 18 years	£40.70
18 years and over	£51.40

Couple

Both under 18 years	£61.35
One or both over 18 years	£80.65

Children As for income support
Premiums As for Income
support except:

Lone parent rate family premium*	£22.05

(*only paid on claims beginning before 6th April 1998.)

Residential/Nursing care (private)

Personal expenses allowance		£14.75
Residential allowance	Greater London	£66.10
	Elsewhere	£59.40

'Preserved rights' residents (before April 1993)

Health condition	Residential care home	Nursing home
Elderly (age 60 or over)	£218	£325
Very dependent elderly	£252	£325
Mental disorder (other than mental handicap)	£230	£326
Drug or alcohol dependence	£230	£326
Mental handicap	£262	£332
Physical disablement under pensionable age	£298	£367

The above amounts are increased by £45 for a residential care home and £50 for a nursing home in Greater London.

Accommodation allowance	Maximum payable
Breakfast per day	£1.10
Midday/Evening meal (per day)	£1.55

Hospital

Single (after 52 weeks)	£13.35
Single (less than 52 weeks)	£16.70
Couple (both in hospital)	£33.40
Couple (one in hospital, reduced by)	£13.35

Working families' tax credit (WFTC)

Fixed applicable amount	£90.00
Maximum working families' tax credit: couple or lone parent:	£49.80
Additional full-time work (30 hrs) credit	£11.05
Children under 11 years	£19.85
Children 11 to 15 years	£20.90
Children 16 years or over	£25.95

Childcare credit 70 per cent of costs up to £100.00 1 child
£150.00 2 or more children

Disabled person's tax credit (DPTC)
Fixed applicable amount:

	Single	£70.00
	Couple	£90.00
Maximum DPTC:	Single	£54.30
	Couple/Lone parent	£83.55
Disabled child		£21.90
Additional full-time work (30 hrs) credit		£11.05
Children	Under 11 years	£19.85
Children	11 to 15 years	£20.90
Children	16 years or over	£25.95

Child care credit 70 per cent of costs up to £100 1 child
£150 2 or more children

Additional earnings disregard where WFTC or DPTC in payment or working 30 hours or more and family premium, disability premium or higher pensioner premium payment.

Capital rules

Disregard	(for IS/JSA/HB/CTB/ FC/DWA)	**£3,000.00
Upper limit	(for IS/JSA/FC)	**£8,000.00
	(for HB/CTB/DWA)	£16,000.00

** For residential/nursing care
(for IS/JSA)

	Disregard	£10,000.00
	Upper limit	£16,000.00

Earnings disregard (for IS/JSA/HB/CTB)

Single person	£5.00
Couple	£10.00
Disability, carers or higher pension premium in payment	£15.00
Lone parents (IS/JSA only)	£15.00
Lone parents (HB/CTB only)	£25.00

Other disregards (for HB/CTB/DWA/FC/WFTC/DPTC)
Maintenance disregard:
for HB/CTB only £15.00
all maintenance disregarded for WFTC/DPTC
Childcare allowance:

For HB/CTB	One child	£60.00
	Two or more	£100.00

Non-dependant deductions
(from HB and IS/JSA housing costs)

Under 25 years on IS/JSA	NIL
Over 25 years on IS/JSA	£7.20
Over 18 years not working	£7.20
Full-time work, gross income under £80.00	£7.20
£80.00 to £117.99	£16.50
£118.00 to £154.99	£22.65
£155.00 to £203.99	£37.10
£204.00 to £254.99	£42.25
£255.00 or more	£46.35

(From CTB)

On IS/JSA (any age)	NIL
Over 18 years not in full-time work	£2.15
Full-time work, gross income under £118.00	£2.15
£118.00 to £203.99	£4.30
£204.00 to £254.99	£5.40
£255.00 or more	£6.50

Second Adult Rebates
(Alternative maximum council tax benefit)

Second adult(s) on IS/JSA	25%
Second adult(s) income less than £118.00	15%
Income £118.00 to £154.00	7.5%

Attendance allowance

Lower rate	£35.40
Higher rate	£52.95

Child benefit

First, only or eldest child:	Ordinary rate	£14.40
	Lone parent rate[†]	£17.10
Each subsequent child		£9.60
Child special or guardians allowance		£11.35

[†] Only paid on claims
beginning for 1st June 1998

Disability living allowance

Care component	Higher	£52.95
	Middle	£35.40
	Lower	£14.05
Mobility component	Higher	£37.00
	Lower	£14.05

Incapacity benefit
Claimant
Long term	£66.75
Short term lower	£50.35
Short term higher	£59.55
Short term over pensionable age	£64.05

Spouse/Adult dependant
Long term	£39.95
Short term lower/higher	£31.15
Short term over pensionable age	£38.40

Dependant child*
All rates	£11.35

Age addition
Incapacity before age 35 years	£14.05
Incapacity age 35 to 44 years	£7.05

Alternative transitional age addition
Incapacity before age 40 years	£14.05
Incapacity age 40 to 49 years	£8.90
Incapacity age 50 to 59 years – men	£4.45
Incapacity aged 50 to 54 years – women	£4.45
Therapeutic earnings limit	£58.00

Industrial death benefit
Widow's pension:	Higher permanent rate	£66.75
	Lower permanent rate	£20.03

Industrial disablement benefit
Maximum 100 per cent	£108.10
Minimum 14 per cent	£21.62
Reduced earnings allowance** maximum	£43.24
Retirement allowance** maximum	£10.81
(** For disablement before October 1990 only.)	

Invalid care allowance
Claimant	£39.95
Spouse/Adult dependent	£23.90
Dependant child*	£11.35
Earnings limit for claimant	£50.00

Jobseeker's allowance (contribution-based)

Aged 18 to 24 years	£40.70
Aged 25 years and over	£51.40
Occupational pension limit	£50.00

Maternity allowance

Lower rate	£51.70
Higher rate	£59.55
Husband/adult dependant	£31.15

Retirement pension

Single person (basic)	£66.75
Spouse/adult dependant	£39.95
Dependant child*	£11.35
Non-contributory (over 80 years)	£39.95
Age addition for over 80 years	£0.25

Severe disablement allowance

Claimant	£40.35
Spouse/Adult dependant	£23.95
Dependant child*	£11.35

Age related additions

Under 40 years	£14.05
40 to 49 years	£8.90
50 to 59 years	£4.45

Statutory maternity pay

Higher rate	90% of average earnings
Lower rate	£59.95
Earnings threshold	£66.00

Statutory sick pay

Standard rate	£59.55
Earnings threshold	£66.00

Widow's benefit

Widows payment (lump sum)	£1,000.00
Widowed mothers allowance	£66.75
Widow's pension (standard rate)	£66.75
Dependant child*	£11.35

(*All child dependant allowance reduced by £1.45 for first child.)

Part 1

Introduction

Chapter 1

∙∙∙

Introduction

This chapter gives a brief overview of community care and the changes that have occurred since 1993 following the NHS and Community Care Act 1990. It looks at the systems in place to deliver the services, and the arrangements you can make yourself to pay for services. It covers

1. What is community care? (p3)
2. Community care changes in 1993 (p5)
3. Systems to deliver services and benefits (p9)
4. Arrangements you can make yourself to pay for services (p14)

---

1. **What is community care?**

Although community care (or care in the community) is a term which has a common usage, it is one of those terms which can mean all things to all people. Some people think of it as excluding residential or nursing care, yet the amendments that were necessary to the social security rules as a consequence of the NHS and Community Care Act 1990 were totally concerned with the rules for benefits in residential and nursing home care. No rule changes were necessary for people living in their own homes. Many residential and nursing home owners go to considerable lengths to ensure that their care home is part of the local community and that residents can make use of local facilities. Equally, staying long term in hospital does not necessarily mean you are no longer part of the community. The hospital itself may be a vital part of the community giving employment to local people and utilising local services.

Others take the view that community care encompasses *anything* which helps older or disabled people remain in their homes for as long as possible. In addition to the services described in the chapters of this *Handbook* they include all the informal care that goes on as part of everyday life. Community care could, therefore, encompass help from friends, relatives, and neighbours. It would include the role of local facilities such as pubs and hairdressers in welcoming older or disabled people. It could also include ways that the local environment supports all people, including paths being in a good state of repair, accessible transport and buildings, and actions which ensure people feel safe to go out – eg, adequate policing and lighting.

The working definition

The previous government in its 1989 White Paper gave the following definition of community care.

> Community care means providing the right level of intervention and support to enable people to achieve maximum independence and control over their own lives. For this aim to become a reality, the development of a wide range of services provided in a variety of settings is essential. These services form part of a spectrum of care, ranging from domiciliary support provided to people in their own homes, strengthened by the availability of respite care and day care for those with more intensive care needs, through sheltered housing, group homes and hostels where increasing levels of care are available, to residential care and nursing homes and long-stay hospital care for those for whom other forms of care are no longer enough.[1]

The White Paper went on to recognise that in reality most care is not provided by statutory bodies but by family, friends and neighbours, so the right level of support for them at the right time is vital. It also confirmed the important role of health care, and the role of the social security system in providing financial support through the benefits system.

It would be fair to say that the aims of community care remain the same under the present government. However, the previous government's introduction of direct payments added a new dimension where, in addition to providing services, people were given the ability to purchase their own services. In its White Paper, the current government outlines planned changes aiming to lead to the following improvements:

- people will be offered a service that is designed not just to keep them going, but to improve their capabilities and allow them maximum possible independence;
- when people need social services help, that help will be arranged in a way that lets them do as much as possible for themselves; and allows them wherever possible to live in their own homes;
- many more people will be able to have real control over their care support through direct payment schemes;
- health and social services will target their support especially on people who are at risk of losing their independence (for instance elderly people living alone during the winter; people who have just left hospital, or who have a visual impairment, and are finding it hard to cope at home), to make sure that special efforts are made to avoid such people having to be admitted to hospital or a care home;
- carers who look after family members, neighbours or friends will be given greater support by social services and other agencies, to allow them to

continue to care where that is what they and the person they are caring for want.[2]

How far the practice of community care lives up to the aims is a source of debate. There is no doubt that some individuals receive excellent services which provide them with the sort of care they need at the time they need it. Equally, the measures that authorities have adopted due to resource constraints described in Chapters 2 and 12 and the extent to which the social security system supports people in need, can leave individuals and their families in a state of high anxiety about whether they will get the services they need, and whether they will be able to afford them.

2. Community care changes in 1993

Although the 1993 changes to the legislation are of paramount importance to the way community care is now delivered, there appear to be two major misconceptions. These are that:
- community care was new in 1993; *and*
- it is only from that date that people have been charged for the services they receive, or for residential or nursing care.

Community care before 1993

The movement to close long-stay hospitals, in particular for those with a learning disability or a mental health problem, had actually started as far back as the 1970s, as a result of a concerns about costs, various high profile cases of abuse, as well as pressure from campaigning groups and staff for these clients to have more normal lives than could ever be achieved in hospital settings.[3]

Measures to enable people to remain in their own homes date back to the National Assistance Act 1948, and statements remarkably similar to the current exhortations on community care can be found periodically since then. The Ministry of Health stated in its Annual Report for 1953 that there was 'universal recognition of the urgency of the task enabling old people to go on living in their own homes as long as possible'.[4]

The services listed in the NHS and Community Care Act 1990 as community care services were not new but arose from legislation enacted between 1948 and 1983. These services are explained in detail in Chapter 2.

Charges for care

Many people are surprised to find that since 1948 charges for residential care have been mandatory, and discretionary for domiciliary care.

There were relatively few changes made in 1993 to the charging regime for residential care as there were already provisions for charging residents who lived in local authority accommodation. Residents in local authority homes who had their own property were expected to sell it in order to pay for the cost of their care, just as they are today.

A number of social services departments charged for domiciliary services before 1993 under the discretionary charging rules. The main change since 1993 is that this number has radically increased. Fewer social services departments charge a low 'flat rate' but instead have charging regimes which reflect the number of hours of care received and are based on a means-test. Also, more services, in particular day care, have become subject to charging.

Charging through DSS benefits

In the early 1980s the Department of Health and Social Security (DHSS) made changes to the supplementary benefit regulations which allowed benefits to be claimed to help with fees in independent residential and nursing homes. There was a huge expansion of independent sector homes when benefits initially meeting the full costs (although they were later capped and set at a national level). At the same time, hospitals were cutting the number of long-stay beds and taking advantage of the fact that many residents could have their fees met by social security benefits. For those who were entitled to benefits, it really made little financial difference whether they were funded in a hospital bed or paid benefits so that they could pay for the residential or nursing care. For many, the more homely environment of a residential or nursing home was far more preferable to a long-stay hospital ward.

However, not all those who were unable to remain in hospital, but who needed residential or nursing care, were able to receive supplementary benefit (or later income support) to help with fees. Those with a high income would have to use it towards their fees. If you had capital rising from £1,250 in 1980 to £8,000 in 1991, and to £16,000 in 1996, you would be expected to pay the full cost of the fees yourself.

Just as now, a person's home was taken into account unless it was disregarded because of someone who lived in it. Six months was allowed for the home to be sold, or longer if necessary. Once it was sold, however, or if capital was over the supplementary benefit/income support capital limits, residents of care homes had to fund themselves until their capital reached the level at which they became entitled to benefit. You were effectively being charged because you had to meet your fees under a direct arrangement with the care home.

The background to the changes

This *Handbook* does not give a detailed analysis of the reasons for the changes that came about in 1993. Some of the main texts on the subject are listed in

Appendix 5. Undoubtedly part of the incentive for change was concern about the rapidly growing costs to the social security budget for residential and nursing home fees – ie, from £10 million in 1979 to over £1,000 million by May 1989.[5] There was concern that with no controls over who went into residential or nursing homes, money which could be spent on helping people to remain in the community was increasingly going into the residential sector.

In December 1986 the government set up a review under the chairmanship of Sir Roy Griffiths to 'review the way in which public funds are used to support community care policy and to advise... on the options for action that would improve the use of these funds as a contribution to more effective community care'. The report was published in March 1988 and the White Paper *Caring For People,* published in November 1989, endorsed many of Griffiths' proposals. The changes were due to come into force in April 1991 but were put back for two years to allow more time for implementation.

The main changes

In essence, what the 1993 changes did was give social services the lead in providing access to services. This was to some extent a new role in relation to residential and nursing home care in the independent sector (although social services had long made decisions about who went into their own residential accommodation). It was a more familiar role in relation to domiciliary services where social services, as the main provider of domiciliary care, had made decisions about whether it was necessary for them to provide it or not.

This 'gatekeeping' role would be done through assessment and care management which were seen as the cornerstones of high quality care and formalised the process of decision-making and the management of cases once services were provided or arranged.

From 1993, in order to have services provided or arranged by social services, you first had to be assessed as needing them. It was not envisaged that social services would necessarily provide the services, but would promote the development of a flourishing independent sector alongside good quality public services. Care management would thus involve budgeting for an individual's care, buying in services from the public and the independent sector. Many social services departments were divided into separate units: purchasers who commission services; and providers who provide the services (eg, home care or local authority homes) as part of the social services functions.

Social services, if they considered that you needed residential care, would either provide it themselves in one of their own homes or buy it from the independent sector. To do that, money was transferred from the DSS, to be allocated to social services. It was calculated on what the DSS would have spent if it had continued to pay benefits at the residential and nursing home rates. Social services could then use the money allocated to provide the most appropriate form of care, either at home or in a care home.

It was hoped that in the long term fewer people would need residential or nursing home care as more received the help they needed in their own homes. The aim was that there should not be any incentive in favour of residential and nursing home care, as there had been under social security.[6]

Social services had previously been allowed to arrange for residential care in the independent sector, but the new provisions allowed them for the first time also to buy care in nursing homes.[7] This was because the DSS had previously paid benefits to people in nursing homes. It was, therefore, seen as part of the transfer from the DSS rather than any major shift from NHS responsibilities. This recently came under the spotlight in a case held in the Court of Appeal and the judgment gives an interesting history of the relationship between nursing care as a health or social service.[8]

The transfer of money from the DSS

The 1993 changes meant that instead of entitlement to benefits to meet the cost of residential or nursing care, social services now had liability for the fees if they decided such care was needed. Charges were then made according to national rules very similar (but not quite the same) as the rules for income support (IS). These rules are explained in detail in Chapters 13, 14, 15, 16 and 17 and 23 and 24.

However, those who were in independent residential or nursing care on 31 March 1993 kept their entitlement to the higher benefit levels that had been paid before April 1993 under preserved rights (see Chapter 22). If you have been in a residential or nursing home care since before 1 April 1993 and now, for the first time, need help with your fees, you should go to the Benefits Agency, not social services.

Even if you went into residential care after April 1993 the DSS still make some payments to you in the form of non-means-tested benefits – eg, your pension or incapacity benefit and any IS to which you might be entitled. The original intention was that the rent element of residential care costs would be met by housing benefit, in the same way as rent at home, but it was generally felt that having a third department involved in funding would be an added complication in an already complex area, and so the residential allowance was added to the IS calculation for those in independent residential and nursing homes. You therefore often need to apply to social services and to the Benefits Agency to get all the help to which you are entitled.

The 1993 community care changes did not affect social security benefits for those living at home.

A formula was worked out to reflect the amount of money which would have been spent by the DSS if it had continued to pay new residents (ie, after April 1993) the higher levels of IS. This money was then passed over to social services in the form of a special transitional grant. There has been much debate as to whether the amount was either correct or adequate, and there are continuing concerns over the levels of funding of community care.

The legislative changes

The 1993 changes were the result of the NHS and Community Care Act 1990. They are contained in nine sections of the Act covering:
- the ability to purchase residential accommodation from independent residential and nursing homes;
- the exclusion of this ability in the cases of people who have preserved rights;
- the setting of a standard charge for those in independent sector homes and the recovery of the charge from the resident based on the ability to pay;
- the requirement to have a community care plan;
- the assessment of needs for community care services;
- inspection of residential premises;
- the setting up of a complaints procedure;
- the default powers of the Secretary of State;
- grants to local authorities for services to the mentally ill.[9]

The Act did not consolidate previous legislation but merely made alterations to it, most notably the National Assistance Act 1948. The Act only outlined the changes with regulations, and policy and practice guidance (see p24) providing the details of how the changes were to be implemented. The 1993 community care legislation made no changes to either health or housing functions, but concentrated entirely on the duties and functions of social services as the lead agency.

In Scotland the National Assistance Act 1948 provides the legal basis for charging for residential and nursing home care. Part IV of the NHS and Community Care Act 1990 amends the Social Work (Scotland) Act 1968 and outlines local authority responsibilities for community care as listed above.

3. **Systems to deliver services and benefits**

If you need help in the form of services or benefits you should normally first contact your local social services or housing department or the Benefits Agency, depending on the nature of your need. If you have a health need you should see your district nurse or GP. If you go to the wrong department or person, they should be able to tell you which department you need.

This section describes briefly the role of central government departments in providing services locally and the structure of those local services. Chapter 2 describes in more detail the individual responsibilities of health, housing and social services and where those responsibilities overlap.

Please note that the terms social services or social services department have been used throughout this handbook. Scottish readers should take these terms to refer to social work departments, the term usually used in Scotland. Similarly the use of the term health authority, should be read as health board in Scotland.

Health services

Responsibility for the overall policy for health services lies with the Department of Health (England), the National Assembly for Wales and Scottish Executive Health Department. They set the framework of policy objectives and resources for the delivery and administration of health services. They issue guidance and circulars to health authorities (health boards in Scotland), NHS and community care trusts and independent providers such as GPs and dentists. In relation to community care, the same guidance is often issued to social services.

Health authorities set policies at local level for the resident population and are responsible for commissioning an appropriate range of health services to meet local needs. Those include hospitals and community nursing and pharmaceutical services, GPs, dentists, and opticians. Although not democratically elected, health authorities are accountable locally and are required to consult their local community.

An area might have both NHS trusts, which provide hospital services, and community health trusts, which co-ordinate the provision of community health services (these are called acute trusts and primary care trusts in Scotland). Since April 1999 all GPs have been grouped into primary care groups (PCGs) (called local health groups in Wales, and local health care co-operatives in Scotland). Together with nurses, a representative from social services and a local lay representative, these groups identify the health needs of the local population and develop community-based health services. Health services for people with mental health problems or learning disabilities remain the responsibility of health authorities, which also retain responsibility for commissioning some public health and specialist services (eg, HIV and AIDS services) across the whole area. It is probable that specialist trusts will be created to take over some of these functions.

From April 2000 under the Health Act 1999 the local groups described above will have greater powers to commission health care for its patients. It is expected that responsibility for commissioning most hospital and community services will be delegated over time from health authorities to locally-based groups.[10]

Local authority services (social services and housing)

Two different government departments in England are responsible for policy-making in the areas of social services and housing: the Department of Health for social services (the Department of Health and Community Care in Scotland) and the Department of Environment, Transport and the Regions for housing (the Development Department in Scotland). These departments issue guidance, circulars and letters to inform, or in some cases instruct, local authorities. The Secretary of State for Health, the National Assembly for Wales or the Scottish Health and Community Care Minister can issue directions to social services which are mandatory. Guidance can also have considerable force if it is issued under Section 7 Local Authority Social Services Act 1970 in England and Wales (see p453). The housing department can also be issued with directions (such as the Code of Guidance on Homelessness).[11]

Central government funding for social services and housing, along with all the other services which local authorities provide, comes from the Revenue Support Grant. The amount each local authority receives is calculated on the standard spending assessment which looks at demographic factors in the area. The standard spending assessment for social services includes such factors as the number of older people in receipt of IS and the number getting attendance allowance (AA). It is advantageous to local authorities to encourage the take up of these benefits, as it can mean they receive a greater proportion of the Revenue Support Grant. However the total amount to be divided remains the decision of government

The local authority can decide how it will divide the money it receives from government between all its departments (although some amounts are ring fenced – eg, the grant for mental health). Some spend less on social services than would be expected from the standard spending assessment, others spend considerably more.

In addition to government money, local authorities top up their funding through locally raised council tax, rents for housing and charges for services (see pp49–54 for a description of social services charges).

Local authority officers are responsible for the day-to-day running of services, but it is elected council members who are responsible for the policies and quality of the services provided. This is why it is sometimes useful to bring your case to the attention of a councillor (see p60).

Different types of local authority

Not all local authorities have both housing and social services functions, although the majority now do. There are four types of local authority:
- County authorities – these are based on fairly large geographical areas and often reflect the historical shires such as Lancashire or Nottinghamshire. There are social services departments in county authorities and they normally have a number of offices so that you do not have to travel too far to the nearest social services office.
- District or borough authorities – within a county area. They do not have any social services functions, but provide housing services.

- Metropolitan district authorities and London borough councils – are based in London and other urban areas and have responsibility for both housing and social services.
- Unitary authorities – were created out of some county and district/borough authorities to form a unitary authority. They are responsible for both social services and housing. Some still retain the title district or borough in their name. All authorities in Wales and Scotland are unitary.

Some authorities which are responsible for both housing and social services have combined their committees and have just one director responsible for both social services and housing.

Social security

The Department of Social Security (DSS) is responsible for policy in relation to benefits, including housing benefit and council tax benefit administered by local authorities. Most benefits, however, are administered by the Benefits Agency, which is an executive arm of the DSS, along with the War Pensions Agency, Child Support Agency and Information Technology Agency. Benefits for the unemployed are administered jointly by Benefits Agency and Employment Services staff at JobCentres. The DSS sets the framework and resources for the delivery and administration of benefits.

Benefits such as income support or incapacity benefit are dealt with at local offices, which together to form a district. The district manager has some freedom about how the district is run, as long as the district stays within budget and specific performance targets are set – eg, accuracy of decisions and clearance times for claims. The payment of benefit, other than the discretionary Social Fund is not limited to budgets. If you are entitled to a benefit, it will be paid.

In some parts of London your claim will be dealt with in Glasgow, Belfast or Makerfield.

Claims for some benefits (eg, attendance allowance or disability living allowance, invalid care allowance and pensions) are processed at central offices. The claim form will tell you which office to send it to, or your Benefits Agency local office will be able to tell you where to make a claim. Information should be passed between local and central offices of the Benefits Agency, but this does not always happen. If you are claiming benefits from both a local and a central Benefits Agency office it may help to speed things up if you inform both offices.

Benefits Agency staff are responsible for making decisions on claims for benefits (see Chapter 10) and are issued with guidance on the interpretation and application of the law. This is called *Decision Makers Guide* and replaced the *Adjudication Officers Guide* in September 1999. Although this guidance is usually strictly adhered to, it is not binding on Benefits Agency staff, and certainly not binding on higher authorities such as tribunals. Staff in local authorities responsible for decisions on housing benefit and council tax benefit also receive guidance. The system is changing and decisions on benefits administered by the Benefits Agency are now made by the Secretary of State (in reality, officers acting on behalf of the Secretary of State who are called Decision Makers).

Working together

In order to achieve good community care services it is essential that all these key players work together. At governmental level, moves have been made to get departments to work more closely together. At Westminster there is now an Inter-Ministerial Group for Older People chaired by a Minister for Older People. Its purpose is to ensure that government strategy and policy affecting older people is effectively co-ordinated, avoids duplication and takes account of the needs of older people.

Working together is not new. For a number of years there have been regular meetings between the Department of Health, the DSS, the Benefits Agency and the Local Government Association (representing local authorities) to try to resolve some of the practical problems arising from DSS benefits being used to pay for charges set by local authorities.

In some cases the government specifies that co-operation at local level between health and social services is necessary, and funding may not be forthcoming unless local agreements have been reached. There are many examples of departments working well together to achieve the best results for individuals. There are also, however, examples where one department tries to pass the cost of care onto another department, which adversely affects the person needing care.

There are different types of local authority and few co-terminous boundaries. This can mean that the health authority may have to reach agreement with a number of local authorities in its area. Or a social services department (especially in shire authorities) can have several health authorities and housing departments within its area and may need to negotiate different ways of working with each. Housing departments in a district or borough council may not always have the same agenda as social services based in a county authority, and each will have its own culture and way of working.

Many local authorities have made service level agreements with Benefits Agency offices at district or local level. An underrated aspect of community care is the importance of prompt and accurate payment of benefit, both from the point of view of the claimant and social services. This is especially true in the case of residential care, where the amount social services charge reflects the amount of benefit paid. As yet there is no national service level agreement between the Benefits Agency and social services, but this is nearing completion.

In addition to working together, statutory agencies need to work with all the other key players who provide or use care services. As the main purchasers of care, social services are in a strong position when setting the price they are prepared to pay for domiciliary or residential/ nursing care. There has been some disquiet expressed by providers of both domiciliary and residential/ nursing care that the prices fixed by social services are too low for the tasks expected. Various initiatives which tend to push prices up, such as the minimum wage, the European working time directive and the constraints within local authority budgets, can create underlying tensions within joint working.

4. Arrangements you can make yourself to pay for your own services

Many people pay for their own care. This means buying your own help or paying the fees for residential or nursing care directly to the owner of the home. You may have too much money to qualify for social services help, or you do not come within social services eligibility criteria for needing help (see p44), or the sort of help you want is not provided eg, gardening or housework. This section looks briefly at some of the practicalities involved in arranging your own care and ways of using your money to pay for your care.

Buying your own care

The points to take into account if you pay for your own residential or nursing care are described on p275.

If you are unable to get help with your care from the state you will need to consider other ways of obtaining help. You may have relatives and friends who will undertake caring tasks or do some gardening for you. However, you may need to pay someone to do these jobs for you. Sometimes you need to buy in extra care over and above that supplied by social services.

Finding a carer

If you have been assessed by social services but found not to need the type of care they offer, they may be able to give you information about local schemes which offer the service you need. Voluntary organisations sometimes provide domestic care, or have gardening or handy-person schemes, so may be a good place to start. Social services may also be able to give you a list of private and voluntary agencies in the area which provide care. At present these agencies are not subject to regulation, but you may prefer to use them rather than find your own worker. As well as the safeguard of having an organisation to which to complain if things go wrong, you should be assured of getting the service even if the person who normally comes to you is unable to do so. If possible, try to use an agency which has been personally recommended.

You may need to advertise for your own carer. You can do this in a JobCentre even if you only want someone a few hours a week (although most people who use JobCentres are looking for full time work) or in local papers, or on a notice board. If you advertise you may want to consider how prospective applicants contact you. If you live alone and feel that you could be vulnerable you may want to think about using a PO box number, or asking a relative or friend if they would have their address or phone number used rather than yours.

Points to consider when paying for your own care

There are national and local organisations which help people who buy their own care using direct payments from social services (see p46) or the Independent Living Fund (see p143). There is also published information to help, particularly about employing your own staff. The National Centre for Independent Living (NCIL) may be able to give you details of this literature – see Appendix 3).

The following are a few considerations to take into account if you are paying for your own care:

- If you are employing your own carer it can be useful to have someone with you when you are interviewing applicants.
- You should always take up written references on someone you plan to employ.
- If you are using an agency or employing someone yourself, you should be very clear exactly what you expect, the number of hours to be worked, and how much you will be paying.
- If you are employing your own staff and do not know how much to pay, the local JobCentre will be able to tell you how much is usually paid for such work.
- If you have not employed people before, it is important to seek advice about your responsibilities as an employer and to check carefully what insurance cover you might need.
- It is useful to put everything in writing before the person starts working for you so you are both clear about the conditions.
- If you use an agency you should ask for a contract (although most agencies will offer you one).
- Currently some agencies are required to charge VAT even if the care they give you is far greater than housework. Others, such as charitable agencies, those which have a qualified nurse in a supervisory role, and small agencies which are below the VAT threshold, will not charge VAT. It is worth

checking which agencies in your area charge VAT and comparing the cost with agencies which do not.

Using your money to pay for care

If you only need small amounts of care you may be able to pay for it without too much difficulty. This *Handbook* describes the various benefits to which you might be entitled and also the powers and duties of the various statutory agencies. Before you arrange to pay for your own care it is useful to check whether it should be provided for you, if this is what you would prefer.

However, the care you need can sometimes be very expensive, especially if you want to remain at home but need a lot of care. Residential or nursing home care can also be very expensive. Therefore, if you have capital which you want to preserve you might want to think of ways to make it last longer.

There are two main ways of using your capital to pay for care: equity release and long-term care insurance. The following is a brief description of some schemes on the market.

Equity release

The most common form of equity release scheme is a 'home reversion scheme' which involves selling your home or part of your home to a 'reversion company'. In return you receive a cash sum (with which you could buy long-term care insurance) or a monthly annuity income. You can remain in the house rent free or for a nominal rent for the rest of your life. When the property is sold, the reversion company receives a share of the proceeds. For instance if you sold a 50 per cent share then the reversion company will receive 50 per cent of the proceeds. However, when you sell your home (or a share of it) to the reversion company you will not receive the full open market value because you retain the right to live there for the rest of your life. The value you receive depends on your age and sex. Older people will get more than younger people and men get more than women.

There are also 'home income plans' where you take out a mortgage loan against your home, usually up to a maximum of £30,000, and the money is used to buy an annuity which pays you a regular income for life. The interest payments on the loan are deducted from this monthly income. Changes to the tax relief on these schemes in the March 1999 budget will probably make them less attractive as the interest payments are no longer eligible for tax relief.

Long-term care insurance

Some insurance companies offer schemes to help pay for long-term care, either in your own home or in a residential or nursing home. You can pay:

- regular premiums or a lump sum to pay for your care in the future (a pre-funded policy); or

- a lump sum to purchase care immediately (an immediate needs plan).

The costs of the policy depend on your age, sex and state of health when you buy long-term care insurance. The premiums are lower the younger you are. Immediate needs policies have the advantage that you know you need the care you are paying for.

An immediate needs policy will start straight away. With a pre-funded scheme, payment will start when you can no longer perform an agreed number of 'activities of daily living'. Your policy will give a precise definition and number. The activities typically include: getting around, bathing, dressing, feeding yourself etc. Mental conditions such as Alzheimer's disease are also covered. Some conditions are not covered, typically depression, schizophrenia, alcohol or drug abuse, and HIV/AIDS. There is often a waiting period before your claim will be paid if you have a pre-funded scheme. Usually this is about 13 weeks but can be adjusted to shorter or longer periods, which will affect your premium.

Getting advice

It is very important to get independent advice when thinking about any scheme which involves your capital. The schemes described above are not as yet subject to financial regulation. Some companies have signed up to a voluntary code of practice (eg, Safe Home Income Plans) and the Association of British Insurers encourages its members to belong to the Insurance Ombudsman, the Personal Insurance Arbitration Service or the Personal Investment Authority Ombudsman Bureau. The Financial Services and Markets Bill is currently going through Parliament and may alter the situation about regulation.

You should always be clear about what you hope to achieve through equity release or long-term care insurance. Then check if those requirements will be met by a particular product.

Notes

1. **What is community care?**

1 Caring for People Community Care in the Next Decade and Beyond 1989, HMSO para 2.2

2 *Modernising Social Services Promoting Independence, Improving Protection, Raising Standards* 1998, DoH page 21. Please note that Wales and Scotland each have their own White Papers.

2. **Community care changes in 1993**

3 See the White Papers *Better Services for the Mentally Handicapped* (1971) and *Better Services for the Mentally Ill* (1975) DHSS

4 *From Poor Law to Community Care*, quoted in Means and Smith, Ministry of Health 1954(b)

5 *Caring for People* (1989) para 1.5

6 *Caring For People* (1989) Key Objectives para 1.11

7 s26(1A) NAA 1948 and s13A SWSA 1968 as amended by the NHS and CCA 1990

8 *R v N and E Devon ex parte Coughlan* (CA) (CCLR) September 1999

9 s42–50 and s51-58 NHS&CCA 1990

3. **Systems to deliver services and benefits**

10 HSC/98/228 DoH para 49

11 s71 HA 1985

Part 2

Care in the community

If you are old, or have any disability which makes it difficult for you to manage without help, you may need a combination of services and benefits in order to be able to remain at home.

This Part explains the rules which apply to services you can get from social services, health and housing, how you might be charged for those services and how to challenge a decision (see Chapter 2). It then covers the rules for the financial support for older or disabled people or their carers paid through social security benefits (see Chapter 3). It goes on to give brief details of other financial assistance that you might be able to get from other sources to help with your costs of care, to make your home more suitable for you to live in, or to help with travel costs (see Chapter 4).

Chapter 5 covers the different types of housing with support that is available but that does not come under the rules for residential or nursing home care. The rules for residential and nursing homes are explained in Part 4 of this book.

Chapter 2

Community care services

This chapter covers the responsibilities of social services, health and housing to provide services for you if you are old, disabled or in ill health. It concentrates on services which you can get in order to stay in your own home (see Chapter 12 for the responsibilities of authorities to provide residential or nursing care). It covers:

1. What are community care services? (p21)
2. The responsibilities of social services, health and housing (p23)
3. Getting the services you need (p40)
4. How far the authority's resources can be taken into account (p44)
5. Getting direct payments instead of services (p46)
6. Charges for your services or equipment (p49)
7. How to complain if you are unhappy about your services (p54)

1. What are community care services?

Although any services that help you remain in the community could be described as 'community care services' they are defined in legislation. The services covered in this *Handbook,* however, are not limited strictly to those services, because other services, in particular those you can get from the NHS and housing, are equally vital in helping you remain at home.

The legislation

England and Wales

The services defined in the National Health Service and Community Care Act (NHS and CCA)[1] as 'community care' services are those which local authorities may provide or arrange under any of the following enactments:
- Part III of the National Assistance Act 1948 (sections 21 and 29);
- s45 of the Health and Public Health Act 1968;
- s21 and Schedule 8 to the National Health Service Act 1977;
- s117 of the Mental Health Act.

2

Chapter 2: Community care services
1. What are community care services?

Scotland

The NHS and Community Care Act 1990 defines community care services as those provided by local authorities under Part II of the Social Work (Scotland) Act 1968[2] or ss7, 8 or 11 of the Mental Health (Scotland) Act 1984. The National Assistance Act 1948 mainly applies to England but it provides the legal basis for charging for residential care (See p273).

These regulations are explained in more detail on p24 where they relate to services which are provided in non-residential settings and on pp259–262 where they relate to residential services.

The non-residential provision which counts as community care services within the legislation spans a wide variety of services, including: practical assistance in the home (home helps or home care); respite care to give you or your carer a break; equipment to help your daily living; adaptations to your home; telephones, televisions, radios; help with travel; facilities for rehabilitation; meals-on-wheels, day centres, recreational activities, outings, and wardens in sheltered housing. It also includes social services advice, support and information.

In some cases social services has the *power* to provide the services and in others it has a *duty* to provide the services. Sometimes this duty is a *general duty* to ensure that the services are available for the local population, and sometimes it is a *specific duty* to you as an individual to provide the services you have been assessed as needing.

Sometimes a service is provided by the NHS (eg, a laundry service or incontinence pads), but in the event of it not providing the service or only providing it inadequately, you may find that social services make these provisions. The Social Fund (see p122) has made a payment for incontinence pads when an applicant failed to meet the health authority's stringent criteria.[3]

There are confusions over who is responsible for adaptations to your home. Assistance in carrying out works of adaptation is listed as a community care service and as such could be the responsibility of the social services department. Grants for facilities to improve housing for disabled people (see p147) are normally the responsibility of the housing department, but social services have a duty to assist where the local housing authority refuses or is unable to approve the application even if housing has established that you need the adaptations.[4]

If you need services you will probably not care which department supplies them. However, there are some vital issues in relation to:
- charging – you will probably be charged for a service if it is supplied by social services;

- your rights – it is important to know when there is a duty to provide you with a service, and how far you can choose the way that service is provided;
- knowing which department to go to or where to complain – it is sometimes not clear which department has responsibility for a service and it is not uncommon to have to complain to more than one department.

In June 2000 the 'long term care charter' in England will introduce a joint charter for social services, health and housing which may help you through the community care maze. The consultation document states that it is essential for people to have information, and that staff are aware of the services provided by other departments and can make appropriate referrals to them.[5] The charter is also expected to indicate how long you may be expected to wait for an assessment or a service and how to complain to each of the departments.

2. The responsibilities of social services, health, and housing

Social services, health and housing authorities each work to different statutes and their respective responsibilities have been the subject of an increasing amount of case law in the courts. Appendix 5 lists books and texts that are essential to any adviser in this area or for individual research on the legislation. The responsibilities of social services, health and housing departments are constantly evolving, with changes being driven by government and case law. Not all the changes need legislation and departments are often informed by circulars about changes in the interpretation of the law or about conditions attached to the money they are allocated. An example of conditions attached to grants are those available (in England only) from April 1999 for three years to promote:

- independence – by providing low level services to prevent or delay loss of independence and to improve quality of life;
- partnership – by getting health and social services to agree a strategy to avoid unnecessary hospital admission, and to work together to improve rehabilitation and hospital discharge arrangements;
- support for carers – to provide more respite care for carers and to work with them on providing the services they need.

Conditions have been attached to such grants to ensure that social services spend the money in the way intended. It is up to each area, however, to decide, in consultation with other key players in the area, how they use the grants to achieve their purpose.[6] Coming at a time when many social services departments are making cuts to community care services, it is useful to be aware of the conditions imposed by government on the spending of these new grants and the types of services they are expected to provide using these grants.

Although Scotland and Wales have not had money ring-fenced in this way, arrangements to encourage independence, partnership and support are being promoted in these countries.

Responsibilities of social services

The prime responsibility for ensuring that community care services are provided rests with social services departments, which also decide, through the assessment process (see p40), who will receive those services. The assessment is part of what is known as 'care management'. A decision that you need services will lead onto the design and setting up of a 'care package' to meet your identified needs. This may include a range of services provided by social services, health, housing, independent providers or family and friends. The care package should be monitored and reviewed to ensure it continues to meets your needs, and changed if necessary.[7]

Social services work to acts, regulations, and directions (which have the force of law) and to guidance from the Secretary of State for Health, or from the National Assembly of Wales, or the Scottish Ministers in Scotland. Guidance can be:

- formal (often called policy guidance);[8] *or*
- general (often called practice guidance).

Formal guidance should be followed and deviation from it without good reason would be a breach of the law.[9] Practice guidance is not issued under the legislation, but even this should not be disregarded by local authorities on a regular basis.[10]

In addition the Social Services Inspectorate (Social Work Services Inspectorate in Scotland) issues advice notes or letters to local authorities.

Community care services which social services can provide or arrange

NB Community care services have a specific legal meaning and are provided under various Acts of Parliament spanning the period from 1948 (see p21). The terms in regulations are therefore often out-dated and can be offensive to modern thinking.

This section looks at the domiciliary services which are part of community care.

Help if you are disabled – Part III National Assistance Act 1948 section 29 (England and Wales)

Section 29 underpins the provision of non-residential care if you are disabled. Although s2 of the Chronically Sick and Disabled Persons Act 1970 gives you stronger rights, it is linked to s29 of the National Assistance Act.[11] S29 gives social services duties in relation to people who are:

- ordinarily resident in the local authority's area[12] (see p261);
- are 18 or over, 'blind deaf or dumb, or suffer from a mental disorder' or are 'substantially and permanently handicapped by illness, injury or congenital deformity or such other disabilities that may be prescribed'. This includes partial sight and hearing.[13]

The *general duties* (which are only powers if you do not ordinarily live in the social services area) are:

- to compile and maintain registers of disabled people (you do not have to be on the register to get a service);
- to provide a social work service and such advice and support as needed for people at home or elsewhere (this can include benefits advice);[14]
- to provide, at centres or elsewhere, facilities for social rehabilitation and to help you adjust to disability including assistance in overcoming limitations of mobility or communication;
- to provide, at centres or elsewhere, facilities for occupational, social, cultural or recreational activities and, if appropriate, payment for work you have done.

These are not individual duties arising from your assessed needs, but just general duties towards the local population.

In addition there are *powers* **to provide holiday homes, travel (free or subsidised if you do not get other travel concessions), help in finding accommodation, contributions to the costs of wardens, information about services available under s29, instruction in overcoming your disability, workshops or work you can do at home.[15] These powers cover you whether or not you are ordinarily resident in the social services area.**

Social services cannot make cash payments (other than for work you have done) under s29. But see p46 for direct payments.

Help if you are disabled – Social Work (Scotland) Act 1968 (Scotland)

In Scotland, the Social Work (Scotland) Act gives local authorities the duty to 'promote social welfare by making available advice, guidance and assistance on such a scale as may be appropriate for their area'. These duties relate to people who are:

- ordinarily resident in the local authority area (see p263);[16]

- 'persons in need'[17] which includes elderly, physically or mentally disabled or suffering from a limiting illness; (disabled is not defined in the legislation).

The social work authority has a general **duty** to promote social welfare through providing:
- advice, guidance and assistance to help promote social welfare;
- providing services in the home to enable a person to maintain as independent an existence as is practicable.

The social work department can give help in the form of practical assistance or cash (see also p46 for direct payments). Under s12 of the Social Work (Scotland) Act cash can only be given in circumstances which amount to an emergency. Practical help can be given in circumstances which do not amount to an emergency – eg, paying a bill. S12 payments are used widely, as the only criteria set down by the Act is that the giving of assistance in either form would avoid the local authority being caused greater expense in the future.[18]

Help if you are disabled – section 2 Chronically Sick and Disabled Persons Act 1970 (England, Wales and Scotland)

Although not listed in the legislation which defines community care services, s2 of the Chronically Sick and Disabled Persons Act 1970 (CSDPA) is linked to s29 of the National Assistance Act. The Chronically Sick and Disabled Persons (Scotland) Act 1972 extended ss 1 and 2(1) of the CSDPA to Scotland. References to functions under s29 of the National Assistance Act 1948 are construed as references to duties to chronically sick and disabled persons (being persons in need) under s12 of the Social Work (Scotland) Act 1968. **The Act places a duty on social services to make arrangements for specific services for you as an individual.** It has been the subject of important community care legal cases, in particular in relation to whether social services can take their own resources into account when deciding whether you need services, whether it will provide services to you, and if so what services[19] (see p44).

You can get any or all of the services listed in section 2 if you are:
- defined as disabled by social services under s29 of the National Assistance Act (see p25). But note it does not specify you have to be over 18;
- ordinarily resident within the social services area[20] (see p263); and
- social services is satisfied that they need to make arrangements for you to meet your needs.

Section 1 of this Act lays a specific duty on social services to establish the number of people who are disabled within their area, to publish what services it provides under s29 (see p25) and to give to existing service users information about other services of which it is aware.

The services listed in section 2 are wide ranging and must be provided if you have been assessed as needing them. They include:

- practical assistance in the home – this can range from housework, to pension collection, to personal care tasks. Many social services departments have concentrated on personal care tasks in recent years and moved away from basic household tasks;
- provision of or assistance in obtaining radio, television, library or similar recreational facilities;
- lectures, games, outings or other recreational facilities outside the home or assistance for you to take advantage of educational facilities;[21]
- facilities for or assistance with travel to and from services provided under s29 or other similar services;
- assistance in carrying out works of adaptation to your home or the provision of any additional facility designed for your greater safety, comfort and convenience. This is a separate duty from that of the housing department to provide grants for facilities to improve housing for disabled people. The guidance makes it clear that social services has the lead role and that the duty to act remains regardless of the housing authority's actions. Additional facilities include fittings such as handrails, alarm systems and hoists;[22]
- help for you to take a holiday either at a holiday home or elsewhere. Case law has established that social services cannot restrict themselves to only providing holidays they have arranged themselves. It has also been found that to only assist with the extra costs caused by disability, not with the ordinary hotel and travel costs, had fettered the authority's discretion and was not consistent with the wording of the Act; [23]
- meals either at home or elsewhere;
- provision of, or help in getting, a telephone or any special equipment to use the phone.[24] Since the Act came into force, technology has changed so it may be possible to consider items such as modems and fax machines.

Help if you are an older person – section 45 of the Health Services and Public Health Act 1968 (England and Wales)

If you are an older person who does not fit into the definition of disabled within s29 of the National Assistance Act, but still need services because of frailty due to old age then you may be able to make use of the general provision which s45 gives to 'promote the welfare of old people'. Directions by the Secretary of State explain that the purpose of s45 is to promote the welfare of older people and as far as possible prevent or postpone personal deterioration or breakdown.[25] The directions merely *empower* social services to provide the following services many of which are *duties* under s2 of the Chronically Sick and Disabled Persons Act 1970. If you are older person who is also disabled your services should be provided under s2 and so you will have some additional rights. The services listed within s45 are:

- meals and recreation in the home and elsewhere;
- information on elderly services;
- assistance to travel to s45 services;
- assistance in finding boarding accommodation;
- social work support and advice;
- home help and home adaptation – including laundry services;
- wardens.

If social services want to provide services outside of the directions, they can do so provided they get the specific approval of the Secretary of State.

Help from social services – National Health Service Act 1977 (England and Wales)

Most of this Act relates to services provided by the NHS, but there are specific responsibilities for social services to make arrangements for:

- expectant mothers;
- the prevention of illness and the care and aftercare of adults suffering from illness; *and*
- the provision of adequate home help services in the area for households with a person who is suffering from illness, is pregnant or lying–in mother, is aged, or disabled by illness or congenital deformity. It is linked to laundry services which can include the provision of washing machines.[26] As there is no age limit it could apply to children.

As with most community care legislation, s21 of the NHS Act is subject to the Secretary of State's Directions. However, the provision of adequate home help and laundry services is not subject to direction and therefore is a *duty*, although it is only a *general duty* to provide for the area.

Social services have *powers* to provide services for expectant and nursing mothers of any age, centres or other facilities with a view to preventing illness or for aftercare, meals at such centres or at home, social work services, advice and support, night sitter services, recuperative holidays, social and recreational facilities, and services specifically for those dependent on alcohol or drugs.[27]

Social services have a *general duty* to those who are, or who have been, suffering from a mental illness to make arrangements:

- for centres for training and occupation;
- for sufficient approved social workers to act under the Mental Health Act 1983;
- to exercise the functions of the authority for those received into guardianship;
- for the provision of social work services to help in the identification, diagnosis, assessment and social treatment of mental disorder and to provide social work support at home and elsewhere.

Help from social services in Scotland

In Scotland there is no equivalent to either s45 (see p27) or to social services provision in the National Health Act 1977 (see above). Local authorities in Scotland have a duty to provide a home help service to 'persons in need' and expectant or lying-in mothers; and a laundry service to people receiving this service. This is a general duty to provide for the area.[28] Under the Mental Health (Scotland) Act social work authorities have a duty to provide aftercare for people who have or have had a mental illness or a learning disability. They must also provide 'suitable training and occupation for people with learning disabilities' and ensure that there is adequate transport to take people to day care or training centres.[29]

If you have previously been detained in hospital – section 117 Mental Health Act 1983 (England and Wales)

Social services and health have a joint responsibility to provide aftercare services if you have been detained in hospital under ss3, 37, 47, or 48 of the Mental Health Act 1983. **This is an individual duty and remains until both health and social services are satisfied that you no longer need such aftercare services.**[30] Some people are subject to aftercare under supervision which may impose conditions on where you live, your attendance at a set time and place for medical treatment, and that the person supervising your care has access to your home.[31]

Aftercare services are not defined in the Act. They would normally include social work support and help with employment, accommodation or family relationship problems, the provision of domiciliary services and the use of day centre and residential facilities[32] (see p268).

Social services have no power to charge you for these services (see p51). Seek advice if you are told you will be charged.

If you have previously been detained in hospital – section 8 Mental Health (Scotland) Act 1984 (Scotland)

The Mental Health (Scotland) Act (s8) places a legal duty on social work departments to provide aftercare for people who are, or have been, suffering from a mental disorder. This means a mental illness or learning disability[33] and would include someone with dementia. In providing aftercare services the local authority must co-operate with the relevant health board. The powers apply regardless of whether the person is, or has been, in hospital. Aftercare is not defined in the Act but could include similar services to examples given for England and Wales (p29). Unlike in England, social work departments in Scotland **can** charge for aftercare services.

Equipment that you can get from social services

Equipment can often be just as vital as services in helping you stay independent and remain at home. The legislation described above gives social services the duty (see p28) or the power (see p28) to provide equipment. Social services can provide an extensive range of equipment that includes:

- help with getting off the toilet – eg, a raised seat or rails;
- help to get in and out of the bath – eg, bath boards, rails or hoists;
- help with getting in and out of a chair – eg, raising your chair, high backed chairs or riser chairs;
- help with dressing – eg, stocking aids and long handled shoe horns;
- help with cooking and eating – eg, safety pans, cooker guards, special cutlery, and non slip surfaces;
- help with reading – eg, magnifiers and page turners.

There are many other ways in which equipment can help. You could be provided with ordinary equipment such as a microwave, washing machine, or TV remote control, although in practice this would be fairly uncommon.

New and improved equipment for disabilities is always being made. It is important, therefore, to ask someone who is knowledgeable if there is a gadget that you don't know about, which will exactly meet your needs. There are various books on the subject of equipment (see Appendix 5).

There are about 40 Disabled Living Centres in the UK (see Appendix 3 for how to find the address of the one nearest to you) which display and demonstrate a wide range of equipment and have staff to give advice. They are open to the public and to professionals and may give advice by phone or letter if you cannot visit. If you are buying equipment it is very important to make sure you get the item that suits your needs.

Social services have a duty to provide general information about the services they provide under the Chronically Sick and Disabled Persons Act. If you are receiving services under this Act, social services also have a specific duty to inform you of other services you might need (see p26). That includes providing information about equipment provided by social services, the NHS, housing or voluntary organisations.

Generally, equipment from social services is provided by occupational therapists (OTs), although it may be provided by physiotherapists, rehabilitation workers for people with sight problems and social workers for people with hearing problems.

In order to get equipment you often need to be assessed (see p40) by qualified staff such as OTs. Social services should have adequate staff to enable them to carry out that function,[34] but the shortage of OTs has been a common problem. If the problem has been acknowledged but not been tackled, contact the Local Government Ombudsman who may find maladministration[35] (see p60). In England, once it has been decided that you need equipment social services should aim to get it delivered within three weeks if it is less than £1,000.[36]

You may be charged for equipment provided by social services (see p49).

Social services responsibilities for planning and providing information

If you need a community care service it is important that you are informed of your rights, what services there are, and that social services have systems to ensure you receive the services you need. Given that most people only approach social services for help at a time of great need and do not know what to expect, information is vital. This was recognised when community care was reformed and various duties were placed on social services departments to plan services and inform people about them.

Planning

Each local authority must prepare and publish a community care plan for its area[37] and it must be updated each year.[38] In drawing up the plans, social services must consult with health, housing and voluntary organisations which appear to the authority to represent groups likely to need services. If a provider organisation writes to ask to be consulted then it must be.[39] Guidance tells social services to identify the following:

- assessment – the care needs of the local population, how those care needs will be assessed, and how identified needs will be incorporated into the planning process;
- services – how priorities for arranging services are made, how they intend to offer practical help and how they intend to develop domiciliary services;
- quality – how they monitor service quality, the role of the inspection unit, and the role of complaints procedures;
- choice – how they intend to increase consumer choice and develop a mixed economy of care;
- resources – the resource implications of planned and future developments and how they intend to improve cost effectiveness;
- consultation – how they intend to consult;
- publishing information – how they intend to inform service users and their carers about services, and how and when they will publish their community care plan for the following year.[40]

The duty to inform

Apart from having to publish its community care plan and complaints procedures (see p57) the only other duties to inform people of the service they can get are set out in the legislation described on p28. Policy guidance states that local authorities must have published information accessible to all potential service users and carers, in formats suitable for those with communication difficulties or differences in language or culture. The information should set out the types of community care services available, the criteria for the provision of services, the assessment procedures and the standards by which care management will be measured.[41]

Local authorities in England are also required to produce community care charters based on a national framework.[42] These should give an indication of the services people can expect to receive, and how quickly they will be provided. Charters do not have any legal effect, but it is possible to complain if standards in a charter are not met. In one case the Local Government Ombudsman found maladministration when a community care charter gave misleading timescales for assessment.[43] It is likely that the Community Care Charter will be replaced in the future by the joint Long term care charter – see p21.

Responsibilities of the NHS

Health services, which are an essential element of community care, are not classified as community care services and are provided under different legislation which was largely unchanged by the community care legislation. Unlike social services, there are no specific duties to individuals who need health care services. If when assessing you (see p40), social services thinks you have a health care need, then in England and Wales it must notify the health authority and invite it to assist in the assessment. The health authority has no duty to respond or co-operate. In Scotland the social work department must notify the health board and ask for what services they are likely to provide and then take this into account in the completed assessments.[44]

Health authorities have only a broad duty to provide services to the extent the Secretary of State (or in Scotland the Scottish Ministers) considers necessary to meet all reasonable requirements. Such services include:
- medical, dental, nursing and ambulance services;
- hospital and other accommodation for services provided by the NHS;
- and facilities for the prevention of illness, care of those suffering an illness and aftercare for those who have suffered and illness which are appropriate for a health service to provide.[45]

Health authorities, therefore, have wide discretion in deciding what meets 'all reasonable requirements', even to the extent of deciding that a particular service will not be provided at all. As long as a decision about the level (or non-provision) of a service is justifiable on the grounds of local priorities and resources, then it would be difficult to challenge.[46]

Guidance has been issued which limits the freedom of health authorities to some extent. For instance a letter was issued about prescribing a particular drug for patients who clinically needed it[47] but a health authority ignored it as they were not convinced about the drug and so did not release money for it. This was found to be unlawful.[48]

There is also guidance about NHS responsibility for continuing health care needs.[49] It covers NHS care in nursing homes (see p262) and NHS care that should be offered at home. It also covers the process of hospital discharge (see p33) to ensure that it runs smoothly and that the necessary services are in place when patients get home. It allows each health authority to decide (in agreement with social services) what health services will be provided. Local policies must be published. The following services must be available in each area:

- specialist medical and nursing care;
- rehabilitation and recovery – local policies should guard against premature discharge and should agree with local authorities any additional social or educational support that may be required as part of an agreed package of rehabilitation;
- palliative health care including support for people in their own homes;[50]
- continuing in-patient care in hospital or nursing home (see p263);
- respite health care;[51]
- specialist health care support for people in nursing homes or residential care homes or in the community. This could include specialist palliative care, incontinence advice, stoma care, diabetic advice, physiotherapy, speech and language therapy, or chiropody. It should also include specialist equipment;
- community health services (such as district nurses) for people in residential care homes (see p263);
- primary health care (ie, the health care from GP surgeries, district nurses, dentists and opticians);
- specialist transport services to and from hospital or other health care facilities, and where emergency admission to a residential care or nursing home is necessary.

The guidance is currently under review and could change early in the New Year. It is likely that Welsh and Scottish guidance will also change.

Given that there are wide differences between areas as to what health services are provided, it is important to find out what is available under the local criteria. From April 2000 in England the long term care charter should provide information about health services in each area.[52]

Hospital discharge

The guidance issued on continuing health care also covers the vexed question of hospital discharge. It is very important that any stay in hospital has a planned discharge so that you do not go home without the services you need. The consultant will normally decide (but should do so in consultation with others) whether or not you continue to need acute care. If your needs are such that you may need intensive support there should be a multi-disciplinary assessment.[53] You, your family and your carer should be kept fully informed so that you can make decisions, and you should be provided with written details of the likely cost of any option you are considering. If services are being arranged by the NHS you should receive information in writing saying what aspects of your care are being funded by the NHS.[54] There is a right of review of discharge decisions (see p56).

In England the framework for the Community Care Charter states that hospital discharge standards should ensure that:

- no one will be discharged until appropriate arrangements have been put in place for their subsequent care; *and*
- these arrangements will begin as soon as the patient is discharged.

There have been numerous complaints made to the Health Service Ombudsman about hospital discharge. If you consider that the hospital has not involved you enough, has not ensured that the services you need are in place, or has failed to follow the guidance, you should complain (see p54).

Equipment you can get from the NHS

As well as providing services, the NHS is responsible for providing certain equipment. You should talk to your doctor, district nurse or health visitor first about any equipment you might need.

The sort of equipment you may be able to get includes:

- wheelchairs;
- commodes (normally for short term use);
- bathing equipment including hoists (if your need is for a medical bath);
- eating and drinking equipment if there is a medical need. This can include food preparation equipment such as a liquidiser if needed for a medical condition;
- bed equipment such as a cradle to keep the bed clothes off you, a back rest, raising blocks, bed rails if your need is defined as a health need rather than a social need. It may include the bed itself if you need a special bed;
- environmental control equipment (on loan);
- walking aids;
- artificial limbs;
- hearing aids;
- low vision aids;
- TENS machines for pain relief;
- special footwear;
- incontinence pads and other equipment;
- environmental control systems.

As with all services provided through the NHS it will depend on the resources available as to whether particular equipment will supplied in your area. If your local area does not supply the item you need, you should complain (see p54).

Equipment issued on prescription

GPs can provide a range of appliances as well as drugs on prescription. These include incontinence devices (this includes pads in Scotland), stoma care appliances, oxygen cylinders, diabetes equipment and elastic stockings.[55]

Home care equipment

Your GP may be able to help you get orthopaedic footwear, breast prostheses, cervical collars, communication equipment, nebulisers, supports for limbs or trunk, hoists, special beds and mattresses, and walking aids.

Help with incontinence

Some equipment for incontinence is issued under prescription including catheter bags, catheters, male urinals, and night drainage bags. Incontinence pads can be supplied by the NHS and usually are, but sometimes their supply can be limited. Guidance has been issued to say that if any changes to incontinence aids are proposed, an assured alternative should be put in place before action is taken.[56]

Pad disposal services are sometimes run jointly by the NHS and social services. Laundry services are normally run by social services but the NHS may have a local laundry service. Some areas will have neither a disposal service nor a laundry service.

Incontinence advisers are now available in many areas and it is important to seek advice about incontinence, which is only a symptom of a variety of physical or mental causes. It is important to find out if there can be any improvement in your situation. A policy review, began in May 1998, is looking at ways of providing a modern incontinence service providing access to high quality, prompt and readily-available assistance. The report is expected in the near future.

Wheelchairs

In addition to a range of ordinary wheelchairs, the NHS now provides outdoor/indoor electric wheelchairs[57] if you are assessed as needing one because you are unable to walk or propel an ordinary wheelchair. Each health authority has its own criteria within the national guidelines, but if you move to another area your wheelchair should not be taken from you without good clinical reason. In Scotland the criteria are set nationally. If you have difficulty being pushed outdoors (ie, because you live in a hilly area or the person pushing you is old or disabled) you may be able to get an attendant-controlled powered wheelchair.

In England there is a voucher scheme in England and Wales which allows you to put extra cash towards a more expensive wheelchair than the NHS will provide.[58]

Recent initiatives on health

Various initiatives are being put into place to encourage joint working between the NHS and local authorities. This section describes what is happening in England but there are similar trends and similar initiatives in Wales and Scotland.

A new Health Act[59] has recently received Royal Assent which will allow more flexibility in the way health services and local authorities work together. For example, in England from April 2000 pooling of budgets will be allowed so that the money can be used strategically. One authority will be able to transfer funds to another and allow that authority to take the lead in arranging services for a particular client or patient group. Social services will be able to provide a range of community health services, and the NHS will be able to provide some social care services. While these are eminently sensible ideas, there is concern that it could lead to further erosion of free NHS services because more services will be provided or arranged by social services. It could also become more difficult to establish under what legislation a service is being provided, which may have charging implications.

Arrangements such as those above, will be part of joint investment plans. Those plans will include joint analysis of current resources, agreed service outcomes and identified gaps in provision.[60]

Further changes are occurring due to the development of primary care groups[61] called local health groups in Wales and local health care co-operatives in Scotland which, led by GPs and nurses, have the task of improving the health of their community, developing primary and community health services and buying-in hospital care for people in their area.

Health authorities now have to draw up health improvement programmes (HImPs) in collaboration with all the various health groups, local authorities and the voluntary sector. The aim is that that health authorities will engage in health improvement at the same time as local authorities carry out new duties to promote the economic, social and environmental wellbeing of their areas across the range of services including housing, transport, education, environment and leisure.[62]

Some areas have become health action zones which provide a framework for the area to tackle the causes of ill health.[63]

Responsibility of housing departments

Housing is a vital part of community care, but like health services it is not listed as a community care service within the legislation. If when assessing you, social services find that you need housing services, they can invite the housing department to assist, but there is no duty for housing to respond.[64] In Scotland the social work department can notify the housing authority and request information from them as to what services are likely to be made available.[65] However, the housing department may be under a duty to make enquiries if you are homeless and in apparent priority need.[66] Priority need is defined as being vulnerable due to old age, mental illness or handicap or physical disability or other reason such as pregnancy or where there are children. It will then have a specific duty towards you as long as you are not intentionally homeless.

Guidance stresses the important role of housing departments and suggests they should be involved in:

- community care planning;
- community care assessments;
- local housing strategies involving co-operation with housing associations and considering special needs housing;
- provisions for homeless people;
- home adaptations.[67]

Different types of housing

Housing departments may assist you in getting accommodation with a housing association or provide the following:

- wheelchair housing – designed to give you access at all times to all principal rooms if you are confined to a wheelchair to get about;
- sheltered housing – this is mainly intended for older people and there is usually a minimum age (often 60). There is almost always an alarm system linked to a 24-hour control service. Some schemes have a resident warden or manager; others have a mobile warden who visits the scheme regularly. A service charge may be included in the rent for which housing benefit may help (see p104);
- extra care sheltered housing - these offer extra care facilities such as help with bathing or dressing, and they will often have a dining room where meals are available. They can be run jointly with social services;
- lifetime homes – a few councils and housing associations build homes which are adaptable to changing needs, including level access and downstairs toilet facilities, wide front door, a living room that can take a bed, kitchens designed for easy use and safety.

Houses in England and Wales built after October 1999 must have basic accessibility features such as a level threshold and downstairs toilet.[68] Scottish Homes, the national housing agency requires all housing funded by them to incorporate barrier free standards.

Home adaptations (England and Wales)

You most likely to live in a house built before 1999, and therefore not built for accessibility. Home adaptations may help you remain at home. They are wide ranging and include handrails, ramps, special bath or shower units, automatic garage doors, downstairs extensions, fixed hoists and widened doors.

Housing authorities can provide some home adaptations to their own housing stock through their general duties and powers,[69] and housing associations can receive revenue or grants from the Housing Corporation (or from Tai Cymru in Wales or Scottish Homes in Scotland) for adaptations to their stock.

Disabled facilities grants (England and Wales)

Housing authorities can provide grants for adaptations if you are disabled or have a disabled child. Social services must be consulted. The housing authority has a *duty* to provide a grant if it accepts that you are disabled (see p26 for a definition) and the adaptations are needed to:

- enable you to have access to and from, and within the house to all rooms that you need;
- make the house safe for you to live in;
- help you to be able to cook;
- improve the heating system or providing a heating system to meet your needs;
- help you to have more control over heating and lighting by moving or providing switches;
- enable you to use a bath or shower and toilet facilities;
- help you to care for someone else (who need not be disabled) if you are disabled.

The housing authority has a *power* to provide a grant for any other purpose to make the dwelling suitable for you to live in if you are disabled.[70] Examples of adaptations quoted in the guidance include: enlarging a home which is already suitable for you, providing a safe play area for a disabled child, or an adaptation which would allow you to receive specialised care or medical treatment in your own home, or enable you to work from home.[71]

Applications must be approved or refused within six months of the date of application. The grant must be given, if approved, no more than 12 months after your application[72] and the 12 month delay should only occur in exceptional circumstances. You must be given reasons if your application is refused.

There are numerous Local Government Ombudsman reports about delays in getting disabled facilities grants (see p41). In particular you should not be prevented from making a formal application. The Ombudsman has stated that authorities should not routinely take up to 12 months simply because the provision allows it. Authorities should process urgent claims more quickly where it would cause hardship – eg, where a person is leaving hospital.[73]

There is a means test which is explained on p147. The maximum grant available is £20,000 in England and £24,000 in Wales. Further help may be obtained from social services if you have been refused a grant or if you have to pay some of the costs and would have difficulty doing so.[74]

Financial help with equipment and adaptations (Scotland)

If you are registered disabled or could be registered disabled you have a right to an assessment of your needs by the social work department, including any need for 'adaptations to your home, or equipment for your use for your greater safety, comfort or convenience'.[75] Following assessment, a social work department should either provide what is needed or provide assistance, including financial assistance to help with the cost of the adaptation. You may be asked to contribute a 'reasonable' amount to the cost. If you are in receipt of benefits this should be very little, if anything (but the local authority will have to look at your individual circumstances).[76]

If you are assessed as in need of housing adaptations the housing department may offer a discretionary improvement grant towards the costs of the works.[77] The grant may cover:

* alteration or enlargement;
* making the house suitable for your accommodation, welfare or employment.

The housing department can pay up to 75 per cent of the approved costs of works, within prescribed limits. Mandatory grants are available to all households for the provision of standard amenities. Even if the house already has one of these amenities, a disabled person may still be entitled to a grant for another if this is essential to her/his needs (eg, a further toilet on the ground floor).[78]

Financial assistance from the social work department is separate from and can be paid in addition to any improvement grant for adaptation – eg, to met the 25 per cent (or more) of the cost not met by the grant.

Home repair assistance (England and Wales)

If you need minor works to your home, housing departments have the *power* to give a grant or materials.[79] To qualify you need to:

* be 18 or over and not a council tenant or landlord;
* have the home as your only residence (this condition is met if you are elderly, disabled or infirm and propose to live somewhere to be cared for);
* be an owner or tenant;
* have a duty or power to carry out the works;
* be on a means-tested benefit or be aged 60 or over, or disabled or infirm, or if the application is to enable you to be cared for.[80]

You can get home repair assistance if you have a mobile home or houseboat. The maximum given is £2,000 per application and a total of £4,000 in three years.

Guidance states that housing authorities may consider assistance with home security for people who are older, disabled or infirm – eg, improved door locks, window locks, or an optical enhanced intercom system.[81] See also p149 for a new scheme in England from April 2000 to assess the security of older people's homes and provide security measures. Other purposes might include minor adaptations, improved heating, or repairs to enable you to continue living in your home.

3. Getting the services you need

If you are having difficulties managing everyday tasks, or are in hospital and think that you will need some help when you leave, you will need to ask social services for a care assessment. Someone else can refer you, although it should always be with your permission unless you are unable to give it because of your mental condition. The care assessment is important as it is the first stage of getting support from social services.

Once you have come to the notice of social services they have a duty to assess and make a decision about whether or not you are entitled to services. If you are, then a care plan will be drawn up, with your agreement, put into place and reviewed on a regular basis to make sure it continues to meet your needs. The care plan could include residential or nursing home care, or a wide range of services to help you stay at home.

The assessment of your needs

Social services must assess you if:
- you appear to them to be in need of a community care service – ie, those listed on p21;[82]
- you are disabled;[83]
- you help look after someone else.[84]

Assessment is a service in its own right.[85]

Most social services operate a screening process to decide who is eligible for an assessment, how quickly it will be provided and the type of assessment you will get. In England, your social services community care charter should give you an indication of how the assessment will be done and how long you should expect to wait. If your need is urgent, social services can provide the services first and assess you as soon as possible afterwards.[86]

Screening for assessment

The practice of screening referred to in policy guidance[87] has been questioned, in particular when it screens people out of an assessment. Even if social services think there is no prospect of providing a service because of lack of resources (see p44) they should still assess you.[88]

Sometimes screening takes place over the phone, and you may have been deemed to have had an assessment without ever seeing anyone or even realising that the phone call was the assessment. You should complain if you feel that you have not been given a proper opportunity to be assessed.

How quickly will the assessment be carried out?

There are no national rules about how quickly an assessment should be carried out. Many local authorities set their own time-scales. In England, the consultation on the Long term care charter suggests urgent requests within 24 hours, high priority requests within five working days and requests requiring less immediate attention within one month to six weeks.[89] Local social services departments may include its time-scales for assessment in its community care charter. An Ombudsman has found maladministration in a case where the local charter set unrealistic time-scales.[90]

Waiting lists for assessments have been the subject of numerous investigations by the Local Government Ombudsman especially in relation to assessments for equipment, which require assessment by an Occupational Therapist. In some cases waits up to four years have been recorded. Because of the large number of complaints in relation to disabled facilities grants, the Local Government Ombudsman has suggested what s/he considers to be 'reasonable times' for awaiting an assessment – ie, two months for urgent cases, four months for serious cases and six months for non-urgent cases.[91] However, these time limits may be too long if your need is very urgent.

If you are in need of drug and alcohol services, there has been guidance on assessment and 'fast track' assessment.[92]

The fact that social services can prioritise the waiting time for your assessment presupposes they have enough information to make a judgement on how long you should wait. It is therefore important when you first contact social services that you make clear the exact nature of your needs and whether your situation is urgent.

The nature of the assessment

There are no set rules about the way an assessment should be carried out and who should do it. If, during the assessment, a need for health or housing services becomes apparent, social services have a duty to notify the relevant department and invite them to assist in the assessment.[93] (See pp32 and 36 for the slightly different wording for Scotland.) There is no duty on either of those to respond, although in practice it is rare for them to refuse.

The type of assessment you get depends on the nature of your needs. Assessments vary from 'simple assessments' – for items like bus passes and disabled car badges which will often be done by reception staff – to 'comprehensive assessments' if you have needs which cut across departments and which are likely to lead to intensive support.[94]

The assessment could take place in your own home or in hospital. You should be fully involved in your assessment, which should look at all of your needs as a whole.[95] This should include your social and psychological needs.[96] It is important to tell the person who is assessing you about all your needs and how you would like to see help arranged.

Carers' assessments

There is a duty to assess your carer, if s/he requests it, at the same time as your assessment.[97] This is not a free standing assessment but is done in conjunction with your own assessment. A carer's assessment is normally only on request, but guidance to social services says they should ensure it is routine practice to inform carers of their right to an assessment.[98] Paid carers and volunteers cannot have a carer's assessment.

A carer is defined as someone who provides or is about to provide a substantial amount of care on a regular basis.[99] It is left to social services to decide what constitutes a substantial amount of care. If your carer is not thought to provide substantial amounts of care, they should still have a role in your assessment.[100]

The result of your carer's assessment must be taken into account when making a decision about services. The object of the assessment is to identify your carers ability to provide and continue to provide care. Practice guidance has made it clear that in assessing your carer's ability to care, social services should not assume her/his willingness to continue caring or to continue to care at the same level.[101]

In England, as part of the National Carers Strategy, carers have been promised that services will be available to help meet their needs as carers. This will require new legislation.

Recording the assessment

You should be told the outcome of your assessment and the decision on service provision.[102] It is unclear whether this should be in writing or verbally. Guidance suggests that in the case of simple needs the outcome of the assessment can be given verbally, but if a continuing service is needed, you should get a written record of your assessment which will normally be combined with your care plan.[103]

If you have difficulty in getting a copy of your assessment (or care plan), you can request a copy of your file under the Access to Personal Files (Social

Services) (Social Work) (Scotland) Regulations 1989. This will soon be a right under the Data Protection Act 1998.

Your care plan

If, having assessed your needs, social services decides that you need services, they should give you a care plan, which should give details of:

- overall objectives;
- specific objectives;
- the services that will be provided and by whom;
- the cost to you;
- other options considered;
- any point of difference between you and the care assessor;
- any unmet needs;
- who will be responsible for monitoring and reviewing; *and*
- the date of the first planned review.[104]

There is no statutory duty to provide a written care plan, and you may find that you are not offered one. If you want to see your care plan then you could ask for access to your file (see above). Lack of care plans, delays or deficiencies in them have been the subject of a number of legal cases and Ombudsman reports.[105]

Your care plan can include a wide range of services, with a mix of social services help, care from the NHS and from your carers. Services can be provided directly by social services or from an independent provider. You could, as an alternative, receive a payment from social services to arrange your own care (see p46).

How soon should services be provided?

The law is silent on how soon services should be provided (except in the case of disabled facilities grants in England and Wales where it can be up to 12 months). Whether or not the delay is excessive will depend on your particular circumstances. Some social services appear to use delays as a way of keeping within their resources (see p44). If you feel that you have been kept waiting too long for your services you should complain (see p54).

Monitoring and reviewing your services

Although there is nothing in the legislation about monitoring and reviewing services, there is guidance. This states that there should be regular reviews to ensure that the objectives of the care plan are being met and to establish whether any changes are required because of changing needs or service delivery policies.

The review should also monitor the quality of the services provided, taking account of your views and the views of your carer.[106] This is important as currently there is no regulation of domiciliary care. If you have concerns about the quality of your care (eg, the manner, the reliability, and trustworthiness of your carer) you should raise this without waiting for a review.

In practice, reviews are not always carried out on a regular basis, and sometimes are only triggered when social services need to make cuts because of resource constraints (see p45). Under the government's 'Fair Access to Care' initiative in England (see p442) the frequency of reviews will be suggested in guidance. The White Paper *Modernising Social Services* suggested the first review should be carried out within three weeks, and then at least annually, although this will depend on various factors.

4. How far the authority's resources can be taken into account

In a perfect world there would be sufficient resources for everyone to have all the help they need. However community care provision is far from perfect, and social services, housing and health must juggle limited resources to best meet the needs of people in their areas.

To a large extent, health is exempt from challenge because the legislation permits it to take account of resources at all times and, other than aftercare services (see p29), there are no specific duties towards individuals. This is not to say it is not worth seeking advice if you have been refused an NHS service.

However, for housing and social services, there are specific duties that arise and there have been various legal challenges to establish whether the local authority's resources can be taken into account.

This section looks at the various ways local authorities try to manage their resources. It also looks at eligibility criteria, when resources can be taken into account in an assessment, and ceilings on home care services. Local authorities often use waiting lists to manage finite resources. Another way local authorities can increase resources is to make discretionary charges (see p49).

Eligibility criteria

After you have been assessed, social services must make a decision about whether your needs are eligible for services.[107] To determine who should get services, social services use 'eligibility criteria'. This process has been described as a 'system of banding which assigns individuals to particular categories, depending on the extent of the difficulties they encounter in carrying out everyday tasks and relating the level of response to the degree of such difficulties. Any 'banding' should not, however, be rigidly applied, as account needs to be taken of individuals circumstances'.[108] A banding system is normally a series of priority groups, and those in low priority may not have their needs met.

Different local authorities will have different criteria, so you could get a service in one area, but if you move to another, you would not be eligible. Where resources are scarce, the eligibility criteria may be tightened so that people who may have been receiving a service are now defined as no longer needing that service.

Your local authority community care plan should give a description of its eligibility criteria. The criteria might also be described in leaflets about community care in your area.

A number of legal cases have confirmed that authorities are free to set their own eligibility criteria and that resources can be balanced against people's needs. Resources should not, however, be the sole factor.[109] The criteria, should not result in legally unreasonable decisions. They should not leave you at severe physical risk.[110]

In England, the White Paper *Modernising Social Services* has stated that there will be guidance under 'Fair Access to Care' which will set out the principles authorities should follow when devising and applying eligibility criteria.

When resources can be taken into account in your assessment

Social services cannot take its resources into account when deciding whether you are *entitled to an assessment*. [111]

When assessing your needs, and the necessity to provide services, resources are taken into account in so far as the local eligibility criteria have been influenced by the local authority's resources. If a local authority tightens its eligibility criteria because of lack of resources, it must assess you against these new eligibility criteria before withdrawing any services you already receive.[112]

Once social services has decided that you need services, resources can no longer be taken into account if the services come under the Chronically Sick and Disabled Person's Act (see p26). There is a duty to provide such services.[113] It is likely that the same principles would apply in a community care assessment under s12 of the Social Work (Scotland) Act 1968. This is equally true of education services[114] and housing services for disabled facilities grants.[115]

Although social services have a duty to provide some services regardless of resources, they can play a part when deciding between various options which would equally meet your assessed need. For example, they could choose the cheaper option of residential care.[116]

Ceilings on home care services

It is quite common, particularly for older people, to find there is a financial ceiling on the amount of home care which will be provided. Sometimes this is expressed in hours. For example, you may find that the maximum social services will provide is 10-15 hours service, as any more home care would make residential care a cheaper option. These ceilings can become even lower if you have to have two carers – eg, under the handling and lifting rules. Sometimes authorities cut by half the number of hours you can receive. In a recent case this was found to be unlawful.[117]

The ceiling may be equivalent to the net or gross cost to social services of providing residential care. The net cost for residential care for older people is, in some areas, only about £100 a week, and that does not buy much help at home. It is known as the 'perverse incentive' for residential care, and one suggestion for tackling it put forward by the government is to transfer the residential allowance to social services so that:

- it becomes more expensive for social services to place you in residential care; *and*
- they will have more money for providing home care.

As yet there has been no consultation on this, so there are unlikely to be any changes in April 2000, the date originally proposed.

The ceilings imposed are particularly noticeable for older people, with many authorities imposing no ceilings (or setting very much higher ones) on support packages for younger people.

Ceilings should not, however, be so rigid as to fetter the discretion of social services. The Local Government Ombudsman has found against an authority which applied a rigid limit of £110 a week and which could show no evidence of ever diverting from that limit. It was also found in the same case that as there was no such limit for younger people there was age discrimination.[118]

If you are told that you need services beyond those that social services are prepared to pay for, you should seek advice. As yet the legality of ceilings has not been challenged, but it is possible they are unlawful. It may also be possible to use the European Convention of Human Rights (see p63).

5. **Getting direct payments instead of services**

Since April 1997, it has been possible to receive a direct payment from social services to buy the services you need rather than have them provided or arranged by social services. It is also possible to have some services provided by social services and some which you buy using your direct payment.[119]

Who can get a direct payment?

Once you have been assessed as needing community care services, you can get a direct payment if you are:
- over 18 and under 65 years of age, although if you were getting a direct payment before reaching 65 it will continue (see below for changes to age limits in England);
- a disabled person as defined by s29 National Assistance Act 1948 (see p25) or a 'person in need' as defined in s94(1) Social Work (Scotland) Act 1968, (see p25);
- willing to manage your direct payment;
- able to manage your direct payment either by yourself or with assistance.

The regulations specify that certain people, whose liberty to arrange their care is restricted by certain mental health or criminal justice legislation, cannot receive direct payments. This will apply if you are:
- on leave of absence from hospital under mental health legislation;
- conditionally discharged but subject to restrictions under criminal justice legislation;
- subject to guardianship or supervised discharge under mental health legislation;
- receiving any form of aftercare under a compulsory court order;
- under a probation order or you have been conditionally released on licence with a requirement to undergo treatment for a mental health condition, or for drug or alcohol dependency.

In England draft regulations have been issued to extend direct payments to people aged 65 or over. These are expected to come into force early in 2000. As a result of the review of direct payments in England, it has also been announced that direct payments will be available to 16/17-year-olds and parents caring for disabled children. This will require changes to legislation. Under planned legislation, carers will in future be able to receive services in their own right (see p443), and this will be extended to the right to receive direct payment in lieu of such services. Scotland and Wales are also reviewing direct payments and announcements are expected early in 2000.

New draft policy and practice guidance issued in England stresses that social services should consider what assistance would enable a prospective direct payment user to manage, rather than assuming the person cannot manage. It suggests that someone with a fluctuating condition may be able to manage if there is greater assistance during the time when the condition has worsened. It also suggests that if you receive a direct payment and have expressed a preference for this within an Enduring Power of Attorney then the direct payment can continue.[120]

The direct payment scheme is not mandatory and currently not all social services departments offer it, or if they do, may offer it only to very small numbers of people or restrict it to particular client groups. Recently, the Department of Health wrote to one authority saying that, 'Whilst local authorities may pursue broad policies they should be careful not to fetter their discretion. Our view has always been that a local authority should consider carefully each application for a direct payment on its own merits'.[121] The draft policy and practice guidance in England reminds social services that schemes which are developed should serve all adult client groups equitably. The government has also suggested it might consider making the direct payments scheme mandatory for all authorities if the case is strong enough.[122]

Local authorities may be concerned by a recent employment tribunal case in Scotland which found that although the contract of employment was between the disabled person and the care worker, the local authority was technically the employer. This case is being appealed and should be heard in 2000.[123]

What can a direct payment be used for

Direct payments can be used to purchase any service or equipment that meets your needs in the way that you want; however, there are some restrictions. Direct payments cannot be used to pay:

- your spouse or partner living in the same house; or
- a close relative, or her/his spouse, if s/he lives in the same house as you (close relative has the same meaning as for benefit purposes – see p97).[124]The guidance says that social services should not allow you to use it to pay a relative who lives elsewhere or a non-relative who lives in your house. This does not apply to using a direct payment to employ a live-in carer. Social services may decide to make an exception if they are satisfied it is the most appropriate way of securing the relevant service;
- for residential accommodation for any period of more than four weeks in a 12-month period. Within this time, periods of less than four weeks separated by periods of more than four weeks will not be added together.[125]

The level of your direct payment

The direct payment should not normally be more than it would have cost social services to provide (or arrange for) the service themselves. It should be enough for you to cover all the legal costs of being an employer – ie, NI, holidays, sick pay, employers' liability insurance. New draft guidance in England states that any consideration of cost effectiveness should consider long-term best value – ie, a direct payment may represent long term savings if it allows a person to remain in their own home.[126] If circumstances warrant it, social services should be prepared to go above the cost they would normally incur in providing the same services.

Problems have been reported by users who want to use a particular home care agency which charges VAT. In some cases social services have limited the payment to what it would cost to use an agency which does not charge VAT. If this happens to you, you should complain.

If you manage to buy services cheaper than expected, your direct payment may be reduced to that level rather than allowing you to use what is left over to buy-in other services for needs that are not specified in your care plan, but which you might still want.

Any charges you would have had to pay if you had been receiving services from the authority will normally be deducted from direct payments (see p49 for a description of domiciliary charges). It is possible, however, for the payment to be made in full and for you to pay the required charges back.

Monitoring

Social services have to monitor the direct payment to make sure you do not misuse it and that your needs are being adequately met. They can recover money if it has not been used for the services for which it was paid, or if you have not kept to conditions that may have been imposed.[127] Social services have been told they should not penalise honest mistakes. They should also consider that there may be legitimate reasons for unspent funds.

Support if you have a direct payment

When setting up direct payment schemes, social services should ensure there is a support group to provide appropriate information, advice, training, and peer support. Such groups often produce leaflets about recruiting someone to care for you (often known as personal assistants), dealing with the administration of the direct payment, being a good employer, and dealing with emergencies. Some produce newsletters. Groups also offer the opportunity to meet with other users of direct payments to talk over issues as they arise. Ask social services about local support groups or the National Council for Independent Living may be able to put you in touch with a local support group (see Appendix 00).

6. Charges for your services or equipment

Not many services you receive either at home or in day centres will be free. There are national rules to calculate charges for housing grants for people with disabilities (see p147) and national charges for health items covered by health benefits (see p137). This section looks at social services charges.

The legal basis for social services charges

Domiciliary services have attracted charges since 1948. The current legislation is the Health and Social Services and Social Security Adjudication Act 1983 (which amended the Social Work (Scotland) Act 1968 in Scotland). If you have services provided under certain enactments you can be charged for them.[128] You can also be charged for services under s2 of the Chronically Sick and Disabled Persons Act (CSDPA) 1970, although it is not listed as an Act which attracts any charges. This is because s2 links with s29 of the National Assistance Act 1948, which is listed.[129] In Scotland a local authority is exercising functions under the social Work (Scotland) Act 1968 when it provides services under the CSDPA 1970.

In England and Wales, you cannot be charged for services provided under s117 of the Mental Health Act as it is a free standing section (see p261).

In Scotland there are no powers to charge for services under s11 of the Mental Health (Scotland) Act 1984. S11 involves a duty to 'provide suitable training and occupation for people with learning disabilities who are over school age'. Nor can social work departments charge for any transport which they provide to these day services. Also guidance states that local authorities should not charge for non-residential aftercare services provided under s8 of the Mental Health (Scotland) Act 1984 if you are a former NHS patient subject to a community care or supervision order. You should also not be charged for social work services, where those services are initiated by an order of the criminal court.[130]

How charges are decided

It is up to each local authority to decide what, if anything, it considers reasonable to charge.[131] If you can show social services that it is not reasonable to expect you to pay that charge then it can be waived or reduced to what is considered reasonable for you to pay.[132]

There has been no guidance in England and Wales to help local authorities decide what is a reasonable charge. Instead there is an Advice Note for the Social Services Inspectorate which suggests that social services should take account of the full cost of the service and how much of that recipients can reasonably be expected to pay. In Scotland, guidance has been issued on charging which sets out the same criteria for establishing a 'reasonable charge'.[133]

The question of reasonableness has been raised in the courts. In one case the 'overriding criterion of reasonableness' enabled social services to make charges long after the person had finished receiving services (in this case when compensation came through).[134] In another case the judge found that it was not necessary to consult about raising charges or when formulating a charging policy as difficulties paying charges can be taken up individually.[135] The case is being appealed to the Court of Appeal.

Which services are charged for?

This will vary from area to area. Most authorities charge for home care, and nearly all charge for meals on wheels and meals in day centres. An increasing number charge for daycare, and some charge for the transport to day care. The number of authorities charging for equipment is relatively small but it is growing. Often the charge for equipment is in the form of a one-off payment which may not always be mean-tested.

Who should be charged

The Advice Note and the Scottish guidance (see above) make it clear that only the person receiving services should be charged. Family members should not be required to pay unless they are acting on your behalf and are responsible for your finances because you are unable to manage them. However, it then qualifies this by saying that there are times when you could have sufficient reliable access to resources not held in your name for them to be considered as part of the means-test.[136] There is some doubt about whether this tallies with the legislation. Practice varies considerably around the country regarding spouses/partners who may be asked for information about their finances, and their income and capital may be included in the calculation of how much you have to pay. If your spouse/partner's resources are being taken into account, you should seek advice.

Taking account of benefits

One of the most controversial aspects of social services charging is in relation to charging people who are on income support (IS) or receiving attendance allowance (AA) or the care component of disability living allowance (DLA). Social services cannot charge against mobility component of DLA.[137]

The Advice Note and the Scottish guidance suggests that there should be no automatic exemption for people in receipt of benefits such as IS, AA, or incapacity benefit. Charging people on IS raises questions of reasonableness, given that this is a basic income and not intended to cover care costs.

There is also concern about the fact that many authorities charge against your AA or DLA, which often means a higher charge than otherwise is imposed. This has been challenged on the grounds of discrimination under the Disability Discrimination Act and is due to be heard in the Court of Appeal.[138]

Taking account of other income and capital

Social services departments vary considerably in the way they look at income and capital. Some have capital cut-off points – some at £8,000 and some at

£16,000, broadly in line with benefits. Many also assume tariff income from that capital. If your area has capital limits, you may have to pay the maximum charge, which may or may not be the full cost of your services. This could run into several hundreds of pounds a week if you require a lot of care services. People in this position can find it is cheaper to buy care from an independent provider as the cost per hour may not be as high as the social services charge.

Taking account of your extra costs of disability

Although the Advice Note and the Scottish guidance say that social services should take account of additional expenditure because of disability, only some do this when working out your charges. Many authorities wait until you ask for a review of your charges on the grounds that you cannot afford them. When filling in the financial assessment form, it may be useful to itemise all the extra costs you have because of your disability. This could include a gardener, taxis, extra heating, special diet, or equipment that you may have to buy.

If you need to buy extra care because some services are no longer offered by social services, or because a ceiling has been imposed (see p46), you should ask that this be taken into account when assessing your charge. You may well have significant extra costs in these circumstances, but not all authorities will automatically take this into account.

You should complain if social services do not take your extra costs into account (see p54).

Information you should receive

Unless your social services department has a flat-rate charge (now fairly uncommon, but some have a single charge for a particular service regardless of your income or the number of hours of care received), you will normally be asked to fill in a financial assessment. This should be done after your needs assessment (see p40) although in practice the two are often done at the same time.

Once your charge has been worked out you should get a written statement explaining how much you need to pay and how to pay it. It should also explain how you can ask for your charge to be waived or lowered.

Social services should offer you a choice of how to pay your charge.[139] If social services are not providing the service themselves but are using an independent provider, they may ask that you pay the charge directly to the provider. You should not be required to do this as, depending on the way your authority's charging system works, the provider could obtain knowledge of your finances, which raises issues of confidentiality.

If you have not received a service for any reason you should not be expected to pay for it unless you have received clear information about charges – eg, you should know how much notice of cancellation you need to give in order not to pay if you are on holiday. You should not have to pay if your carer does not turn up. Some computer systems have difficulty in dealing with all the changes that can occur in a care plan. Complain if you think you have been charged for services you have not received.

If you cannot afford your charge

You should ask social services to look at your situation again and give them as much detail as possible to support your case – eg, extra costs you have because of disability.

Some people withdraw from the service because of the cost. Before you do this you should make sure the authority will not waive the charge. Failing that, ask for a reassessment of your needs to establish that you will not be left at severe risk if you no longer receive, or have less, services.

Social services cannot withdraw your service if you are unable, or refuse, to pay the charge. As social services have a duty to provide the service you need, this cannot be overruled by the power to charge. The Advice Note and the Scottish guidance make it clear that services should not be withdrawn.

Social services can, however, recover the charge as a civil debt through the magistrates courts (or Sheriff Court in Scotland).[140] During 1999 one or two authorities were prepared to suggest they might take this action against groups which have refused to pay the charges on principle.

Charging practices around the country

Although charges have been imposed for some time, it is during the 1990s that the practice has become a major issue. Care packages requiring extensive services, mean that some charges can be very high, and many authorities have moved away from flat-rate charges to a banded system which relates to the number of hours of care received and your resources. It may appear that charges are introduced, or raised above inflation, and hurriedly introduced, at any time during the year, as a reaction to an immediate resource crisis within social services. Often charging systems which had remained steady for a long time have been radically changed several times within a matter of a few years, leading to huge increases for some individuals.

Charges, tightened eligibility criteria, and ceilings on the amount of home care that social services will provide can mean that you end up paying more. If you are no longer offered a service because you now fall outside of eligibility criteria which have been tightened because of resources (see p44) you may well end up having to buy in that care privately. If the authority imposes a ceiling on the amount of home care it provides, you could be buying in large amounts of care over and above what social services provides.

However it is the disparity between authorities that has caught the most attention. The Audit Commission has done research into the charging policies of most local authorities in England and Wales to look at the extent of the differences. Its report is due in Spring 2000 and the Government has said it will consider how to improve the situation. The Government believes that the scale of variation in the discretionary charging system, including the difference in how income is assessed, is unacceptable.

7. How to complain if you are unhappy about your services

Social services and the NHS each have standard complaints procedures. Housing has no specific procedures other than the normal local authority complaints procedure, which may be similar in practice to that of social services, certainly in the initial stages. There is, however, a national appeals process regarding homelessness and guidance on this, which housing departments have to follow.

This section looks at how to complain to social services and to health authorities. It then looks at what other steps you can take if you are not satisfied.

Complaining about health services

A new complaints procedure was introduced into the NHS in 1996, as there were many concerns about how difficult it was to know who to complain to about something that had happened within the NHS. The new legislation was brought in to unify all the various channels for complaints about both clinical (such as a complaint about medical treatment) and non-clinical (such as the failure of the ambulance service to arrive promptly) issues.[141] It does not cover disciplinary matters or criminal offences. If your complaint is about negligence then the complaints procedure can be used unless you have explicitly indicated an intention to take legal action. As well as directions, guidance was issued setting out the procedures which are explained below.[142]

Each sector within the NHS must produce a written complaints procedure which must be published. You can complain if you are a user or former user of the NHS. Other people may complain on your behalf if they have your consent, and there are specific considerations if the patient lacks mental capacity or has died.

The complaint should be made as soon as possible after the event, and in any case within six months. There is discretion to extend the time limit where it would be unreasonable in the circumstances not to, and where it is still possible to investigate the facts of the case.

If you are considering making a complaint you may find it helpful to speak to your local community health council (health council in Scotland).

The first stage – local resolution

There should be clear complaints procedures to try to resolve the complaint locally on an informal basis. There should be a complaints manager who is responsible for ensuring complaints are responded to and that this first stage is properly carried out. There are differences between trusts, health authorities and GPs. In the case of trusts, written complaints must receive a response in writing from the chief executive. GPs have to comply with minimum standards in their practices. They must publicise the complaints procedure and ensure that patients know where to log a complaint. An initial response should be made within two working days, and the person nominated to investigate complaints should make all necessary enquires and respond within two weeks.

The whole of this first stage can be conducted orally. If you want to take it further, guidance suggests that you should be sent a letter which also indicates your right to seek an independent review panel.

The second stage – the independent review panel

If you are still dissatisfied you can ask for an independent review panel to be set up. Any request for an independent review panel must be passed to the panel's convenor within 28 days. It is not automatic that your case will be heard at a panel. A decision will be made by the convenor based on a signed statement by you. The convenor will:

- decide whether all opportunities to resolve the complaint have been explored at the first stage;
- consult with an independent lay chairman to get an external independent view; *and*
- take appropriate clinical advice.

A decision will be given within 20 working days from the date the convenor received the request. If you are refused a review you can ask the convenor to reconsider, and as a last resort you can complain to the Health Service Ombudsman if you are refused (see p62).

The independent review panel normally comprises three people:

- an independent chair who must not be a past or present employee of the NHS, nor a member of the clinical profession, nor have had formal links with the trust or health authority;
- the convenor;
- and either a representative of the purchaser (in the case of an NHS trust), or an independent person.

If the complaint is about clinical matters there will also be two independent clinical assessors.

The panel should be convened within four weeks of the decision to convene it and should complete its work within 12 weeks. It should be an informal process, and although you cannot have legal representation, you can be accompanied by a person of your choice.

A draft of the panel's report will be sent to the relevant parties 14 days before it is formally issued, in order to check its accuracy. Following the final report, the chief executive must inform you in writing of what action will be taken as a result of the panel's deliberations and of your right to take your case to the ombudsman.

Asking for a review of the decision that you should be discharged from hospital (England and Wales)

There is a separate procedure[143] if you think you should not leave hospital. It can only be used while you are a patient in a hospital, hospice or nursing home. If you are no longer an in-patient you should use the complaints procedure described above if there were aspects of your discharge that you want to complain about.

You, your family, or any carer have the right to ask for a review of the decision that you no longer need in-patient care. During this review you should remain as an in-patient, although the request should be dealt with urgently and you should have an answer within two weeks. This can be extended if there are exceptional circumstances which make the time-scale impossible.[144]

In reaching a decision the health authority should seek advice from an independent panel which will consider your case and make a recommendation. The health authority has the right not to convene a panel if your need falls well outside its eligibility criteria for continuing in-patient care (see p262). If it is decided not to convene the panel you should be given the reasons in writing.

This review procedure cannot be used to challenge the health authority's eligibility criteria. You can only challenge the way the criteria have been applied to you. Neither can it be used to review the type of in-patient care and, where it is offered, the content of any alternative care package or any other aspect of your treatment in hospital. It cannot be used for resolving funding disputes between the health authority and local authority. In all these cases you can use the complaints procedure.

The review procedure can only be used to:
- check that the procedures have been followed correctly in reaching the decision; *and/or*
- ensure that the eligibility criteria have been properly and consistently applied.

The health authority is required to appoint a designated officer to check that all the informal channels have been used and collect information for the panel, including interviewing you and any family or relevant carers.

The panel consists of an independent chair and representatives from the health and local authorities. It has access to an independent clinical adviser to advise the panel on the original clinical judgement and how it relates to the eligibility criteria.

The role of the panel is advisory but the expectation is that its recommendations will be accepted in all but the most exceptional circumstances. You must be given reasons if its recommendations are rejected.

The panel must produce a report each year on the number of cases it has considered and the outcomes.

The right to appeal against the decision to discharge you (Scotland)

If you are in hospital in Scotland you have the right to appeal against the clinical decision to discharge you from continuing NHS care.[145]

Information on this procedure and any advocacy services must be available from hospital staff on request. The appeal is in two stages. Once the consultant has decided that you can be discharged, you or your carer/advocate have ten days to request a review of the decision by the Director of Public Health. This should be completed within two weeks. If it is decided that you should be discharged, you have the right to request a second opinion from an independent consultant from another health board area.

You cannot be discharged during the appeal process. The aim of this appeal process is to ensure that the criteria set out in the guidance has been correctly applied. It cannot be used to complain about the content of the criteria. The appeal procedure is separate from the NHS complaints procedure and there is nothing to stop you using both procedures at the same time.

Complaining about social services

Social services must have a complaints procedure in place, and information about it must be published.[146] As well as Directions there is policy and good practice guidance, *The Right to Complain* (*A Right to Complain* in Scotland). To have the right to complain you must be a 'qualifying individual' – ie, social services has a power or duty to provide you with services and your needs or possible needs for service have come to the attention of social services. Although you cannot complain if social services has no power or duty to provide you with a service, they can use their discretion deal with your complaint even if you are not a qualifying individual.[147]

Each authority must have a designated complaints officer.[148]

The stages of your complaint

Social services complaints procedures are carried out in three stages:
- stage 1 – informal problem–solving stage;
- stage 2 – the formal stage;
- stage 3 – the review stage.

Stage 1 – the informal stage

If you have a complaint social services must attempt to resolve it informally. Your complaint does not need to be in writing. The good practice guide states that just because a complaint is informal it does not mean it is casual. There does not need to be a written record, as this stage is one of negotiation and conciliation. There is no time-scale, which can cause problems if a complaint drags on without resolution. If at this stage your problem has not been resolved within what you think is a reasonable time (which may well depend on the gravity of your situation), you should insist that you are allowed to go on to the next stage of the complaints procedure.

Stage 2 – the formal stage

At this stage you need to formally register your complaint in writing. It is possible to go straight to stage 2, without going through the informal stage 1. Social services must offer you assistance (or let you know where you can get assistance – eg, advocacy) on the use of the complaints procedure. They could help you make sure you have covered all the points you want to make in your formal complaint.

Once it has received your complaint, social services must investigate your complaint and respond to you within 28 days. In England and Wales, if the investigation will take longer, you must be told why (before the 28 days is up) and how long it is likely to take. The response must be within three months.[149]

These response times are often not met, especially in complex cases where a number of people need to be interviewed. If you think the authority is being slow in the way it is handling your complaint you should point out the time limits and ask for reasons why they are not being met. There have been a number of Local Government Ombudsman reports on excessive delays in the complaints procedure.

Social services must notify you in writing of the outcome of your complaint. They should also notify any other person who has sufficient interest. They do not need to give reasons for the decision.

Stage 3 – the review stage

If you are still unhappy with the outcome of your complaint you can, within 28 days of receiving the decision, ask for your complaint to be referred to a review panel.[150] This panel should hear your complaint within 28 days of your request, and you should be told ten days beforehand of the time and place the panel will meet. In Scotland the review committee has to make its recommendation within 56 days of your request.

The panel should be made up of three people. The chair must be an 'independent person' who is not a member of, or employed by, social services, or the spouse of such a person. The other two members can be any individuals whom the authority considers suitable. Often social services appoint a councillor as one wing member and an officer as the other. This can bring into question the independence of the panel.

The panels should be as informal as possible. It can be helpful to take someone along with you for support or to help present you case but it must not be a barrister or solicitor acting in their official capacity. There may be social services officers present in addition to the three panel members (you should be told in advance who they will be) and it may feel intimidating if, like most people, you are not used to such hearings. You can put your complaint in writing or talk to the panel. If you plan to give an oral submission it is worth making notes to make sure you keep to a structure and include all the points you want to make.

The panel should look at all the facts and re-examine the previous decision. It must reach its decision within 24 hours of the hearing and give its recommendations and reasons to you, the local authority and to anyone who is considered to have sufficient interest. If the decision is split between the three panel members this also must be recorded.

The panel should not take into consideration irrelevant factors. In one case the Ombudsman found against an authority where the panel came to the decision that, although the person had lost over £4,200 in benefit due to misleading advice, only a small amount of compensation should be offered as the panel thought it was not appropriate to reimburse lost benefit. This was considered to be an irrelevant factor.[151]

The social services department has 28 days (42 in Scotland) to decide what action to take, to notify you and all those who received the panel's recommendations, and to give reasons for its decision. It must have very good reasons for departing from the panel's recommendations. [152]

Other remedies

At the same time as, or instead of, a complaint to health, housing, or social services you may want to think of other action you can take. Sometimes it is difficult to decide which course of action will have the best outcome. It is useful to talk this over with someone experienced in community care issues. Most national organisations for older or disabled people have helplines and they may be able to suggest the options you could consider to remedy your situation.

Local action

There are other actions which could be pursued at the same time as a formal complaint or as a way of attempting to resolve your situation without recourse to the complaints procedure.

Getting in touch with a local advice group, your councillor or MP/MSP/National Assembly Member

Sometimes you can get help in resolving your problem with the authority by contacting a local advice group, your councillor or MP/MSP. In Wales you can also write to your National Assembly Member (AM). Some gentle querying of a decision by a knowledgeable adviser may get to the root of the problem far faster than the complaints procedure. Councillors and MPs will often take up your case. Sometimes your MP/MSP/AM will pass your complaint to the minister responsible for Health. This can sometimes lead to resolution, as officials will look at the complaint and, where necessary, take it up with the local authority or health service, although this is only likely to happen where the authority is clearly outside the law.

Local (or national) newspapers

Although you may want to think twice about going to the papers, sometimes in an urgent or very difficult situation it can resolve your problems. It has proved quite an effective remedy against waiting in hospital for funding for residential care, or against withdrawal of services.

Contacting the local authority monitoring officer

This is one of the lesser known remedies which can at times be very speedy and effective. Each local authority is required to have an officer (often it is the Chief Executive) to ensure that the authority's policies and decisions are within the law.[153] If you think that a decision has been made which does not follow the law then a letter or fax to the monitoring officer will ensure that the legal department looks at it. It may be worth making sure you are right before taking this action, but in an emergency it can produce a very swift response if you have not been able to persuade the officers dealing with your case to think again about a decision they have made.

Using the ombudsman

There is an ombudsman for health authorities and for local authorities. They can investigate cases of maladministration, which can be quite widely defined. The Local Government Ombudsman has issued 42 principles of good administration. These include:

- staff understanding the law and local policies;
- establishing the relevant facts;
- communication of policies and consistent application of policies;

- giving reasons for decisions;
- adequate record keeping;
- avoiding misleading statements;
- ensuring that decisions and actions are taken within a reasonable time.

You should make your complaint to either the health authority or local authority ombudsman within 12 months of the action which you are complaining about. This time limit can be extended if it is reasonable to do so.[154] An investigator will examine your case, look at the relevant papers, interview you if necessary and interview the officers. Sometimes the investigations are discontinued either because it becomes apparent there was no maladministration or because the authority settles the dispute.

Some cases are reported. If that is to be done, you and the local authority or health authority will have an opportunity to comment on the report for factual correctness before it is finalised. If the case is reported, the authority will be named, but your name will be changed and the officers identified by a letter of the alphabet. Although Ombudsman decisions do not have the force of law, some can be very influential and become well known throughout local authorities and health services. They can occasionally lead to changes in law or to guidance. Sometimes they can influence practice not only in your area but others.

Complaints to the Ombudsman have the great advantage of being free, so can be very useful if you cannot get legal aid to pursue your complaint through the courts. Their great disadvantage is that they can take a very long time; 18 months to 2 years is not uncommon.

The Local Government Ombudsman

The Local Government Ombudsman can look into maladministration in any department of the local authority. S/he will look at the way a decision has been made, and if maladministration is found, may suggest financial compensation. In some cases this can be a considerable sum.

Many decisions have covered delays by housing (in particular disabled facilities grants and housing benefit) and social services – eg, waiting times for assessment or services. Sometimes decisions cover issues such as fettering of discretion, which could also be pursued through the courts.

You cannot complain to the Ombudsman without first having given the local authority the opportunity to answer your complaint.[155] Usually this will mean going through the complaints procedure. However, the Ombudsman will intervene earlier than this if the complaint is taking a long time, in which case this delay itself may be taken up as part of your complaint to the Ombudsman.

The local authority is not obliged to follow the recommendations of the Ombudsman, but if it refuses it can be compelled to publish an agreed statement in a local newspaper.[156]

The Health Service Ombudsman (Health Service Commissioner)

The Health Service Ombudsman is known as the Health Service Commissioner. S/he can investigate complaints about the failure of a service, the failure to provide a service where there is a duty, clinical matters and maladministration. You must have already given the health service opportunity to investigate your complaint.[157]

You can also use the Commissioner to complain against GPs, dentists, opticians who provide NHS services, and chemists.

The Commissioner can make suggestions for remedies if s/he upholds your complaint. You could get a decision changed or repayment of costs incurred. Sometimes the Commissioner recommends changes to procedures so that other people will not be similarly affected.

Secretary of State's default powers

If either social services or the NHS fail to carry out their duties the Secretary of State can declare them to be in default of their duty[158] and direct them to do so. In Wales these powers have devolved to the First Secretary of the National Assembly for Wales. In Scotland these powers have now transferred to the Scottish ministers. In practice that step has never been taken, but if you write to the Secretary of State asking her/him to use her/his default powers, an investigation by officers of the relevant department may informally resolve your problem if the facts show that the authority is clearly in breach of the law.

Judicial review

The main legal remedy in cases which involve public bodies such as local authorities and the NHS is judicial review. Until recently fairly rarely used, there is now an increasing body of case law and there have been some very important test cases addressing some of the most contentious community care issues.

The most common grounds for judicial review are:
* the decision is illegal (*ultra vires*);
* the authority has misunderstood the relevant law;
* it is unreasonable given the facts;
* it shows an improper exercise of discretionary power – for instance fettering its discretion;
* it has taken into account an irrelevant consideration.

To take your complaint to judicial review you will need to seek legal advice and in particular discuss the costs, as it can be very expensive if you are not eligible for legal aid. Judicial review can be a lengthy process, but at times, when your situation is very urgent, action can be taken within days and sometimes on the same day.

There are strict time limits and you must start your case within three months of the decision relating to your complaint. Normally your solicitor will write a 'letter before action' which tells the authority the grounds of the complaint and indicate that unless it is resolved, an application will be made to the courts to grant leave for a hearing.

Sometimes this letter itself will resolve the problem (often because the authority's legal department sees the case for the first time and realises there are flaws in the decision, or because a decision is made not to get involved in litigation).

If this does not happen you seek leave to the High Court for a full hearing. Sometimes your case will get settled before the full hearing. The court can put into place the following remedies:

- overturn the decision and order the authority to take the decision again (*certiorari*). This can sometimes mean the authority could still make the same decision, but this time may make it correctly;
- forbid the authority to do something (injunction). This is often used as an interim way of making sure services are put back in place while waiting for the hearing by forbidding them to be withdrawn;
- oblige the authority to take positive action (*mandamus*);
- forbid the authority to do something inconsistent with its legal power (prohibition);
- make a statement about your rights and the general legal position (declaration).

Your case may go on to the Court of Appeal either on the grounds that there is a realistic prospect of success on a point of law or that the case is of public interest and so merits a hearing in a higher court. Eventually your case could go to the House of Lords.

In Scotland a similar process for judicial review exists through raising action in the court of session in Edinburgh. These are other (seldom used) remedies under Scottish law: consult an adviser or a lawyer for details.

European Court of Human Rights and Human Rights Act 1998

The European Court of Human Rights and Human Rights Act 1998 are beginning to have an effect on decisions made in the field of community care. Currently cases can be taken to Europe under the Convention on Human Rights. However, the UK has now passed the Human Rights Act which will mean that the same basic set of rights will be able to be considered in UK courts. Although the Act does not come into force until 2 October 2000, there is already evidence that the courts are taking it into consideration in their decisions.[159]

The articles in the Convention on Human Rights that are of significance in community care are:

- the right to life (article 2);
- the right not to be subject to torture or degrading treatment or punishment (article 3);
- the right to liberty and security of the person (article 5);
- the right to a fair hearing by an independent and impartial tribunal (article 6);
- the right to respect for family life, home and correspondence (article 8).

The Convention also includes the right to an effective remedy if a violation of any right has been committed by a public body. It also requires that your rights and freedoms are secured without discrimination.

Local authorities and health services are gearing up to the changes the Act will bring and are scrutinising decisions on the basis of whether they impinge on any of these rights.

- This is a remedy which is likely to become increasingly common over the next few years and the extent of these rights will be tested in the courts. As yet it is not clear how far they can be used.

Notes

1. **What are community care services?**
   1 s46(3) NHS and CCA 1990
   2 s5A(4) SW(S)A 1968
   3 *R v Social Fund Inspector ex parte Connick* 8 June 1993.
   4 DoE Guidance 17/96
   5 DoH /DETR CD 'You and Your services'.

2. **The responsibilities of social services, health, and housing**
   6 LAC (99)13 and LAC (99)14
   7 *Community Care in the Next Decade and Beyond* – Policy Guidance – 1990. Assessment and are management SWSG11/1991

8 s7 (1) LASSA 1970; s5(1) SW(S)A 1968
9 *R v North Yorkshire County Council ex parte Hargreaves* CCLR December 1997 and *R v Islington LBC ex parte Rixon* (CCLR) March 1998
10 *R v Islington ex parte Rixon* (CCLR) March 1998
11 *R v Powys CC ex parte Hambidge Court of Appeal* (CCLR) September 1998
12 LAC (93)7 WOC 41/93
13 LAC (93)10 WOC 35/93 Appendix 4
14 There have been a number of Ombudsman Reports on the extent of advice and the accuracy of such advice. Nos 91/C/1246, 94/B/2128, and 93 /A/3738

15 LAC (93)10 WOC 35/93 Appendix 2

16 SWA 1968 / SWSG 11/96

17 s94 SWSA 1968

18 s12(2) SWSA

19 *R v Gloucestershire CC ex parte Barry* (CCLR) December 1997

20 LAC (93)7 WOC 41/93

21 *R v Haringay ex parte Norton* (CCLR) March 1998. because these words are in the Act social services have to assess you for them if you are a disabled person.

22 Guidance is given in LAC (90)7 SDD40/1985

23 *R v Ealing LBC ex parte Leaman* (TLR) 10 February 1984 and *R v N Yorkshire ex parte Hargreaves* (no 2) (CCLR) June 1998

24 The AMA/ACC issued a joint circular in 1971 but there has been no government guidance.

25 DHSS Circular 19/71 is the only and still current circular.

26 s21 NHSA 1977 and Sch 8

27 LAC (93)10 WOC 35/93 Appendix 3

28 s14 SWSA 1968

29 s8 and 11 MHSA 1984

30 s117(2) MHA 1983 and *R v Ealing District Health Authority ex parte Fox* 1993, all ER 170 QDB

31 LAC (96)8/HSG(96)11WHC(95)6

32 *Clunis v Camden and Islington Health Authority. Court of Appeal* (CCLR) March 1998

33 s1(2) MHSA 1984

34 s6 LASSA 1970; s3 SWSA 1968

35 LGOR 92/A/4108

36 This is one of a range of performance indicators used to measure the performance of social services. It is mentioned in the draft 'Long term care charter – You and Your Services'.

37 s46 NHS and CCA 1990; s5(A) SWSA 1968

38 CCPD LAC 91/16; CCP SW1/91

39 CCCD LAC (93)4 WDC 16/93/SW4/93

40 Community Care and the Next Decade and Beyond – Policy Guidance 1990 para 2.25; SWSG 11/1 para 7

41 Policy Guidance 1990 para 3.56 SWSG 11/91

42 LAC (94)24 WDC/6/92

43 LGOR 97/A/4069.

44 s47(3) NHS and CCA 1990; s12A(3) SWSA 1968

45 s3 NHSA 1977 and Part III NHSSA 1978

46 See *R v N and E Devon ex parte Coughlan* (CA) CCLR September 1999 which discusses the duties of the Secretary of State to provide nursing.

47 EL (95) 97

48 *R v North Derbyshire Health Authority ex parte Fisher* (CCLR) March 1998

49 HSG (95)8 LAC (95)5 WHC (95)7 WOC 16/95 NHS MEL(1996) 22 para 10 but please note that this guidance may change early in 2000

50 Further guidance on palliative care is found in EL(93)14 and EL (94)14 MEL (94) 104

51 Further guidance on respite care was issued in EL(96)89 following concerns about restrictions being imposed on respite care.

52 DoH and DETR Consultation Document – You and Your services

53 HSG (95)8 LAC (95)5 WHC (95)7 / WOC 16/95 NHS MEL (1996)22 para 17

54 Ibid para 25

55 NHS (GPS) Reg 1992

56 EL (91) 28 Management Executive Continence Services and the Supply of incontinence aids.

57 HSG(96)34 MEL 92/67

58 HSG (96)53 and HSC 1998/004

59 HA 1999

60 EL (97)62

61 HSC 1998/228

62 HSC 1998/167

63 EL(97)65

64 s47(3) NHS and CCA 1990

65 s12A(3) SWSA 1968

66 Part VII HA 1996; part II HSA

67 DoE Guidance 10/92 SWSG 7/94

68 Building Regs Part M 1991 Access and facilities for disabled people. Approved document 17 1999

69 ss9 and 10 HA 1985; part 1 HSA 1987

70 s23 HGCRA 1996

71 DoE 17/96

72 ss33 and 36 HGCRA 1996

73 DoE 17/96

74 s2 CSDPA 1970

75 s2 CSDPA 1970

76 s87 SWSA 1968
77 HSA 1987 Part XIII
78 SOC SDD 40/1985. Provision of aids equipment and house adaptations for disabled people living at home.
79 s76 HGCRA 1996
80 s77 HGCRA 1996
81 DoE Guidance 17/96

3. Getting the services you need

82 s47(1) NHS and CCA 1990; s12(A) SWSA 1968
83 s47(2) NHS and CCA; s12(A) SWSA 1968; and s4 DPSCRA 1986
84 ss4 and 8 DPSCRA1986 and s1 CRSA 1995. s2 of this Act added a new s3A into the SW(S)A 1968
85 Community Care in the next Decade and Beyond – Policy Guidance 1990, para 3.15
86 s47(5) NHS and CCA 1990; s12(5) SWSA 1968
87 Community Care into the Next Decade and Beyond –Policy Guidance 1990 para 3.20; Assessment and Care Management (SW11/1991) para 5.2 and Practice Guidance-Care Management and Assessment 1991.
88 *R v Bristol ex parte Penfold* (CCLR) September 1998
89 DoH Consultation – You and Your Services.
90 LGOR 97/A/4069
91 LGOR 94/C/1165 and 94/C/0805
92 LAC (93)2 SWSG 14/93
93 s47(3) NHS and CCA 1990; s12A(3) SWSA 1968
94 Practice Guidance Care Management and Assessment 1991 (jointly issued England, Wales and Scotland)
95 Community Care into the Next Decade and Beyond – Policy Guidance 1990 para 3.9; Assessment Care Management (SW11/1991) para 5.
96 *R v Haringay ex parte Norton CCLR March 1998* and *R v Avon CC ex parte M* (CCLR) June 1999
97 s1(1)A CRSA 1995
98 LAC (96) 7 WOC 16/96 para 20 SWSG 11/96
99 s1(1)V CRSA 1995
100 Policy Guidance 1990 para 3.27 – 3.29
101 Practice Guidance 1991 para 9.8

102 Policy Guidance 1990 para 3.56 EW.S SW11/1991 para 5.9
103 England, Wales and Scotland Practice Guidance 1991 para 3.5
104 England, Wales and Scotland Practice Guidance 1991 para 4.37
105 *R v Islington ex parte Rixon CCLR, March 1998, R v Sutton ex parte Tucker* (CCLR) June 1998; LGOR 93/A/2071.
106 Policy Guidance 1990 para 3.52 SW11/1991 para 19.2

4. How far the authority's resources can be taken into account

107 s41(1)(b) NHS and CCA 1990; s12A(b) SWSA 1968
108 CI (92)34 known as the Laming letter. Although cancelled in 1994 this letter is still used and quoted in legal judgments.
109 *R v Gloucestershire ex parte Barry* (CCLR) December 1997
110 *R v Gloucestershire ex parte Mahfood* (CCLR) December 1997
111 *R v Bristol ex parte Penfold* (CCLR) September 1998
112 *R v Gloucestershire ex parte Barry* (CCLR) December 1997
113 *R v Gloucestershire ex parte Barry* (CCLR) December 1997
114 *R v Sussex ex parte Tandy* (CCLR) June 1998
115 *R v Birmingham ex parte Mohammed* (CCLR) September 1998
116 *R v Lancashire ex parte Ingham (R v Gloucestershire ex parte Barry Court of Appeal)* (CCLR) December 1997
117 *R v Birmingham City Council ex parte Killigrew* (CCLR) December 1999.
118 LGOR 96/C/4315

5. Getting direct payments instead of services

119 CCDPA 1996.
120 Direct Payments – Draft Policy and Practice Guidance Consultation 1999
121 Quoted in CCLR June 1999
122 White Paper 'Modernising Social Services'
123 Employment Tribunal Scotland – Case No S/103022/97
124 CCDP Reg 3
125 Reg 4

126 Draft Policy and Practice Guidance Consultation 1999
127 s2 CCDPA

6. **Charges for your services or equipment**
128 s29 NAA 1948; s45 HSPHA; s8 NHSA 1977, and meals and recreation provided under Sch 9 para 1 part II of HASSASSAA; s87 SWSA 1968 councils can charge for services provided under the 1968 Act and ss7 and 8 MHSA 1984
129 *R v Powys CC ex parte Hambidge 1* (CA) (CCLR) September 1998
130 SWSG1/97 para 8 and 9
131 s17(1) HASSASSAA 1983; s87(1A)6 SWSA this was inserted by s18 HASSASSAA
132 s17(3) HASSASSAA 1983; s87 SWSA 1968
133 SWSG1/97
134 *Avon CC v Hooper* (CCLR) September 1998
135 *R v Powys CC ex parte Hambidge (2)* (CCLR) September 1999
136 SSI Advice Note Discretionary Charges for Adult Social Services paras 18 and 19 SWSG 91/97 para 29
137 s73(14) SSCBA 1992.
138 *R v Powys CC ex parte Hambidge 2.* (CCLR) September 1999
139 The Local Government Association has produced a Good Practice Guide for Discretionary Charges.
140 s17(4) HASSASSA; s87 SWSA 1968

7. **How to complain if you are unhappy about your services**
141 Directions were made under the NHSA 1977; NHSSA 1978 and HCPA1995
142 EL (95)121, EL(96) 19, and EL (96)58 (in Scotland, 'Listening, acting, improving' Guidance on the implementation of the NHS complaints procedure 1996)
143 LAC (95)5, HSG (95) 8 WOC 16/95 WHC (95)7 (but note that this guidance may change early in 2000
144 LAC (95)17, HSG (95)39 WHC (95)7
145 NHS MEL (1996) 22
146 s7B LASSA 1970 and Complaints Procedure Directions 1990; s5B SW(S)A 1968 and SW(RP)(S)D 1996

147 Policy Guidance 1990 Para 6.5
148 Direction 4(1) England and Wales Direction 3A Scotland
149 Direction 6(1)
150 Direction 7(2) England and Wales Direction 8(3) Scotland
151 LGOR 93/A/3738
152 *R v Islington ex parte Rixon* (CCLR) March 1998 and *R v Avon CC ex parte M* CCLR June 1999
153 s5 LGHA 1989
154 ss 26 LGA 1974; s9 HSCA 1993; s25 LGSA 1975
155 s26 LGA 1974; s25 LGSA 1975
156 s31 LGA 1974
157 HSCA 1993
158 s7D LASSA 1970, s85 NHSA 1977; s211 LGSA 1973
159 *R v N and E Devon ex parte Coughlan* (CCLR) September 1999

3

Chapter 3

Social security benefits in the community

This chapter outlines the main social security benefits which are available to people living in the community. It explains which benefits can and cannot be paid at the same time, and the main conditions relating to each benefit. This chapter covers:
1. Which benefits you can claim (p69)
2. Non-means-tested benefits (p70)
3. Means-tested benefits (p93)
4. People in hospitals (p125)
5. Increasing your entitlement to benefit – examples (p130)

General rules about income, capital, claims and appeals are covered in Chapters 6 to 11. Special rules which apply to some benefits if you are living in a care home, are covered in Chapters 21 and 22. Special rules which apply if you are in hospital are explained on pp125–30. You may be excluded from benefit if you are classed as a 'person from abroad' (see Chapter 9). Proposed changes to some benefits are set out in Chapter 25.

With community care services increasingly becoming subject to charges (see Chapter 2), it is important to ensure you are receiving all the benefits you are entitled to, so that you can afford to pay for the care you need. Many people do not claim their full entitlement, partly because the rules are so complex. This chapter gives only an outline of the rules but should help you identify the benefits you can claim. If you need further details, you can consult CPAG's *Welfare Benefits Handbook* (see Appendix 5). If you are unsure whether you are receiving your correct entitlement, or you are refused benefit, you should seek advice (see Appendix 2).

It is important to understand the conditions of all the benefits which may apply to your circumstances, as you may have to claim more than one benefit in order to maximise your income. Some typical examples of where claimants have been able to maximise their incomes are set out on p130. For details of problems commonly encountered when claiming benefits, and how to overcome them, see Chapter 11.

1. **Which benefits you can claim**

Types of benefits

There are two main types of benefits:

- **Means-tested benefits**. These are payable if you have less than a set amount of income and capital. The amount of benefit you are entitled to depends on your financial and family circumstances. The main means-tested benefits are described on p93.
- **Non-means-tested benefits**. These are payable in specified circumstances – eg, if you are disabled, widowed, retired, or a carer. Set amounts are payable, mostly regardless of your means (some benefits are affected by earnings or occupational pensions). Some benefits are only payable if you have made sufficient national insurance (NI) contributions. The main non-means-tested benefits are described on p70.

Combinations of benefits

You can generally claim any combination of benefits to which you are entitled. In particular:

- All **means-tested benefits** such as income support (IS), housing benefit (HB) and council tax benefit (CTB) can be paid with any other benefit. IS is commonly claimed to 'top up' non-means-tested benefits such as retirement pension and incapacity benefit. If you are entitled to IS, you are automatically eligible for maximum HB and CTB, and as social fund payments, and other sources of financial assistance.
- All **non-means-tested benefits** can be paid with means-tested benefits. Although most count as income when calculating entitlement to means-tested benefits, some result in additional payments of means-tested benefits in the form of premiums (see p97). Attendance allowance (AA) and disability living allowance (DLA) are particularly valuable benefits because they can be paid on top of any other benefit, they do not count as income for means-tested benefits and they can entitle you to premiums as well.

Note, however, that if you are entitled to more than one of the following overlapping non-means-tested benefits, you can only be paid the highest amount for which you qualify:[1]

- retirement pension;
- widow's pension;
- widowed mother's allowance;
- incapacity benefit;
- severe disablement allowance;
- invalid care allowance;
- maternity allowance;

- contribution-based jobseeker's allowance.

When identifying which benefits you could claim, check:
- whether you are entitled to any of the overlapping benefits listed above; *then*
- whether you are entitled to any other non-means-tested benefits, in particular AA or DLA; *then*
- whether you qualify for any means-tested benefits.

Example

Mrs Anelka is aged 62 and lives alone. She has become severely disabled. She receives a widow's pension of £66.75 a week and an occupational pension of £20 a week. She is also entitled to severe disablement allowance but receives no payment because of the overlapping benefit rules. She has £2,500 savings. She claims DLA and is awarded the higher rate care component of £52.95 a week. This enables her to claim IS of £35.25 a week (because she now qualifies for a severe disability premium – see p97). She has more than doubled her income from £86.75 to £174.95 a week.

Most of the benefits described below are administered and paid by the Benefits Agency. Claim forms are available at your local Benefits Agency office. General rules about claiming (including appointees), getting paid and challenging decisions are covered in Chapter 10. From April 2000 you may be required to attend an interview to claim some benefits (see Chapter 25).

2. Non-means-tested benefits

Retirement pension

Retirement pension is paid to people over pensionable age. For most types of pensions, eligibility and the amount payable are dependent on NI contribution conditions. Retirement pension is taxable (apart from increases for children).

Who can claim

There are three main categories of retirement pension. Despite the name, you do not have to retire to claim a pension and if you continue to work your earnings will not reduce your pension. Pensionable age is currently 60 for a woman and 65 for a man.[2]

Category A pension

You qualify for a Category A pension if:[3]
- you satisfy the NI contribution conditions (see below); *and*
- you are over pensionable age (see above).

Category B pension

You qualify for a Category B pension if you are a married woman and:[4]
- your husband satisfies the NI contribution conditions (see below); *and*
- you and your husband are both over pensionable age (see above); *and*
- your husband is entitled to a Category A pension (see above).

You qualify for a Category B Pension if you are a widow and:[5]
- your husband satisfied the NI contribution conditions (see below) or died from an industrial injury or disease (see p89); *and*
- you were over 60 when he died or you were entitled to a widow's pension when you became 60.

You qualify for a Category B pension if you are a widower and;[6]
- your wife satisfied the NI contribution conditions (see below); *and*
- you became 65 after 5 April 1979; *and*
- your wife died when you were both over pensionable age.

Category D pension

You qualify for a Category D pension if:[7]
- you are aged 80 or over; *and*
- you have been resident in Great Britain for at least 10 of the 20 years which include your 80th birthday; *and*
- you are not entitled to a higher category pension.

National insurance contribution conditions[8]

National insurance contributions are payable on earnings above a certain limit. You can also be credited with contributions during periods of unemployment or incapacity for work.

To qualify for a full Category A or B retirement pension, contributions must have been paid or credited for all the years of your 'working life' (less an allowance of up to five years). A minimum number of contributions must have been paid during at least one tax year. Your working life normally runs from the age of 16 up to pensionable age or the year of death (if earlier) but does not include years spent out of the labour market while bringing up a child. If the conditions were met for a proportion of your working life, a reduced-rate pension may be payable. It may be possible to enhance your contribution record by paying Class 3 voluntary contributions at a later date (you should always get advice before doing this). Widows, widowers and divorcees may be able to use the contribution record of their late or former spouse to help them qualify for a Category A pension.

Amount
Full basic pension[9]

Category A / Category B (widow/widower)	£66.75 a week
Category B (married woman)/Category D	£39.95 a week

Adult dependants[10]
You are entitled to a weekly increase of Category A retirement pension of up to £39.95 for a spouse (depending on your NI record) if s/he is 'residing with' you, or you are contributing to her/his maintenance at a weekly rate of at least the amount of the increase. You still count as 'residing with' your spouse during temporary absences or while either of you is in hospital. You are not entitled to an increase, however, if your spouse is receiving one of the overlapping benefits listed on p69, or if s/he has weekly earnings and/or a private pension exceeding £51.40 (or exceeding the amount of the increase if s/he is not residing with you). For full details of how earnings are calculated (including child care allowances), see CPAG's *Welfare Benefits Handbook*. You are only entitled to an increase for your husband if you were previously getting an increase in incapacity benefit for him (see p74).

If you are not receiving an increase for a spouse, you can claim an increase for another adult who is looking after a child for whom you are responsible. You must be residing with, or maintaining the adult (the rules are as for a spouse – see above), or employing her/him at a weekly cost of at least £39.95. The overlapping benefit and earnings rules which apply to spouses (see above) also apply to other adult dependants. If you are employing an adult dependant, however, the earnings rule only applies if s/he is living with you and the amount you are paying her/him is ignored.

Other additions
There are a number of other additions which may be payable with the basic pension:
- You may qualify for a weekly increase of Category A or B pension of £9.90 for your eldest child and £11.35 for other children, but entitlement is affected if your partner has weekly earnings and/or a private pension exceeding £145.[11] For further details of the conditions see CPAG's *Welfare Benefits Handbook*.
- You may be entitled to additional pension under the State Earnings-Related Pension Scheme (SERPS) depending on your (or your spouse's) earnings and NI contributions from 1978 (this will not apply if you were contracted out of SERPS because you were in an occupational or personal pension scheme).[12]
- You may be entitled to graduated retirement benefit based on your NI contributions from 1961 to 1975.

- You can qualify for extra pension by not claiming (deferring) your entitlement for up to five years.[13] You should always take advice before doing this, as it may not be in your best interest.

How to claim

The Benefits Agency should send you a claim form (BR1) about four months before you reach pensionable age. You must make a separate claim for increases for any dependants as they are not paid automatically. You can get a pension forecast of your likely entitlement by completing form BR19. You should claim a Category D pension on form BR2488.

Widows' benefits

Widows' benefits are paid to women whose husbands have died. There is currently no equivalent benefit for widowers – but see p445 for future proposals.

Who can claim

There are three types of widows' benefits (see below). You can get a widow's payment and either widowed mother's allowance or widow's pension. Entitlement is not affected by any earnings or savings you have. Widow's payment is not taxable. Widow's pension and widowed mother's allowance are taxable (apart from any increases for children).

You count as a widow if were legally married to a man when he died. The law is complex and you should seek advice if:

- you lived with your late partner as husband and wife for a long time but were never married; *or*
- your marriage was polygamous; *or*
- the Benefits Agency decides your marriage was not valid under UK law or does not accept that your husband is dead.

You are not entitled to widows' benefit if you remarry or while you are living with another man as husband and wife.[14]

Widow's payment

You qualify for a one-off, lump sum widow's payment of £1,000 if:[15]

- your late husband paid a minimum number of NI contributions in any one tax year or died after 10 April 1988 from an industrial injury or disease (see p89); *and*
- when he died, you were either under 60 or he was not entitled to a Category A retirement pension (see p70).

Widowed mother's allowance

You qualify for widowed mother's allowance if:[16]
- your late husband satisfied the NI contribution conditions (the conditions are as for retirement pensions – see p70) or died after 10 April 1988 from an industrial injury or disease (see p89); *and*
- you are pregnant by your late husband (or by artificial means if you were residing with your husband when he died), or you are entitled to child benefit for a 'qualifying child' (ie, a child of yours and your late husband) or a child for whom either of you were getting child benefit when your husband died (you must have been residing with your husband if you were the one getting child benefit).

Widow's pension

You qualify for widow's pension if:[17]
- your late husband satisfied the NI contribution conditions (the conditions are as for retirement pensions – see p70) or died after 10 April 1988 from an industrial injury or disease (see p89); *and*
- when he died or when you stopped being entitled to widowed mother's allowance (see above) you were aged 45 to 65 (40 to 65 if he died before 11 April 1988).

If you are entitled to widowed mother's allowance, you cannot qualify for widow's pension until your entitlement ceases. Widow's pension is only payable until you are 65.

Amount[18]

Basic amount

Widow's payment	£1,000	
Widowed mother's allowance	£66.75	a week, plus
	£9.90	for your eldest qualifying child and
	£11.35	for other qualifying children (see p74 for who counts as a qualifying child)
Widow's pension	£66.75	a week

Additional amounts

You may be entitled to additional widowed mother's allowance and widow's pension based on your late husband's earnings and NI contributions under SERPS (see p71).

Reductions

Your widowed mother's allowance or widow's pension may be paid at a reduced rate if your husband's NI record was incomplete (see p78 – but note that you may be able to increase your entitlement by paying Class 3 contributions).

Your widow's pension is reduced if you were under 55 when your husband died, or when your widowed mother's allowance stopped (under 50 if your husband died before 11 April 1988). Your basic and additional (SERPS) pension is reduced by 7 per cent for each year you were under the age of 55 (or 50).

How to claim

You should claim on form BW1. You must claim a widow's payment within three months of your husband's death and your claim for widowed mother's allowance or a widow's pension can only be backdated for up to three months.[19] The time limits may be waived if you were unaware of your husband's death. You should seek advice if this applies to you.[20]

Incapacity benefit

Incapacity benefit (IB) is paid to people who are incapable of work and have made sufficient NI contributions. IB is taxable, apart from the short-term lower rate (see p78).

Who can claim

You qualify for IB if:[21]
- you are 'incapable of work' (see p76); *and*
- you satisfy the NI contribution conditions (see p78); *and*
- you are under pensionable age (see p70) if you are claiming long-term IB (see p78) or not more than five years over pensionable age if you are claiming short-term IB (see p78).

You should also note the following points:
- If you are an employee you will normally be entitled to statutory sick pay (SSP) from your employer for up to 28 weeks while you are off sick (see p92). You cannot be paid IB while you are entitled to SSP.[22]
- You must be incapable of work for at least four consecutive days (a 'period of incapacity for work') to qualify for IB. Periods of incapacity which are separated by eight weeks or less are treated as single period (in some circumstances, the linking period can be extended to one or two years if you have been working or training). IB is not payable for the first three days of a period of incapacity ('waiting days').[23]
- You may be entitled to IB without satisfying the normal NI contribution conditions, if you are a widow, widower or pensioner (see p78 if you are a

pensioner). The rules are complex and you should seek further information or advice.

'Incapable of work'

Two tests are used to decide whether you are incapable of work:

- The 'own-occupation-test' applies for the first 28 weeks of incapacity if you have been working for at least 16 hours a week for more than 8 weeks in the 21 weeks before your claim. You satisfy the test if you are incapable of carrying out your last job because of illness or disablement (physical or mental). All that is normally required is a medical certificate (Med 3) from your doctor.[24]

- The 'all-work' test applies when the own occupation test does not, or ceases to, apply.[25] Details of the test are set out below.

The 'all-work-test' measures your ability to perform a range of physical and mental activities which are laid down in regulations.[26] These include walking, using stairs, sitting, standing, bending, reaching, lifting, speaking, hearing, seeing, controlling your bladder and bowels, coping with pressure and everyday tasks and interacting with people. Each activity is sub-divided into a series of 'descriptors' which measure the varying degrees of difficulty a person may have in relation to that activity – eg, unable to walk a few steps/50 metres/ 200 metres/400 metres, without stopping or severe discomfort. Each descriptor is allocated a fixed number of points. To satisfy the test, you must score at least 15 points for the physical descriptors, or 10 points for the mental descriptors or 15 points for both.[27] For a full list of the descriptors and details of their application, see CPAG's *Welfare Benefits Handbook*.

You are normally assessed for the 'all-work-test' in two stages:[28]

- You are sent a questionnaire (form IB 50) which you must complete. The questionnaire takes you through the physical descriptors and asks you to identify which ones apply to you and why. If you unable to carry out an activity repeatedly, or not without pain or discomfort, you should explain this on the form. The questionnaire also asks if you have any mental health problems – eg, depression. When the 'all-work-test' is first applied, you will be asked to submit a Med 4 certificate from your doctor with your questionnaire.

- You may then be required to attend a DSS medical examination by a Medical Services doctor. The doctor will complete a medical report form for the Benefits Agency, including details of which descriptors apply to you.

You may be re-assessed at any time and you should not assume that you will be found incapable of work because you have previously satisfied the all work test.[29]

You are treated as incapable of work without having to satisfy the all work test in the following circumstances:

- You are waiting to be assessed. It can take weeks or months before you are sent a questionnaire and required to attend a DSS medical. You are treated as incapable of work in the meantime as long as you continue to submit medical certificates and you have not been found capable of work in the previous six months (unless you are suffering from a different or worsened condition).[30]
- You are receiving the highest rate care component of disability living allowance (see p81), or are registered blind, or terminally ill, or 80 per cent disabled for the purposes of severe disablement allowance (see p79) or disablement benefit (see p91).[31]
- You are suffering from certain severe conditions including tetraplegia, paraplegia, dementia, persistent vegetative state; a severe learning disability, mental illness or neurological or muscle wasting disease; inflammatory polyarthritis, severe cardio-respiratory impairment, dense paralysis on one side, severe damage to the brain or nervous system, severe immune deficiency, or a certified contagious or infectious disease.[32]
- You have failed the 'all-work-test' but are suffering from a severe, life threatening condition, or you are likely to undergo major surgery or therapy within three months of a Medical Services examination.[33]
- You are in hospital, or are having renal dialysis, total parenteral nutrition, plasmapheresis, chemotherapy or radiotherapy.[34]
- You have been receiving benefit on the basis on incapacity since 12 April 1995 (you must be aged 58 or over, or receiving severe disablement allowance – see p79).[35]

Work you may do while claiming

You are not entitled to benefit for any week in which you actually do any work. The following work, however, does not count and has no effect on your benefit:[36]

- 'therapeutic work' for less than an average of 16 hours a week, which pays less than £58 a week. 'Therapeutic work' is work carried out on the advice of your doctor to help improve, prevent, or delay deterioration of your condition;
- voluntary work, caring for a relative, or work in a sheltered work scheme or as part of a treatment programme under medical supervision.

Note: The above rules and procedures relating to incapacity for work also apply to severe disablement allowance (see p79), IS (see p93) and the payment of the disability premium (see p97) with IS, housing benefit (see p102) and council tax benefit (see p111). A decision that you are incapable of work for the purposes of one benefit is conclusive for the purposes of subsequent claims for other benefits, so you do not have to be re-assessed separately for each benefit claim.[37] You can appeal against any decision that you are capable of work (see p224) and you may be able to claim IS until your appeal is decided (see p94). For further details of the 'all-work' test and how to challenge decisions, see CPAG's *Welfare Benefits Handbook*.

National insurance contribution conditions

You must have paid a minimum number of national insurance (NI) contributions in any one tax year (April to April) and you must have paid or been credited with a minimum number of contributions during each of the last two tax years before the start of the calendar year in which your period of incapacity for work (see p79) began.[38]

Amount

Basic amount

There are three rates of IB:[39]

- The lower rate of short-term IB is £50.35 a week. It is paid for the first 28 weeks of entitlement.
- The higher rate of short-term IB is £59.55 a week. It is paid after you have been receiving the lower rate of IB or SSP (see p92) for 28 weeks.
- The long-term rate of IB is £66.75 a week. It is paid after you have been receiving the higher rate of short term IB for 28 weeks (ie, after a year of incapacity).

If you are terminally ill or entitled to the highest rate care component of disability living allowance, you are entitled to the long-term rate of IB after six months, rather than a year, of incapacity.[40] Previous periods of incapacity may link to your current period to entitle you to a higher rate of IB (see p75).

Additional amounts

- If you are over pensionable age (see p70), short-term IB is paid at an enhanced rate of £64.05 (lower rate) or £66.75 (higher rate). You only qualify if you are less than five years over pensionable age, your period of incapacity (see p76) began before you reached pensionable age and you have deferred entitlement to a Category A or B retirement pension (see p70).[41] You do not need to have satisfied the normal NI conditions for IB (see p78).
- You are entitled to a weekly age addition of £14.05 with long-term IB if you were under 35, or £7.05 if you were under 45, when your period of incapacity began (see p76).[42]
- You may qualify for an extra £31.15 a week short-term IB (£38.40 if you are over pensionable age), or £39.95 long-term IB, for a spouse aged 60 or over, or for an adult who is looking after your child. The rules are the same as for

Category A retirement pension (see p70) except that your spouse must be aged 60 or over, or you must be residing with her/him and responsible for a child. The earnings/private pension limit is £31.15 a week for short-term IB and £51.40 a week for long-term IB.[43]

- You may qualify for a weekly increase of short-term higher rate IB (and lower rate if you over pensionable age) and long term IB of £9.90 for your eldest child and £11.35 for other children but entitlement is affected if your partner has weekly earnings and/or a private pension exceeding £145 (less some childcare costs in certain circumstances).[44]

- If you were receiving invalidity benefit on 12 April 1995 and have remained incapable of work , you may be entitled to 'transitionally protected' higher amounts of IB.[45]

How to claim

You should claim on form SC1. If you are an employee and are not, or no longer, entitled to SSP, your employer should give you a form SSP1, which includes the SC1 claim form. You will normally be required to submit a Med 3 certificate from your doctor with your claim. You must make a separate claim for any increases for dependants – they are not paid automatically.

Severe disablement allowance

Severe disablement allowance (SDA) is paid to people who have been incapable of work for at least 28 weeks but cannot qualify for IB because they have not made sufficient NI contributions. People whose incapacity began after the age of 20 must also be assessed as at least '80 per cent disabled'. SDA is not taxable.

Who can claim

You qualify for SDA if:[46]

- you are incapable of work (see below) and have been continuously incapable of work for at least 28 weeks prior to your claim; *and*

- your incapacity began before you were 20, or you are assessed as 80 per cent disabled (see below); *and*

- you are aged 16 or over and under 65 (see note below); *and*

- you are present and ordinarily resident in Great Britain, have been here for 26 weeks in the past year and have no limitation or condition on your right to be here (see p219).

You should also note the following points:
- You can continue to get SDA after the age of 65 if you were entitled to it when you become 65 (you should seek advice when you reach pensionable age about whether you might be better off claiming retirement pension or IB).

- You are not entitled to SDA if you are aged 16, 17 or 18 and are attending a course of education for 21 hours or more a week (but any part of the course which is only suitable for people with a disability does not count).[47]
- You cannot be paid SDA while you are entitled to statutory sick pay (SSP) (see p92) but days on SSP count towards the 28 week qualifying period.
- If you break your claim for SDA for less than eight weeks, you can re-qualify immediately (in some circumstances the linking period can be extended to one or two years if you have been working or training).[48]

'Incapable of work'

The rules and procedures are the same as for incapacity benefit (see p75). Note that you are exempt from the 'all-work' test if you are assessed as 80 per cent disabled or you have been receiving SDA since 12 April 1995.

'80 per cent disabled'

You are treated as 80 per cent disabled if:[49]

- you receive the highest rate care component of disability living allowance (see p81); *or*
- you are registered blind, or have an invalid carriage or car allowance from the DSS; *or*
- you have been assessed as 80 per cent disabled for disablement benefit or a war pension (see p93), or you are receiving a vaccine damage payment.

If you do not fit into any of the above groups, you will normally be required to attend a DSS medical examination to assess whether you are 80 per cent disabled due to a loss of physical or mental faculty.[50]

Amount

The basic SDA is £40.35 a week.[51] You may also be entitled to the following weekly additions:

- an age addition, depending on your age when your period of incapacity began;[52]

Age	Weekly addition
Under 40	£14.05
40 – 49 incl.	£8.90
50 – 59 incl.	£4.45

- £23.95 for your spouse or an adult who is looking after your child and £9.90 for your eldest child and £11.35 for your other children. The rules are the same as for long-term IB (see p75).

How to claim

You should claim on form SDA1. Claims for dependants should be made on form IB10.

Disability living allowance

Disability living allowance (DLA) is paid to people who need help with personal care or have difficulty getting around. Claimants must be under the age of 65 when they claim DLA, but once an award is in payment it can continue after the age of 65. There are no NI contribution conditions and DLA is not taxable. DLA is a particularly valuable benefit because it can be paid in addition to any other benefit, does not count as income for means-tested benefits, and can entitle a claimant to premiums of means-tested benefits.

Who can claim

You qualify for DLA if:[53]

- you are under the age of 65 when you first claim (if you have been awarded DLA you can continue to receive it after the age of 65); *and*
- you are present and ordinarily resident in Great Britain and have been present for 26 weeks in the past year (disregarding temporary absences of up to 26 weeks), and your immigration status is not subject to any limitation or condition (see p219); *and*
- you satisfy one or more of the 'disability conditions' (see below), have done so throughout the three months prior to your claim and are likely to continue to do so for at least another six months (unless you are 'terminally ill' – see p84).

The 'disability conditions'

DLA consists of a 'care component' paid at three different rates and a 'mobility component' paid at two different rates (see below for details). You can qualify for one or both components but only for one rate of each component. You can be given an award for a fixed period, or for life.[54]

The care component[55]

Higher rate care component

You qualify for the higher rate care component if you are so severely physically or mentally disabled that you require:

- frequent attention throughout the day in connection with your bodily functions, or continual supervision throughout the day to avoid substantial danger to yourself or others; *and*
- prolonged or repeated attention at night in connection with your bodily functions, or another person to be awake at night for a prolonged period or at frequent intervals to watch over you.

If you are terminally ill (see p84), you are treated as satisfying the above conditions.

Middle rate care component

You qualify for the middle rate care component if you satisfy either the 'day' or 'night' condition described above. You may also qualify automatically if you undergo regular renal dialysis.

Lower rate care component

You qualify for the lower rate care component if:

- you are aged 16 or over and are so severely physically or mentally disabled that you cannot prepare a cooked main meal for yourself if you have the ingredients; *or*
- you are so severely physically or mentally disabled that you require attention in connection with your bodily functions for a significant portion of the day, whether during a single period or a number of periods.

Additional rule for children

Children under 16 only qualify for the care component if they have attention or supervision requirements which are 'substantially in excess' of the normal requirements of children of the same age, or which children of the same age in normal health do not have.[56]

Meaning of terms

- 'Attention' means service of a close and intimate nature from another person, involving personal (but not necessarily physical) contact.[57] 'Frequent attention throughout the day' means help which is needed several times (not once or twice) at intervals spread throughout the day (not, for example, just in the early morning or evening).[58] 'A significant portion of the day' means about an hour.[59] 'Prolonged' attention at night means about 20 minutes. 'Repeated' simply means more than once.[60] You may, therefore, qualify if you need help to go to the toilet once in the night, which takes 20 minutes, or twice which only takes five minutes.
- 'Bodily functions' include breathing, hearing, seeing, eating, drinking, walking, sitting, sleeping, getting in and out of bed, dressing, undressing, using the toilet and moving around. They do not generally include domestic tasks such as cooking, shopping, cleaning or laundry.[61]
- 'Supervision' and 'watching over' involves keeping an eye on somebody to prevent substantial danger. It can be precautionary, without resulting in actual intervention.[62] 'Continual supervision' means frequent or regular, rather than continuous, supervision.[63] 'Prolonged' watching over at night is probably about 20 minutes.
- 'Requires' means 'reasonably requires' and not 'medically requires'.[64] Attention which you need in order to live as normal a life as possible (including having a social life) should count.[65] The test is whether you *need* attention or supervision, rather than whether you actually *receive* it. If you

can only manage to carry out a 'bodily function' with great difficulty, you can argue that you 'reasonably require' attention in connection with it.
- The 'cooking test' for the lower rate is an abstract test of whether your disabilities would prevent you from preparing a labour-intensive main meal for one, freshly cooked on a traditional cooker (it is irrelevant whether you actually cook or know how to cook).[66] You should qualify if you are unable to peel and chop vegetables, or cope with hot pans, or use a conventional oven and turn taps, or read labels and instructions, or tell whether food is clean or cooked, or if you lack the motivation or concentration to plan and cook a main meal.

The mobility component

There are two rates of the mobility component. Note that you cannot qualify for either rate if it is impossible for you to go out or be taken out (eg, you are in a coma or cannot be moved).[67] If you are awarded the higher rate mobility component, you will also be entitled to certain transport concessions (see p141).

Higher rate mobility component

You qualify for the higher rate mobility component if:[68]
- you are unable to walk or 'virtually unable to walk' (see below for meaning) because of a physical disability; *or*
- you are unable to walk out of doors without help because you are both blind and deaf; *or*
- you have no feet; *or*
- you are severely mentally impaired, have severe behavioural problems and qualify for the higher rate care component.

You are only treated as being 'virtually unable to walk' if:[69]
- your ability to walk out of doors is so limited, as regards the distance, speed, or length of time you can walk without severe discomfort, that you are virtually unable to walk; *or*
- the exertion required to walk would constitute a danger to your life or would be likely to lead to a serious deterioration in your health.

Note that you must be unable or virtually unable to walk for a physical, rather than a purely psychological reason, although many behavioural and mental problems have an organic or physical cause.[70] The test is applied as if you were using any artificial aid (eg, a stick) which would be suitable for you.[71] The test is whether you can walk out of doors, taking into account uneven surfaces and other obstacles and weather conditions.[72] There is no specific distance below which you qualify as 'virtually unable to walk'. Your stamina, speed, manner of walking and recovery time should be taken into account. Any walking you can only do with 'severe discomfort' must be ignored.[73] Severe discomfort can include pain, breathlessness and tiredness.[74]

Lower rate mobility component

You qualify for the lower rate mobility component if you are able to walk but are unable to take advantage of your walking ability outdoors, apart from on familiar routes, without guidance or supervision from another person for most of the time.

Any walking you can do on familiar routes is ignored. 'Guidance' can include being physically led or directed, being helped to avoid obstacles and being persuaded or reassured. 'Supervision' can include being monitored and encouraged. You may qualify for the lower rate if you are blind or deaf, or suffer from panic attacks, agoraphobia or epilepsy.[75]

Additional rules for children

The mobility component cannot be paid for a child under 5 (but see p.000 for future changes).[76]

Children under 16 can only qualify for the lower rate mobility component if they need substantially more guidance or supervision than children of the same age in normal health, or guidance or supervision which such other children would not need.[77]

Terminal illness

You are regarded as 'terminally ill' if you are suffering from a progressive disease and can reasonably be expected to die within six months as a result of that disease.[78] Claims for DLA on the basis of terminal illness are dealt with under 'special rules'. You automatically qualify for the higher rate care component if you are terminally ill and you do not have to satisfy the three and six month qualifying conditions in respect of the mobility component (see p81).[79] You also do not have to have been in Great Britain for 26 weeks in the last year to qualify for DLA.[80] You do not have to complete the sections of the claim form relating to care needs (see below) but you do need to submit a special form called a DS1500, which has to be completed by your doctor, giving details of your medical condition. Somebody can claim DLA for you without your knowledge or authority if you are terminally ill.[81]

Amount[82]

Higher rate care component	£52.95 a week
Middle rate care component	£35.40 a week
Lower rate care component	£14.05 a week
Higher rate mobility component	£37.00 a week
Lower rate mobility component	£14.05 a week

How to claim

You can only claim DLA in respect of your own care and mobility needs. If your partner also qualifies, s/he should make a separate claim. A claim for a child under 16 must be made by an appointee (normally a parent). A claim can be made on your behalf by an appointee if you are unable to manage your own affairs (see p226).

A claim for DLA must be made on form DLA1. There is one claim pack for adults and one for children under 16. You can get a claim pack by contacting your local Disability Benefits Centre, or by using the tear-off slip on leaflet DS704 (available form you local Benefits Agency office), or by ringing 0800 882200. The pack should be date stamped and you can be awarded benefit from the date on the form, provided the Benefits Agency receive your completed application within six weeks.[83]

The forms are long and difficult to complete and the information you give will largely determine the outcome of the application. You should always consider getting advice, therefore, if you are unsure about how to complete the forms. You should give as much information as possible about your difficulties. The questions on the forms are designed to test whether you satisfy the legal criteria for the care and mobility components set out above. When answering the questions about your care needs you should bear in mind that the test concerns the help you need, and you can legitimately say you need help even though you may not always get it. When answering the questions about your mobility problems, remember that the test is how far you can walk *without severe discomfort* (see p83). When completing the claim pack for children, you need to give as many examples as possible of the extra attention, supervision and guidance they need compared with a healthy child of the same age.

Claims are initially dealt with by a regional Disability Benefit Centre. You may be required to undergo a medical examination by a visiting doctor if further information is needed to decide your claim.[84] It can be several weeks before you receive a decision but claims on the basis of terminal illness (see p84) should be dealt with more quickly (normally within 10 days).

Attendance allowance

Attendance allowance (AA) is paid to people aged 65 or over who need help with personal care (whether or not they have a carer). There are no NI contribution conditions and AA is not taxable. AA is a particularly valuable benefit to claim because it can be paid in addition to any other benefit, does not count as income for means-tested benefits and can entitle a claimant to premiums of means-tested benefits.

Who can claim

You qualify for attendance allowance (AA) if:[85]

- you are aged 65 or over; *and*
- you are present and ordinarily resident in Great Britain and have been present for 26 weeks in the past year (disregarding temporary absences of up to 26 weeks), and your immigration status is not subject to any limitation or condition (see p219); *and*
- you satisfy one or more of the 'disability conditions' (see below) and have done so throughout the six months prior to your claim, or you are terminally ill (see below).

The 'disability conditions'

AA is paid at two rates. The conditions for the higher rate of AA are the same as those for the higher rate care component of DLA (see p81). The conditions for the lower rate of AA are the same as those for the middle rate care component of DLA (see p82).[86] See the section on DLA for guidance on the rules. There is no equivalent in AA of the lower rate of care component of DLA, or the mobility component.

Terminal illness

You are regarded as 'terminally ill' for AA as for DLA (see p84). If you are terminally ill, you automatically qualify for the higher rate of AA without having to satisfy the six month qualifying period.[87] You also do not have to have been in Great Britain for 26 weeks in the past year to qualify for AA.[88] The same rules relating to claims apply to AA as for DLA (see p84).

Amount[89]

Higher rate	£52.95 a week
Lower rate	£35.40 a week

How to claim

You can only claim AA in respect of your own care needs. If your partner also qualifies, s/he should make a separate claim. A claim can be made on your behalf if you are unable to manage your own affairs (see p96), or if you are terminally ill (see p84).

A claim for AA must be made on form DS2. You can get a claim pack by contacting your local Disability Benefits Centre, by using the tear-off slip on leaflet DS702 (available form you local Benefits Agency office), or by ringing 0800 882200. The pack should be date stamped and benefit is payable from the relevant date, provided the Benefits Agency receive your completed application within six weeks.[90]

The forms are long and difficult to complete and the information you give will largely determine the outcome of the application. You should always consider getting advice, therefore, if you are unsure about how to complete the forms. You should give as much information as possible about your difficulties. The questions on the forms are designed to test whether you satisfy the legal criteria. When answering the questions about your care and supervision needs you should bear in mind that the test concerns the help you need, and you can legitimately say you need help even though you may not always get it.

Claims are initially dealt with by a regional Disability Benefit Centre. You may be required to undergo a medical examination by a visiting doctor if further information is needed to decide your claim.[91] It can be several weeks before you receive a decision but claims on the basis of terminal illness should be dealt with more quickly (normally within 10 days).

Invalid care allowance

Invalid care allowance (ICA) is paid to people who are caring for a severely disabled person. There are no NI contribution conditions but ICA is taxable (apart from increases for children).

Who can claim
You qualify for ICA if:[92]
- you are 'regularly and substantially' caring for a 'severely disabled person' (see below); *and*
- you are present and ordinarily resident in Great Britain and have been present for 26 weeks in the past year (disregarding temporary absences of up to four weeks, or longer if you have gone abroad with the disabled person to look after her/him), and your immigration status is not subject to any limitation or condition (see p219); *and*
- you are aged 16-64 inclusive when you claim ICA (**note:** you can continue to get ICA if you are receiving it when you become 65, even if you are then no longer caring for a disabled person, or you are earning more than £50 a week – see below); *and*
- your net earnings from any employment do not exceed £50 a week (see p88); *and*
- you are not attending classes at a university, college or school for more than 21 hours a week.

'Regularly and substantially' caring for a 'severely disabled person'
To qualify for ICA for any week, you must spend at least 35 hours in that week, caring for a person who is receiving AA or the middle or higher rate care component of DLA (see pp81 and 85).[93] Care is not restricted to help with bodily functions and could include providing assistance (of any sort), supervision and even just company, as well as time spent preparing and clearing up meals. You can have temporary breaks from caring without losing

your ICA, as long as they do not add up to more than four weeks in any six months (or 12 weeks if you or the disabled person has spend at least eight of those weeks in hospital).[94] You should also note the following rules:

- You cannot qualify for ICA during any week in which you are caring for somebody for less than 35 hours a week, even if you spend more than 35 hours on average looking after her/him.[95]
- You also cannot satisfy the 35 hour rule by adding together the hours you spend looking after more than one disabled person.[96]
- If you are looking after two or more people for more than 35 hours a week each, you can only qualify for one award of ICA. If two people each spend more than 35 hours a week looking after the same person, only one of them can receive ICA.[97] One person may be better off claiming ICA than another (see ICA and other benefits – below).

Net earnings[98]

Your net earnings are your gross earnings from paid work, less tax, NI contributions and half of any contributions you make towards a pension scheme. If you have to pay someone, other than a close relative (see below), to look after the person you are caring for while you are working, the amount you pay can be deducted from your earnings, up to a maximum of 50 per cent of your net earnings. 'Close relative' means a parent, son, daughter, brother, sister, or partner of yours or of the person you are caring for. Certain childcare costs can also be deducted from your earnings. For more details of this and how your earnings are calculated see CPAG's *Welfare Benefits Handbook*.

ICA and other benefits

The relationship between ICA and other benefits can be complex and it is not always in your interest to claim ICA. You should particularly bear in mind the following points. If you are unsure whether you would be better off by claiming ICA, you should seek further advice.

- ICA counts as income for means-tested benefits (see p169) but can entitle you to a carer's premium (see p97).
- ICA cannot be paid at the same time as another overlapping benefit (see p69). It can still be worth claiming, however, because you are entitled to a carer's premium if you are entitled to ICA, even though you are not receiving it because you are getting an overlapping benefit (see p69).
- If you are receiving ICA, the person you are caring for is not entitled to a severe disability premium (SDP) with her/his means-tested benefits (see p97). In some circumstances, it may be better for the disabled person to get the SDP rather than you getting ICA. Where, for example, you are receiving a means-tested benefit, your ICA will be fully taken into account as income and you will only gain financially from the carer's premium, which may be worth considerably less than the SDP. Note, however, that if you have

claimed ICA but are not receiving it because you are getting an overlapping benefit (see p69), the person you are caring for remains entitled to the SDP and you can also get the carer's premium. Backdated payments of ICA do not affect payments of SDP which have already been made.

- If you give up or fail to claim your entitlement to ICA in order to qualify for, or get more, means-tested benefit, the Benefits Agency can treat you as if you were receiving it and deduct it from your means-tested benefit entitlement. This rule does not apply, however, if you give up ICA so that the person you are caring for can get the SDP, as long as s/he is not a member of your family for benefit purposes (see p182).

Amount[99]

The basic allowance is £39.95 a week.

You may also be entitled to a weekly increase of £23.95 for your spouse or an adult who is looking after your child. The rules are the same as for Category A retirement pension (see p70) except that you must be residing with the person to get the increase, and the earnings/private pension limit is £23.95 a week. You may also qualify for weekly additions of £9.90 for your eldest child and £11.35 for other children but entitlement is affected if your partner has weekly earnings (less certain allowable childcare costs) and/or a private pension exceeding £145 a week. For full details of the rules see CPAG's *Welfare Benefits Handbook*.

How to claim

You should claim on form DS700. You must make a separate claim for any increases for dependants as they are not paid automatically.

If the person you are caring for has claimed AA or DLA, you should not wait until her/his claim is decided before you claim ICA. Although your claim for ICA will be refused, if you reclaim it within three months of her/him being awarded AA or the middle/higher DLA care component, your claim for ICA can be backdated to the date of your original claim, or the date from which AA/DLA is awarded (whichever is the later date).[100]

Industrial injuries benefits

Industrial injuries benefits are paid to people who are disabled as a result of an accident at work or a prescribed industrial disease. There are no NI contribution conditions and industrial injuries benefits are not taxable. There are actually three industrial injury benefits. The main benefit is called disablement benefit, which pays a weekly allowance depending on the extent of a claimant's disablement. You can claim it even if you are still working. The other two benefits, reduced earnings allowance and retirement allowance, are meant to compensate for loss of earnings. They are gradually being phased out, however, as they are only paid to people who became disabled prior to 1 October 1990.

Who can claim

You qualify for industrial injuries benefits if:[101]

- you suffered personal injury caused by an accident which arose 'out of and in the course of' your employment as an 'employed earner', or you are suffering from a 'prescribed disease' as a result of working in a 'prescribed occupation' (see below for meaning of terms); *and*
- as a result, you have suffered a 'loss of faculty' which has caused 'disablement' (see below for meaning).

In addition, you must satisfy the following rules to qualify for the different types of industrial injury benefit:

- To qualify for **disablement benefit**, your disablement must normally be assessed as at least 14 per cent (see below) and 90 days (excluding Sundays) must have elapsed since the accident or onset of the disease.[102]
- To qualify for **reduced earnings allowance**, you must have had an accident or contracted a prescribed disease before 1 October 1990 and be assessed as at least one per cent disabled. You must also be under pensionable age (see p70), unless you are in regular employment, and be incapable of following your regular or equivalent employment because of the accident or disease. The rules are complex and you should seek advice if you think you may qualify.[103]
- To qualify for **retirement allowance**, you must be over pensionable age and getting reduced earnings allowance when you gave up regular employment.[104]

Meaning of terms

- 'Personal injury' encompasses both physical and psychological damage.[105]
- An 'accident' is an 'unlooked for occurrence' or 'mishap'.[106] There can be difficulties if you become injured over a long period. The Benefits Agency may decide this is a 'process' rather than an 'accident'. Seek advice if this applies to you.
- The accident must arise 'out of and in the course of' your employment. This means it must have had some connection with your work and happened at a time and place you could reasonably be expected to be working.[107] You should be covered during normal breaks on your employer's property.[108] You are not generally covered while you are travelling to and from work, unless this can be seen as part of your job.[109]
- 'Employed earner' covers most employees but excludes most self-employed people (although agency workers, office cleaners and taxi drivers should be covered).[110]
- A 'prescribed disease' means a disease listed in regulations, which is known to have a link with a particular 'prescribed occupation', which is also so listed. You must show that you are suffering from the disease as a result of

working in a relevant prescribed occupation.[111] A full list is included in Appendix 8 of CPAG's *Welfare Benefits Handbook*.

- A 'loss of faculty' means damage or impairment to the body or mind. 'Disablement' is any resulting inability to carry out a function.[112] Loss of faculty and disablement are assessed by 'adjudicating medical authorities' (AMAs) comprising one or two doctors who will examine you on behalf of the DSS and decide the percentage of your disablement. Some disabilities have prescribed percentages, set out in regulations (see Appendix 7 of CPAG's *Welfare Benefits Handbook* for a full list) but others are left to the discretion of the AMA to decide.[113] If your disablement is only partly due to an accident or prescribed disease there may be an 'offset' or addition to your percentage disablement. The rules on this and if you have suffered two or more accidents or diseases are complex and you should seek advice if this applies to you.[114] The AMA also decides the period of your assessment, which can be fixed or for life.[115] If your condition deteriorates, you should request a reassessment.

Amount

Disablement benefit

The amount you get depends on the extent of your disablement (see above).[116]

% Disablement	Amount pw
14-24	£21.62
25-34	£32.43
35-44	£43.24
45-54	£54.05
55-64	£64.86
65-74	£75.67
75-84	£86.48
85-94	£97.29
95-100+	£108.10

Note: The amounts payable are less if you are under the age of 18.

You may also qualify for two increases of disablement benefit:
- **Constant attendance allowance** of up to £86.60 a week is payable if you are assessed as 100 per cent disabled and need constant attendance.[117]
- **Exceptionally severe disablement allowance** of £43.30 a week is payable if you are entitled to at least £43.30 constant attendance allowance and are likely to permanently require constant attendance.[118]

Reduced earnings allowance

You are entitled to the difference between the earnings you would receive in your previous regular occupation and the earnings you currently receive, or could receive in a job you could do. The calculation is a complex one and open to argument and you should seek advice if you are unhappy with your assessment. The maximum you can receive, however, is £43.30 a week and the total amount of your disablement benefit and reduced earnings allowance cannot exceed £151.34 a week.[119]

Retirement allowance

You are entitled to £10.81 a week or 25 per cent of the reduced earnings allowance you were getting, whichever is the lower.[120]

How to claim

You should ask for the appropriate claim form at your local Benefits Agency office. Leaflet NI6 has details about claiming disablement benefit. You can apply for a declaration that you have had an accident on form BI 95, in readiness for a subsequent claim for disablement benefit.

Other non-means-tested benefits

Other non-means-tested benefits are briefly described below. The amounts payable are set out on p86. For further details see CPAG's *Welfare Benefits Handbook*.

Statutory sick pay

Statutory sick pay (SSP) is paid to most employees (earning more than £66 a week) for up to 28 weeks of incapacity for work. There are no NI contribution conditions. SSP is paid by the employer with the employee's wages and is taxable. Disputes are dealt with by the Inland Revenue.

Maternity benefits

Statutory maternity pay (SMP) is paid to pregnant employees (earning more than £66 a week) for up to 18 weeks. SMP is paid by employer to employees who have been working for them for at least 26 weeks and is taxable. Disputes are dealt with by the Inland Revenue.

Maternity allowance is paid by the Benefits Agency to pregnant women who are not entitled to SMP but have been working for at least 26 weeks in the 66 weeks before they are due to give birth. It is not taxable.

Child benefit and guardian's allowance

Child benefit can be claimed by anyone who is responsible for a child who is under 16, or aged 16-18 in full-time non-advanced education. Guardian's allowance can be claimed by anyone bringing up a child whose natural parents are dead (or one is dead and the other is missing, or in prison for at least five years). Neither benefit is taxable and there are no NI contribution conditions.

Contribution-based jobseeker's allowance

Contribution-based jobseeker's allowance (JSA) is paid for up to six months to people who are unemployed (or working less than 16 hours a week) and who have satisfied NI contribution conditions. Claimants must be capable of work, available for work and actively seeking work to qualify. Contribution-based JSA is taxable.

War pensions

Various levels of war pensions and additions can be paid to forces personnel disabled by war service, civilians disabled by war injury and war widows. For further details, contact the War Pensions Directorate, Norcross, Blackpool FY5 3TA or the War Pensions Helpline on 01253-858858. War pensions are not taxable.

Vaccine damage payment

A tax-free lump sum payment of £40,000 is payable to anyone who is severely disabled as a result of specified vaccinations. For further details contact the Vaccine Damage Payments Unit, Palatine House, Lancaster Road, Preston PR1 1HB.

Christmas bonus

A tax-free Christmas bonus of £10 is paid to most pensioners and people with disabilities who are receiving qualifying benefits at the beginning of December.

3. Means-tested benefits

Income support

Income support (IS) is a tax-free benefit paid to specified categories of people who are not required to be available for work and whose income and capital is below set levels. People on IS are eligible for maximum housing and council tax benefit (see p102), social fund payments (see p117) and other sources of financial assistance (see p137). People who are not eligible for IS may be able to claim income-based jobseeker's allowance (JSA) instead, if they are available for and actively seeking work (see p125).

Who can claim

You qualify for IS if:[121]

- you are aged 16 or over; *and*
- you fall into one of the categories of people who are eligible to claim (see below); *and*
- neither you nor your partner (see p96) are working 'full-time' (see p95 for details and the exceptions to this rule); and you are not studying full-time (but see p95 for exceptions); *and*
- you are not treated as a person from abroad (see p219 – this includes anyone who is not habitually resident in the UK, but note that some persons from abroad are entitled to urgent cases payments of IS); *and*
- you are not receiving contribution-based JSA (see p93) and your partner is not receiving income-based JSA (see p125); *and*
- your income (see p167) is less than your applicable amount (see p96); *and*
- your savings and other capital are less than £8,000, or £16,000 if you live in a residential or nursing home (see p190 for details of how your capital is calculated).

Special rules apply to prisoners, people without accommodation, 16/17-year-olds and people affected by a trade dispute (see CPAG's *Welfare Benefits Handbook* for details). If you live in residential or nursing care home, see p343 and p377. If you are in hospital, see p125.

If you qualify for IS, you can claim for yourself, your partner and your children (see p96 – claiming for others). If you do not qualify but your partner does, s/he could be the claimant for your family. You can also 'swap' claimants if this would be advantageous (see p101). Where there is a choice of claiming IS or income-based JSA, you may be better off if you or your partner claims IS, as you may be entitled to more benefit and you will not have to be 'available for work' and 'actively seeking work'.

Categories of people eligible to claim IS

You are eligible to claim IS if:[122]

- you are aged 60 or over; *or*
- you are 'incapable of work', or treated as incapable for work, under the same rules and assessment procedures that apply to incapacity benefit (see p76 and the note on p78), or you are entitled to SSP (see p92); *or*
- you are appealing against a decision that you are not incapable of work under the 'own occupation' or 'all-work' test (see p76 – your IS personal allowance is reduced by 20 per cent while you are appealing against an all work test decision); *or*
- you are a 'disabled worker', or are working while living in a residential or nursing care home (see p95); *or*
- you are registered blind; *or*

- you are a carer and you are receiving invalid care allowance (see p87), or you are looking after somebody who is receiving AA (see p85) or the middle or higher rate care component of DLA (see p81), or who has claimed these benefits in the last 26 weeks and is waiting for a decision (you can also continue to claim IS for eight weeks after these conditions cease to apply); *or*
- you are a single parent who is responsible for a child under 16; *or*
- you are looking after your partner or child because they are temporarily ill, or you are looking after a child whose parent is ill or temporarily away, or you are fostering a child and do not have a partner; *or*
- you are a disabled student who can claim IS (see below); *or*
- you are a person from abroad (see p220) who is entitled to urgent cases payments of IS.

People working full-time

You are not generally entitled to IS if you are working (for payment) 16 hours or more a week, or if your partner is working 24 or more hours a week.[123] If both of you work less than this, you can claim IS but most of your earnings will be taken into account (see p97). Even if you or your partner are working more than the prescribed hours, you are not excluded from IS under the full time work rule if:[124]

- you are a 'disabled worker' – ie, you are mentally or physically disabled and as a result your earnings or hours of work are 75 per cent or less of what a person without your disability would expect from the same or comparable employment; *or*
- you are a carer who is eligible to claim IS (see above); *or*
- you are working at home as a childminder, or you are being paid by social services or a health authority or voluntary organisation to foster a child or care for a person in your home; *or*
- you are living in a care home.

People studying full-time

You are not generally entitled to IS if you are studying full time but there are exceptions. The rules are complex and for further details, you should consult CPAG's *Welfare Benefits Handbook*. You are not excluded from IS under the full-time student rule if:[125]

- you are under 19, in non-advanced education and so severely disabled that you are unlikely to get a job in the next 12 months; *or*
- you are 19 or over or in advanced education and you qualify for a disability or severe disability premium (see p97), or you have been incapable of work for 28 weeks, or you qualify for a disabled student's allowance because you are deaf; *or*
- you are a lone parent or over pensionable age.

Claiming for others

When you claim IS, your claim is assessed for the whole of your 'family' (see below) who share your 'household' (see below):

- Your 'family' means yourself, your 'partner' (if you have one) and any 'dependent children'. 'Partner' means someone of the opposite sex to whom you are married or with whom you are living as if you were married. 'Dependent children' (not necessarily your own) usually means anyone you are responsible for who is under the age of 16, or aged 16-19 and in full-time non-advanced education.[126]

- 'Household' is not defined in the law but involves people living together in a domestic establishment that has some degree of independence and self-sufficiency. If you separate permanently from your partner, you no longer count as members of the same household and you can only claim IS as single claimants. If you are temporarily separated from your partner, you continue to count as members of the same household, unless you have no intention of living together again, or you are likely to be apart for more than 52 weeks (this period can be extended if you or your partner are in hospital, or in a care home, provided the period of your separation is not 'substantially' longer than 52 weeks).[127]

Amount

IS is a means-tested benefit and the amount you are entitled to depends on your circumstances. There are three steps involved in working out your IS. An example is given on p99.

Step one: Calculate your 'applicable amount'. This represents the weekly income the government decides you need to live on. It is made up of fixed amounts, depending on your age, the size of your family and other circumstances. Details of how to calculate your applicable amount are set out below.

Step two: Calculate your income. Details of how to calculate your income are set out in Chapter 6. Note that not all your income counts when working out your IS. Any AA and DLA (see pp85 and 81) you receive, for example, are ignored but incapacity benefit and invalid care allowance (see pp75 and 87) count in full. Some of your earnings are disregarded. If you have capital over £3,000 (£10,000 if you live in a care home) you are treated as having a 'tariff income'.

Step three: Deduct your income from your applicable amount. The resulting amount is your IS.[128] If your income exceeds your applicable amount, you are not entitled to IS.

Applicable amount

Your applicable amount is made up of three elements:

- personal allowances for you and your family;

- premiums in specific circumstances;
- housing costs, primarily for mortgage interest payments (rent payments are covered by the housing benefit scheme – see p102).

Personal allowances[129]

These are set amounts for single people, lone parents, couples (ie, people with partners – see p96) and dependent children. There are different rates for people of different ages. The rates are set out on p86.

Premiums

Premiums are set allowances intended to help with extra expenses associated with age, disability or children. You can qualify for one or more premiums but you can only receive one of the disability premium, the pensioner premium or the higher pensioner premium (the highest you qualify for).[130] The rates of the premiums are set out on p86.

Family premium

You are entitled to a family premium if your family includes a child under 16, or under 19 and in full-time non-advanced education.[131] Only one premium is payable, regardless of the number of children you have.

Pensioner premium

You are entitled to the normal rate of pensioner premium if you or your partner are aged 60-74 inclusive and to the enhanced rate if either of you are aged 75-79 inclusive. The couple rate is paid even if only one partner fulfils the conditions.[132]

Higher pensioner premium

You are entitled to the higher pensioner premium if:[133]

- you or your partner are aged 80 or over; *or*
- you were getting the disability premium (see below) when you became 60 (or in the eight weeks before) and have been getting IS since; *or*
- you or your partner are aged 60-79 inclusive and either of you is registered blind or receiving a 'qualifying benefit' – ie, AA (see p85), DLA (see p81), severe disablement allowance (see p79), disabled person's tax credit or disability working allowance (see p115), long-term IB (see p75) or retirement pension if this replaced your long term IB and you have been getting IS since.

The couple rate is paid even if only one partner fulfils the conditions.

Disability premium

You are entitled to the disability premium if:[134]

- you are aged under 60 and are registered blind, or receiving a qualifying benefit (see above), or have been incapable of work (see p75 and below) for a continuous period of 52 weeks (or 28 weeks if you are terminally ill); *or*
- your partner is aged under 60 and is registered blind or receiving a qualifying benefit.

The couple rate is paid if either condition is satisfied. Note that only the *claimant's* incapacity for work can qualify a couple for the premium (this is particularly relevant where there is a choice of claimant – see p101). Note also that you can only satisfy the incapable of work condition, if you have claimed IB (whether you are entitled to it or not) or if you are entitled to SSP (see pp75 and 92). You may be able to establish that you have been incapable of work for a past period by submitting a backdated medical certificate from your GP.

Severe disability premium
You are entitled to the severe disability premium if:[135]
- you are receiving AA (see p85) or the middle or higher rate care component of DLA (see p81); *and*
- you have no non-dependant, aged 18 or over, normally residing with you (see below); *and*
- no one is being paid invalid care allowance (ICA) for looking after you (see p87 – note that a person is not treated as receiving ICA if s/he is not getting it because of the overlapping benefit rules – see p69).

If you have a partner you must both satisfy the above rules. If you do, the couple rate is paid. If your partner does not satisfy the first condition but is registered blind, or if only one of you has a carer receiving ICA, you are entitled to the single person's rate.

A 'non-dependant' is anybody aged 18 or over who normally lives with you (whether in their house or yours) and with whom you share accommodation, apart from a bathroom, toilet, or common access area, or a communal room in sheltered accommodation.[136] This could include your grown-up son or daughter, or your parent. The following people do not, however, count as non-dependants:[137]
- anyone receiving AA or the middle or higher rate care component of DLA;
- anyone registered blind;
- anyone who is a member of your family for IS purposes (see p104);
- anyone engaged by a charitable or voluntary organisation to care for you or your partner, for which you pay a charge;
- anyone (or a member of their household) who makes payments to you on a commercial basis (eg, rent) for occupying your dwelling or to whom you make such payments to occupy their dwelling, apart from a close relative – ie, parent, parent-in-law, son, son-in-law, daughter, daughter-in-law, step-

parent, step-son, step-daughter, brother, sister or partner of any of the above;
- anyone (and their partner) who jointly occupies your home and is either a joint owner or joint tenant with you or your partner (apart from a close relative (see above), unless you were joint owners or tenants prior to 11 April 1988, or before you moved in);

If a non-dependant comes to live with you for the first time to care for you or your partner, you can keep your entitlement to the severe disability premium for 12 weeks. After that, you will lose the premium and the carer should consider claiming ICA. In other situations, however, you should be aware that if somebody is receiving ICA for looking after you, you will lose your entitlement to the severe disability premium and this may leave you considerably worse off (see p88).

Disabled child premium
You are entitled to a disabled child premium for each child in your family who gets disability living allowance or who is registered blind, as long as the child has less than £3,000 capital.[138]

Carer's premium
You are entitled to the carer's premium if you or your partner are getting ICA (see p87), or would get it but for the overlapping benefit rules (see p69). You remain entitled to the premium for eight weeks after you stop getting ICA. If both you and your partner satisfy the conditions for a carer's premium, you are entitled to double the normal rate.[139]

Housing costs
The final element of your applicable amount is housing costs.[140] These are paid to home owners to help meet the costs of:
- mortgage interest payments;
- interest payments on loans for specified home repairs and improvements;
- service charges, other than for specified repairs and improvements.

Housing costs for mortgage interest payments are usually paid directly to the lender.

The rules and conditions relating to IS housing costs are complex (see CPAG's *Welfare Benefits Handbook* for more details) Note, particularly, the following restrictions:
- You may not be entitled to help with interest payments on a mortgage taken out while you were getting IS or income-based JSA but this rule does not apply if the loan was taken out to buy a more suitable home for the needs of a disabled person – ie, somebody could satisfy the conditions for a

disability, disabled child, enhanced pensioner of higher pensioner premium (see pp97–99);

- Your housing costs may be restricted if excessive (but the needs of disabled members of your family must be considered). There is also an absolute ceiling of £100,000 on eligible loans.
- If you or your partner are aged 60 or over you will be paid all your housing costs straight away. Most other claimants who took out a loan after 1 October 1995 are not entitled to housing costs until they have been receiving IS for 39 weeks. If you took out your loan before 2 October 1995 or you are receiving ICA or are caring for somebody getting AA or DLA middle or higher rate care components, you are not entitled to any housing costs for the first eight weeks of your IS claim, after which you can get 50 per cent of your housing costs for the next 18 weeks and then full housing costs after 26 weeks. If you have not been able to qualify for IS because you have been receiving IB or SSP, periods spent on these benefits can count towards the waiting periods.
- Deductions may be made from your housing costs if you have a non-dependant living with you (see p97). The amounts deducted are the same as apply to housing benefit (see p109 for details). Note that, as for housing benefit, no deductions are made for non-dependants if you or your partner receive AA or DLA or are registered blind.
- You can only get help with interest payments, not capital repayments and insurance premiums, on eligible loans. Unless your rate of interest is less than 5 per cent, your standard rate of interest is used, which may be less than the rate you are actually paying.

Housing costs are payable in respect of the dwelling you normally occupy as your home.[141] If you are temporarily away from home, you can normally continue to get housing costs for 13 weeks.[142] This also applies if you are in a care home for a trial period.[143] If you are in a care home for short-term or respite care, you can continue to get housing costs on your normal home for up to 52 weeks.[144] The 52 week rule also applies if you are in hospital, or receiving medical treatment or convalescence, or providing medically approved care to another person. The 52 week period may, however, be extended if the reason for your temporary absence is that essential repairs are being carried out on your home.[145]

In either case, once you return home, even if this is only for a weekend or even a day, you may claim housing costs for a new 13 or 52 week period of temporary absence.[146]

You may be paid housing costs for two homes for up to four weeks if you have moved into a new home and cannot avoid having to pay for the other one as well, or indefinitely if you have left your home because of domestic violence, provided it is reasonable for the costs of both homes to be met.[147]

You may also be paid housing costs for up to four weeks before you move into a new home if your move is delayed because it is being adapted for a disabled person or because you are waiting for a social fund payment, and you are entitled to a disability or pensioner premium.[148]

• •

Example of an IS calculation

Mr and Mrs Earnshaw, both aged 35, have two children aged 8 and 10. They live in rented accommodation. Mr Earnshaw has a severe mental illness and Mrs Earnshaw spends a lot of time looking after and supervising him. Mr Earnshaw receives the middle rate care component of DLA. Mrs Earnshaw receives ICA and CB. The family have no other income and no savings. Mrs Earnshaw claims IS as a carer.

Step one: Applicable amount

Personal allowance for a couple	£80.65
Personal allowance for first child	£24.90
Personal allowance for second child	£24.90
Family premium	£13.90
Disability premium	£31.25
Carer's premium	£13.95
Total applicable amount	£189.55

Step two: Income (note DLA is ignored as income)

Invalid care allowance (including dependants' additions)	£85.10
Child benefit for first child	£14.40
Child benefit for second child	£ 9.60
Total income	£109.10

Step three: Deduct income from applicable amount

Applicable amount,	£189.55
Less income	-£109.10
= IS	= £ 80.45

Mrs Earnshaw is entitled to £80.45 a week IS.

• •

How to claim

You should claim IS on form SP1 (for pensioners), or form A1 (for other claimants), from your local Benefits Agency office. You can also get the forms by completing the tear-off slip in leaflet IS1, which should be available from post offices. You must fully complete the form and supply any documentation required (eg, proof of savings and payslips) for your claim to be valid. If you are claiming because you are incapable of work you must also submit an SC1 form. If you have a mortgage you should ask your lender to complete form MI12, which comes with the claim pack.

You claim IS for yourself and your family (see p96). If you and your partner are both eligible to claim, you can choose who should be the claimant. You will sometimes be better off if one of you claims rather than the other, where, for example, this would qualify you for the disability premium based on the claimant's incapacity for work (see p97). Sometimes one member of a couple is eligible to claim IS and the other is eligible to claim income-based JSA. You may be better off on IS if this enables you to qualify for the disability premium.

Housing benefit

Housing benefit (HB) is paid to people with a low income and less than £16,000 capital, to help with their rent payments. It can be claimed by people who are working or unemployed. HB is paid and administered by local authorities.

Who can claim

You qualify for HB if:[149]

- you or your partner (see p104) are liable to pay rent on the dwelling you occupy as your home (see below); *and*
- you do not fall within any of the categories of excluded people listed on p103; *and*
- your income (see p104) is low enough to qualify (see p104 – Amount); *and*
- your savings and other capital do not exceed £16,000 (see Chapter 7 for details of how your capital is calculated).

Liability to pay rent for your home

'Rent' includes any payments you make for the use and occupation of premises, including service charges and payments for hostel, bed and breakfast and other types of accommodation.[150] Some payments, however, including some types of service charges, are not eligible for HB (see p104 – Eligible rent).

To qualify for HB, you or your partner must be liable to pay rent under a legally enforceable agreement, although the agreement does not have to be in writing.[151] If you are not legally liable to pay rent but have to do so to keep your home because the liable person has stopped paying, you can be treated as liable.[152] Some people are excluded from HB, however, even though they are liable to pay rent (see p104). If you live with a partner (see p103) only one of you can claim HB.[153] If you are jointly liable to pay rent with other people who are not members of your family (see p103) you can claim HB for your proportion of the rent.[154]

HB is only usually payable in respect of your normal home. If you are temporarily absent from your home, you can get HB for up to 13 weeks or 52 weeks. The rules are the same as for IS housing costs (see p99).[155]

People excluded from housing benefit

You are excluded from HB if you fall into one of the following categories:

- You are treated as a 'person from abroad' (see p220 – this includes anyone who is not 'habitually resident' in the UK).[156]
- You are a full-time student.[157] Some full-time students are eligible for HB, however, including those who qualify for IS (see p95), lone parents, pensioners, people who have been incapable of work for 28 weeks and those who qualify for the disability or severe disability premiums (see p97).[158] See also p104, Eligible rent.
- You move permanently into an independent care home or a local authority care home which provides and charges for meals (see Chapter 5 for the rules relating to less dependent residents in local authority care homes where board is not provided).[159] You may be able to claim IS and apply to social services for help to pay for home fees (see Chapters 12 and 21).
- You own your home, or have a lease of more than 21 years, or are receiving IS housing costs for your accommodation.[160]
- Your rental agreement is not commercial, taking into account, in particular, whether the terms are legally enforceable.[161] Note that the fact that you are paying less than the market rent, or that you are renting from a friend or relative does not necessarily mean that your agreement is not commercial.
- You pay rent to a 'close relative' of yours or your partner's who shares your accommodation.[162] 'Close relative' means parent, parent-in-law, son, son-in-law, daughter, daughter-in-law, step-parent, step-son, step-daughter, brother, sister or partner of any of the above.[163] You do not count as sharing accommodation if you only share a bathroom, toilet or common access area, or communal rooms in sheltered accommodation, and the rule may not apply if you have exclusive occupation of one or more rooms.[164]
- You are renting a home from your ex-partner, or partner's ex-partner, which you formerly shared with them.[165]
- A child belonging to the person you are renting from is living as part of your family.[166]
- You or your partner previously owned the accommodation you are renting, unless you can show that you had to relinquish ownership to keep your home – eg, because of mortgage arrears.[167]
- You were previously a non-dependant (see p109) of someone living in your accommodation, or you pay rent to a company or trust which has a connection with your partner, ex-partner, child or close relative (see p104) with whom you live, unless in either case you can show that your rental agreement was not created to enable you to claim HB.[168]
- None of the above apply, but the local authority decides that your agreement to pay rent was created to enable you to claim HB.[169] You should seek advice if this rule is applied to you.

Claiming for others

As with IS, you claim HB for yourself and your family, including your partner and dependent children. The amount you receive depends on the circumstances of your family.[170]

Amount

HB is a means-tested benefit and the amount you are entitled to depends on your 'applicable amount', your 'income' and your 'eligible rent' (see below for details).

If you are receiving IB (see p93) *or income-based JSA* (see p125) you are entitled to maximum HB, which is your weekly eligible rent less any non-dependant deductions (see p109).[171]

If you are not receiving IS or income-based JSA you are entitled to maximum HB (see above) less 65 per cent of the difference between your income and applicable amount. If your income is less than your applicable amount, you are entitled to maximum HB.[172]

Examples of HB calculations are given on p110.

Applicable amount

Your 'applicable amount' is worked out as for IS[173] (see p96) except that:
- the personal allowance for a person aged 16-24 is £40.70;
- for the purposes of the severe disability premium, any joint tenant or owner, or a landlord or tenant of yours who lives with you, counts as a non-dependant if s/he falls into one of the categories of people who are excluded from HB (see p103);[174]
- IS housing costs are not included in your applicable amount (you are not entitled to HB if you are receiving them – see p103).

Income

Details of how to calculate your income are set out in Chapter 6. Note that not all your income counts when working out your HB. For example, any AA and DLA (see pp85 and 81) you receive are ignored, but IB and ICA (see p75 and 88) count in full. Some of your earnings are disregarded. If you have capital over £3,000, you are treated as having a 'tariff income'.[175]

Eligible rent

Your 'eligible rent' is the amount of rent (including service charge) which is taken into account when calculating your HB. It may be significantly less than the rent you actually pay because of the deductions and restrictions described below. This means that HB may not cover the whole of your rent payments even if you are entitled to maximum HB (see p96). If you are a full-time student who can claim HB your eligible rent may be subject to special fixed deductions (see CPAG's *Welfare Benefits Handbook* for details).[176]

Service charges for which housing benefit is not paid

The following charges are not eligible for HB and are deducted from the rent you pay, when calculating your eligible rent.

Fuel charges[177]

If your rent includes a specified amount for fuel, that amount is deducted when calculating your eligible rent. If your rent includes an unspecified amount for fuel, the following fixed weekly amounts are deducted:

- £9.25 for heating
- £1.15 for hot water
- £0.80 for lighting
- £1.15 for cooking

If you (and your family) occupy only one room, only £5.60 is deducted for heating, or heating plus hot water and/or lighting. Fuel charges for common access areas and for communal rooms in sheltered accommodation are eligible for HB, as are specified charges for the maintenance of a heating system.[178]

Water charges[179]

Any water charges which are included in your rent are ineligible for HB.

Charges for meals[180]

If you pay for meals, the following fixed weekly deductions are made when calculating your eligible rent, regardless of the charge you actually pay:

- £18.35 for each member of your family aged 16 or over and £9.25 for each child who receives at least three meals a day;
- £2.20 for each member of your family who receives breakfast only;
- £12.20 for each member of your family aged 16 or over and £6.15 for each child in other cases – ie, half board.

Certain other service charges[181]

Charges for the following items are also ineligible for HB:

- personal laundry (but charges for use of a laundry room or machines are eligible – see below);
- cleaning your room(s), unless no one in your household is able to do it (see below);
- TV rental and licence fees, transport and most leisure and sports facilities;
- nursing or personal care, medical expenses and emergency alarm systems (unless the alarm system is provided in specially designed or adapted accommodation – see below).

If you are jointly liable for rent which includes ineligible charges, proportionate deductions are made from your share of the rent.[182]

Service charges for which housing benefit may be paid (until April 2000)

Charges for other services not specified above may be paid for by HB (under an *interim* HB scheme – see p107), but only if:

- your liability for the service charges is a condition of occupying the accommodation (rather than, for example, an optional extra, or if the service is provided by another person or agency and it is not done so on behalf of the landlord)[183]; *and*

- the charge is not excessive (in which case HB will only be paid up to a reasonable amount estimated according to the cost of comparable services)[184]; *and*

- the service is for:

  –the provision of adequate accommodation. Such services include general management costs, gardens, children's play areas, lifts, entry phones, communal telephone costs, portering and rubbish removal. TV and radio relay is covered, but only for ordinary UK channels and not satellite dishes or decoders. Cable TV is also excluded unless it is the only practicable way of providing you with ordinary domestic channels;[185]

  –laundry facilities (eg, a laundry room in an apartment block), but not charges for the provision of personal laundry – see above);[186]

  –furniture and household equipment (but not if there is any agreement that it will eventually become yours);[187]

  –cleaning of communal areas;[188]

  –cleaning within your own accommodation (but only if no one living in the household is able to do it – see above);[189]

  –emergency alarm systems in accommodation designed or adapted for elderly, sick or disabled people, or which is otherwise suitable for them, taking into account factors such as size, heating system or other facilities. In all other cases, alarms are ineligible;[190]

  –general counselling and support services, but only to the extent that they are:

  –necessary for the provision of adequate accommodation.[191] This concerns only keeping the accommodation fit for use and does not cover counselling designed to ensure that you do not break the terms of your occupation of the accommodation[192] (but see below); *or*

  –provided on a '50 per cent' basis.[193] This test requires the service to be provided by someone (whether a landlord or her/his employee) who spends the majority of time during which services are provided providing services which are not within the list of ineligible services set out on p105; *or*

  –provided in 'supported accommodation'[194] (see below).

'Supported accommodation' is currently defined as accommodation that is provided by a local authority, housing association, or charity or similar voluntary body where care, support or supervision is given to the occupants; or accommodation provided by the Resettlement Agency; or similar accommodation which does not have to be referred to a rent officer (this applies to occupants who have been getting HB since 1 January 1996 and partners or family members who claim HB within four weeks of taking over the occupation due to death, imprisonment or desertion). In all cases, accommodation only counts as supported accommodation if it was used for the same purpose on 18 August 1997 (unless it was only closed for refurbishment, cleaning or pest control).[195]

Service charges for which housing benefit may be paid from April 2000[196]

HB for general counselling and support services is currently only payable under an *interim* HB scheme which has applied since 18 August 1997. This was introduced in order to relax a strict interpretation by the courts of earlier rules while the government reviewed funding arrangements for supported accommodation.[197] From April 2000 the *interim* scheme will be replaced by a *transitional* HB scheme (see below) which will apply until 2003, when it will be replaced by more fundamental changes to the funding arrangements for supported housing (see Chapter 25).

The *transitional* HB scheme[198] will continue to provide for HB to meet the cost of all reasonable charges for the *provision of adequate accommodation* which is a condition of occupation (as now, see p106). The existing rules on service charges for which HB is not paid (see p105) will also continue to apply. No other service charges (except for charges for cleaning the outside of windows if no one living in the household can do it) will, however, be met by HB unless they are provided in *'supported accommodation'* and for *'eligible services'* as re-defined below.

From April 2000, *'supported accommodation'* will include only:

- accommodation provided by a local authority, housing association, or charity or similar voluntary body where care, support or supervision is given to the occupants; or accommodation provided by the Resettlement Agency (as under the *interim* scheme); *or*
- accommodation which is occupied by someone for whom social services have undertaken a community care assessment (see p40) which confirms that the occupant needs the services which are eligible for HB (see below) *and* that the landlord (or someone acting on her/his behalf) is capable of providing the occupant with those services.

From April 2000, *'eligible services'* will include (as well as services relating to the provision of adequate accommodation as under the *interim* scheme referred to above) only those charges which are conditions of occupation of the 'supported accommodation' and which are for:

- *general counselling and support* to assist the claimant with:
  – maintaining the security of the home (eg, reminding her/him to lock up, or controlling access);

– maintaining the safety of the home (eg, checking, arranging services for, and ensuring safe use of, appliances which could pose a safety risk);
– complying with those conditions of occupation which are concerned with nuisance, payment of rent, and maintaining the interior of the home in an appropriate condition; *and*

- *other services provided by a warden* (who is either resident or on alarm-call) in a group of dwellings normally let to people in need of general counselling and support services *and* the warden provides those services wholly or mainly for those occupiers (eg, help with shopping or errands and other 'good neighbour' tasks); *and*

–*window cleaning and room cleaning* (if no one in the household can do it); *and*

– *emergency alarm systems.*

From April 2000, service charges will no longer be referred to a rent officer (see below) and will no longer be covered by the 'exceptional hardship' provisions (see p110).

Rent restrictions

If you are a private tenant, your eligible rent may be restricted to an amount determined by the local rent officer. This will not apply to you if:[199]

- you live in local authority or registered housing association accommodation; *or*
- you live in accommodation provided by a housing association, registered charity or voluntary organisation where care, support or supervision is provided; *or*
- you have receiving HB for the same accommodation since 1 January 1996.

If you fall into one of the above categories, the local authority can still restrict your eligible rent if it decides your home is too big or expensive.[200] If this happens, you should seek further information and advice (see CPAG's *Welfare Benefits Handbook*).

If you do not fall into one of the above categories, the local authority will refer your HB claim to an independent local rent officer who will use set criteria to determine whether your eligible rent should be restricted because your home is too large or expensive, or because you are under 25 (see below).[201] See CPAG's *Welfare Benefits Handbook* for further details about the procedure.

The local authority is bound by the rent officer's determinations.[202] In practice, this means that in most cases, your eligible rent cannot exceed the average local rent for the size of accommodation you need. If you are under 25, your eligible rent will be restricted to the average local rent for one room only (plus shared kitchen and toilet), unless you are entitled to the severe disability premium (see p97), or you are under 22 and were formally in care, or you have a non-dependant (see below) living with you. You should seek advice if you wish to challenge a rent restriction (see also p110). If you are considering renting private accommodation, you can ask the local authority for a 'pre-tenancy-determination' to find out whether the eligible rent will be restricted for HB.[203]

Non-dependant deductions

If you have a non-dependant living with you, a deduction is made from your HB on the assumption that s/he is making a contribution towards your rent (whether s/he is or not).

A non-dependant is anyone who normally resides with you, does not have a normal home elsewhere, and shares accommodation with you apart from a bathroom, toilet, or common access area, or a communal room in sheltered accommodation.[204] The following people, however, do not count as non-dependants:[205]

- anyone who is separately liable to pay rent or other housing costs;
- a member of your family (see p104);
- a person employed by a charitable or voluntary organisation as a resident carer for you or your partner;
- anyone who pays you, or to whom you pay, rent on a commercial basis;
- anyone who jointly occupies your home and is either a co-owner or joint tenant.

Anyone falling into the last two categories, however, will count as a non-dependant if they are excluded from HB under the rules set out on page 000 (apart from students and 'persons from abroad').

No non-dependant deductions are made if:

- you or your partner receive AA (see p85) or DLA care component (see p81), or are registered blind; *or,*
- a non-dependant is aged under 18, or is aged under 25 and receiving IS (see p93) or income-based JSA (see p125), or has been in hospital for more than six weeks.

The amount deducted depends on the income of the non-dependant.[206] If the non-dependant is working for more than 16 hours a week the deductions are as follows:

Weekly gross income	Weekly deduction
£255 or more	£46.35
£204-£245.99	£42.25
£155-£203.99	£37.10
£118-£154.99	£22.65
£80-£117.99	£16.50

If the non-dependant is not working more than 16 hours a week, or has a weekly income of less than £80, the deduction is £7.20 a week.

A deduction is made for each non-dependant but only one deduction is made for a non-dependant couple.

Extra housing benefit in exceptional circumstances

You can be paid extra HB if:[207]

- you are entitled to less than maximum HB (see p104) or subject to a non-dependant deduction (see p109) and your 'circumstances are exceptional'; *and/or*
- your rent has been restricted under the rules described on p108 and you or a member of your family will suffer 'exceptional hardship' unless you receive more HB.

'Exceptional circumstances' and 'exceptional hardship' are not defined and you should always consider asking for extra HB if you will experience hardship without it. The maximum you can be paid is your contractual rent less ineligible charges.

Examples of HB calculations

Example one

Mr and Mrs Khan are in receipt of IS. They live with their son, aged 28, who has learning difficulties and receives IS and DLA. Their rent is £70 a week, including all their fuel costs. No restrictions are imposed by the rent officer.

1. Eligible rent = £70 less £12.35 deduction for fuel charges (see p105) = £57.65
2. HB = £57.65 eligible rent less £7.20 non-dependant deduction (see p109) = £50.45

Example two

Mrs Cole is aged 70 and lives alone. She receives AA, retirement pension and an occupational pension. She has £10,500 savings. Her rent is £50 a week and does not include any service charges. No restrictions are imposed on her eligible rent by the rent officer.

1. Her weekly income is:

£80	retirement pension
£40	occupational pension
£30	tariff income from savings (see p104)
£150	

(Note: AA is ignored as income when calculating HB)

2. Her applicable amount is:

£51.40	personal allowance
£30.85	higher pensioner premium
£39.75	severe disability premium
£122.00	

3. £150 income less £122 applicable amount = £28 x 65 per cent = £18.20
4. HB = £50 eligible rent less £18.20 = £31.80

How to claim

Claim forms are available from your local authority and should be returned to the HB section of the authority. If you are claiming IS (see p93) or income-based JSA (see p125), there is a special HB claim form (NHB1) included in the claim pack, which can be submitted to the Benefits Agency, which will forward it to the local authority, together with confirmation that you are entitled to IS or income-based JSA.

You claim HB for yourself and your family (see p104). Either you or your partner can be the claimant and, as with IS, you can sometimes be better off if one of you claims rather the other (see p101).

HB is paid for a period of up to 60 weeks, after which you have to re-claim.[208] If you are a local authority tenant, your HB will be paid by reducing your rent (rent rebate). If you are a private tenant, your HB will usually be paid to you (rent allowance) but in specified circumstances, it can be paid directly to your landlord.[209]

Council tax benefit

Council tax benefit (CTB) is paid to people with a low income and less than £16,000 capital, to help with their council tax. It can be claimed by people who are working or unemployed. CTB is paid and administered by local authorities.

Who can claim

You qualify for CTB if:[210]

- you are liable to pay council tax (see below); *and*
- your income (see Chapter 6) is low enough (see p113); *and*
- your savings and other capital do not exceed £16,000 (see Chapter 7 for details of how your capital is calculated); *and*
- you are not a full-time student (there are exceptions, however, as for HB, see p103); *and*
- you are not treated as a 'person from abroad' (see Chapter 9) this includes people who are not habitually resident in the UK).

In certain circumstances, you can instead qualify for CTB in the form of a 'second adult rebate' regardless of your income or capital if you have a non-dependant living with you who has a low income and who is not disregarded for council tax discount purposes (see below).[211] For more information see CPAG's *Welfare Benefits Handbook*.

Liability to pay council tax

Council tax is payable on most residential dwellings. There are eight different 'bands' (or levels) of council tax, depending on the valuation of the dwelling. However, some dwellings are exempt from council tax, and for other dwellings liability may be reduced by a discount scheme (which applies to dwellings where less than two adults are considered to be resident) and/or a disability reduction scheme (which applies if any resident is considered to be 'substantially and permanently disabled'). The rules about who is liable to pay the tax and which dwellings are taxable are complex and these, and the rules on applications, backdating and appeals are explained in detail in CPAG's *Council Tax Handbook*. The following points, however, are of particular importance:

- Unless an exemption or disregard applies (see below), you are liable to pay council tax in respect of your 'sole or main residence'[212], even if you are temporarily absent from it. You should remain eligible for CTB as long as you remain liable to pay council tax, including while you are away from home in the circumstances during which IS housing costs remain payable (see p99).[213]
- Some dwellings are *exempt* from council tax, including:[214]
- Dwellings which are unoccupied because the former resident(s) has moved
  - (either temporarily or permanently) into a care home; *or*
  - (permanently) into a hospital, *or*
  - (permanently) into the home of another person (which could be a relative or a friend) in order to provide or receive personal care for old age, disablement, illness, mental disorder, or drug or alcohol dependence;
- (in England and Wales) 'granny flats' occupied by elderly or disabled relatives;
- dwellings occupied solely by people who are 'severely mentally impaired'.
- The *disability reduction scheme*[215] will apply if your dwelling has an additional kitchen or bathroom for the use of a 'substantially and permanently disabled' person, or another room used predominantly for her/his needs, or enough space for the use of her/his wheelchair. If this applies, your council tax bill is reduced to the valuation band below that for your dwelling (eg, your bill may be reduced from Band D to Band C). If is already in the lowest band (band A), no reduction will apply until April 2000, when new rules will provide for it to be reduced by one-sixth of your bill.[216]
- The *discount scheme*[217] will apply so as to reduce your bill by 25 per cent if there is only one adult resident in the dwelling, or 50 per cent if there are no adult residents. Some people are disregarded as residents, including anyone who is:
  - receiving care or treatment in a care home (or in a hostel if the owner is liable for the council tax); *or*
  - 'severely mentally impaired'; *or*

– a carer who:
- provides at least 35 hours care a week for a person who is not their partner or parent and who receives the higher rate of the DLA care component or AA; *or*
- provides care and/or support for at least 24 hours a week, and is employed by the person being looked after and was introduced to that person by, or provides the care or support on behalf of, a local authority, government department or charity and in either case is paid no more than £36 a week for the work;
- under the age of 18 or a student.

- Only one council tax bill is payable in respect of each dwelling. A 'hierarchy of liability' determines which resident is liable to pay the bill. In general, owner-occupiers are primarily liable, then tenants, then licensees, then other residents. Partners, joint owners and joint tenants are normally jointly liable. Owners of care homes (and some hostels) and houses in multiple occupation are usually liable rather than the residents.

Claiming for others

As with IS, you claim CTB for yourself and your family, including your partner and dependent children, and the amount you receive depends on the circumstances of your family.[218]

Amount

CTB is a means-tested benefit and the amount you are entitled to depends on your circumstances. CTB is paid in the form of a rebate – ie, reduction in your bill.

If you are receiving IS (see p93) *or income-based JSA* (see p125), your council tax is fully rebated, apart from any non-dependant deductions which you will have to pay (see below).

If you are not receiving income support or income-based JSA, your weekly council tax liability is reduced to 20 per cent of the difference between your income and your applicable amount (see below), plus any non-dependant deductions which you have to pay (see p114). If this figure exceeds your council tax liability you are not entitled to any CTB. If your income is less than your applicable amount your council tax is fully rebated.[219] Your income and applicable amount are worked out in the same way as for HB (see p104), except that the categories of people who do not count as non-dependants for the purposes of the severe disability premium (see p97) are slightly different (see below).[220]

Examples of CTB calculations are given on p114.

You should also note the following points:
- If you are jointly liable for council tax with someone other than your partner (see p113) your CTB will be calculated on your proportionate share of the bill.[221]

- If your home is in council tax valuation band F or above, your CTB may be reduced by a set proportion.[222]
- Your CTB can be increased if your 'circumstances are exceptional' – eg, you will suffer hardship without an increase.[223]
- If you qualify for a second adult rebate (see p111) your council tax is rebated by up to 25 per cent, depending on the income of your non-dependant.[224]

Non-dependant deductions

If you have a non-dependant living with you, a deduction is made from your CTB and will not form part of your rebate, on the assumption that s/he is making a contribution towards your council tax (whether s/he is or not).

The rules about non-dependant deductions are the same as for housing benefit (see p109), apart from the following differences

- The last two categories of people on p109 who do not count as non-dependants for HB do not apply to CTB. For CTB, a joint occupier who is jointly liable for council tax, or a person other than close relative who is liable to pay you rent on a commercial basis, does not count as a non-dependant unless her/his liability was created to take advantage of the CTB scheme.[225]
- No non-dependant deduction is made for anyone who is receiving IS or income-based JSA (not just those under 25 as for HB), or anyone who is disregarded for council tax discount purposes (see p111).[226]
- If the non-dependant is working more than 16 hours a week, the amount of deduction is as follows:[227]

Weekly gross income	Weekly deduction
£255 or over	£6.50
£204-£254.99	£5.40
£118-£203.99	£4.40
£117.99 or below	£2.15

- If the non-dependant is not working more than 16 hours a week, the weekly deduction is £2.15.[228]

Examples of CTB calculations

Example one

In the case of Mr and Mrs Khan, whose circumstances are set out on p110, they would be entitled to a full rebate of their council tax (there would be no non-dependant deduction for their son because he is in receipt of IS).

Example two

In the case of Mrs Cole, whose circumstances are set out on p86, her council tax liability would be reduced to £28 x 20 per cent = £5.60

How to claim

The procedure is the same as for HB (see p111). Application forms are available from your local authority, or you can claim on form NHB1, if you are claiming IS or income-based JSA. CTB is paid by rebating your council tax liability.

Disabled person's tax credit

Disabled person's tax credit (DPTC) has replaced DLA from October 1994 and is paid to people with a disability who are working for 16 hours or more a week and whose income and capital are below set levels. DPTC is calculated and administered by the Inland Revenue and from April 2000 will normally be paid with the claimant's salary. It is not taxable, but counts in full as income when calculating entitlement to other means-tested benefits, including HB/CTB (see p169). If you cannot qualify for DPTC, you may be entitled to working families' tax credit (WFTC) if you have a dependent child (see p125).

Who can claim

You qualify for DPTC if:[229]
- you are working for an average of at least 16 hours a week; *and*
- you are present and ordinarily resident in Great Britain and are not subject to any restrictions on your immigration status (see Chapter 9); *and*
- you are, or have been, receiving a qualifying benefit (see below); *and*
- you and your partner have less than £16,000 capital (your capital is calculated in a similar way as for other means-tested benefits – see Chapter 7 and CPAG's *Welfare Benefits Handbook* for details); *and*
- your income is low enough for you to qualify (see p116).

Qualifying benefits

To qualify for DPTC, you must either;
- be receiving DLA (see p81) or AA (see p85) (including constant attendance allowance paid with a war pension or industrial injuries benefit); *or*
- have been receiving one of the following benefits at any time in the 26 weeks before you claimed DPTC;
  - incapacity benefit (IB) at the short-term higher rate or long-term rate (see p75);
  - severe disablement allowance (SDA – see p79);
  - IS, income-based JSA, HB or CTB, if your applicable amount includes a disability premium or higher pensioner premium paid in respect of you (see p97).

You can also qualify if you were on a 'training for work' course in the eight weeks before you claimed DPTC and you were receiving IB (at one of the above rates) or SDA in the eight weeks before your course began.

Amount

DPTC is a means-tested benefit and the amount you are entitled to depends on your circumstances. Your claim is assessed for your family (the rules on who counts as your family are the same as for IS – see p96). Your entitlement is calculated as follows:

Step one: Work out your maximum DPTC
Add up the following amounts to arrive at the maximum weekly payable DPTC:

- £54.30 if you are a single claimant, or £83.55 if you have a partner or are a lone parent;
- £19.85 for each dependent child aged up to 11
- £20.90 for each dependent child aged 11-15
- £25.95 for each dependent child aged 16-18.
  Note: Ages apply from the first Tuesday in September following the actual birthday;
- £21.90 for each child who gets DLA or who is blind;
- childcare costs of up to £70 if you have one child and £105 if you have more children (see CPAG's *Welfare Benefits Handbook* for details of who qualifies and how costs are calculated);
- £11.05 if you or your partner are working for at least 30 hours a week.

Step two: Calculate your weekly income
Your income is calculated in a similar way as it is for other means-tested benefits (see Chapter 6 and CPAG's *Welfare Benefits Handbook* for details of differences). It includes your net earnings and most benefits (but not AA, DLA or CB) but not maintenance payments.

Step three: Amount of DPTC payable
- If your weekly income is less than £70 (if you are single) or £90 (if you have a partner or are a lone parent), you are entitled to your maximum DPTC (see step one, above).
- If your weekly income is more than the above amounts, your maximum DPTC is reduced by 55 per cent of the excess.

Example of a DPTC calculation

Mr and Mrs Evans have one child aged 7. Mr Evans receives DLA and works for 24 hours a week, taking home £180 weekly earnings. Mrs Evans receives CB. They have no other income or savings.
Step one: Maximum DPTC: £83.55 for a couple plus £19.85 for a child = £103.40
Step two: Weekly income: £180 (DLA and CB are ignored)

Step three: DPTC: £180 income, *less*
£90
=£90 excess income x 55 per cent = £49.50
£103.40 maximum DPTC, *less*
£49.50 excess income
=£53.90
Mr Evans will be entitled to £53.90 DPTC a week.

How to claim

You should claim on form DPTC1, which is included in a claims pack available from Benefits Agency offices, JobCentres and tax offices. You can also get a pack by telephoning 0845-605-5858 (text phone: 0845-6088844).

From April 2000, most employees will receive DPTC with their salary (the Inland Revenue will inform employers how much you are entitled to but not any other details of your claim). Until then, the Inland Revenue will pay you directly by order book, or into your bank account. Awards are made for 26 weeks and are generally not affected by any changes of circumstances – eg, changes in your income. After 26 weeks, you must re-apply for a further award.

Social fund payments

The social fund (SF) is a government fund which makes payments to people on low incomes to meet specified needs. The fund is administered by the Benefits Agency. There are two types of payments available from the social fund:

- *Funeral grants, maternity grants and winter payments.* You are legally entitled to these payments if you satisfy the rules.
- *Community care grants, budgeting loans and crisis loans.* You are eligible for these payments if you satisfy the rules but awards are discretionary and budget-limited.

Funeral grants

Funeral grants are paid to people to help with the cost of a funeral of a close relative or friend.

Who can claim

You qualify for a funeral grant if:[230]

- you or your partner have been awarded IS (see p93), income-based JSA (see p125), HB (see p102), CTB (see p111), DPTC (see p115) or WFTC (see p125) when you claim a funeral grant; *and*
- you or your partner are in one of the categories of people who are eligible to claim (see below); *and*

- you have accepted responsibility for paying the cost of a funeral (ie, you are liable to pay the cost because, for example, the funeral director's bill is in your name); *and*
- the deceased was ordinarily resident in the UK when s/he died and the funeral takes place in the UK (or, in certain circumstances, in an EC state); *and*
- you do not have too much capital (see p118).

People eligible to claim

You can claim a funeral grant if you or your partner fall into one of the following categories:[231]

- You were the partner of the deceased when s/he died. Partner means spouse, or someone you were living with as husband and wife.[232]
- The deceased was a child for whom you were responsible (you may be excluded if the child had an absent parent who was not getting one of the qualifying benefits listed above);
- You were a 'close relative' or close friend of the deceased and it is reasonable for you to accept responsibility for the funeral costs, given the nature and extent of your contact with the deceased.[233] 'Close relative' means parent, parent-in-law, son, son-in-law, daughter, daughter-in-law, step-parent, stepson, stepson-in-law, stepdaughter, stepdaughter-in-law, brother, brother-in-law, sister and sister-in-law.[234] You are excluded from getting a grant as close relative or close friend, however, if the deceased has a partner, parent or adult son or daughter (unless the parent, son, or daughter is receiving one of the qualifying benefits listed above, or was estranged from the deceased when s/he died, or is a student, or prisoner).[235] You are also excluded if there is a close relative of the deceased who was in closer contact with her/him than you were.[236]

Amount

The following amounts can be paid, subject to the deductions below:[237]
- the costs of burial or cremation (including documentation); *plus*
- specified transport costs; *plus*
- up to £600 for other costs – eg, funeral directors' fees, flowers, religious costs.

The following amounts are deducted from an award of a funeral grant:
- any capital you or your partner have in excess of £500 (£1,000 if either of you is aged 60 or over);[238]
- any of the deceased's assets available to you without probate or letters of administration.[239] Note that the Benefits Agency can recover a funeral grant from the deceased's estate;[240]

- any payment made on the death of the deceased from an insurance policy, pre-paid funeral plan, burial club, charity or relative of yours.[241]

How to claim

You should claim a funeral grant on form SF200 from your local Benefits Agency. You must claim within three months of the date of the funeral.[242]

Maternity grants

Maternity grants of £100 are paid to help with the cost of maternity expenses.

Who can claim

You qualify for a maternity grant if:[243]
- you or your partner have been awarded IS, income-based JSA, DPTC or WFTC when you claim a maternity grant; *and*
- you or a member of your family (as defined for IS – see p104) are pregnant, or have given birth in the last three months (including stillbirth after 24 weeks of pregnancy), or have adopted a baby under 12 months old, or have a parental order for a surrogate child; *and*
- you do not have too much capital (see below).

Amount

The maternity grant is £100 for each child.[244] Any capital you or your partner have in excess of £500 (£1000 if either of you is aged 60 or over) is deducted form the grant.[245] This means if you have capital of more than £600 (or £1,100) you will not get a grant.

How to claim

You should claim on form SF 100 obtainable from your local Benefits Agency. You must claim in the 11 weeks before the expected week of birth or in the three months after the birth, adoption or parental order.

Winter payments

Winter payments are made to help with the cost of fuel bills.

Who can claim

There are two types of winter payments:
- *Cold weather payments* are made if the average temperature in your area falls below 0 degrees Celsius for at least a week. You qualify for a payment if you are receiving IS or income-based JSA and either you have child under five, or you are receiving a pensioner, higher pensioner, disability, severe disability of disabled child premium (see p97).[246]
- *Winter fuel payments* are made to people over pension age who are receiving retirement pension (see p70), widows' benefits (see p73), AA (see p85), DLA

(see p81), incapacity benefit (see p75), severe disablement allowance (see p79), industrial injuries benefits (see p89) or war pensions (see p93); and to people aged 60 or over who are receiving IS (see p93) or income-based JSA (see p125). You must be in receipt of one of the above benefits in the week commencing the third Monday of September.[247] The European Court of Justice, following an opinion of the Advocate General,[248] is expected to find that restrictions relating to pension age are unlawfully discriminatory. If you are a man aged 60-64 and you are not awarded a payment you should seek expert advice (see Appendix 4).

You are generally excluded from a payment if you receive IS while you live in a care home.

Amount

Cold weather payments are £8.50 for each qualifying week. Winter fuel payments are one-off grants of £100 a household.

How to claim

There is no need to make a claim for winter payments as they should be paid automatically if you qualify. All payments should be issued by the middle of December. If you do not receive a payment you are entitled to, you should telephone the special helpline on 0645-151515 (text phone 0191 2187280).

Community care grants

Community care grants (CCGs) are paid to help people on IS or income-based JSA to live independently in the community.

Who can claim

You are eligible for a CCG if:
- you are receiving IS (see p93) or income-based JSA (see p125) when you claim a CCG, or you are due to leave institutional or residential care within six weeks of claiming a CCG and are likely to get IS or income-based JSA when you leave;[249] *and*
- you do not have too much capital (see p122); *and*
- you do not want the CCG to obtain an 'excluded item' (see p122); *and*
- you need the CCG;
  – to help you or a member of your family, or someone for whom you or a member of your family will be providing care, to become established in the community following a stay in institutional or residential care, or to remain in the community rather than enter such care; or
  – to ease exceptional pressures on you and your family; *or*
  – to help you set up home as part of a planned re-settlement programme; *or*
  – to help you care for a prisoner or young offender on temporary release; *or*

– to help you with travel expenses to visit someone who is ill, attend a relative's funeral, ease a domestic crisis, or move to a more suitable accommodation.[250]

There is no legal entitlement to a CCG. Payments are discretionary and each Benefits Agency district office is given a fixed annual budget for CCGs. Guidance is issued by the DSS (the *Social Fund Guide*) and by each district on the circumstances in which a CCG should be awarded. The guidance is not legally binding, however, and decisions must take into account all the circumstances of each application, including the nature, extent and urgency of the need.[251] The guidance suggests that priority should be given where there is mental or physical disability, illness, general frailty, abuse or neglect, unstable family circumstances, an unsettled way of life and drug or alcohol misuse.

You should also note the following points:

- You must specify the items for which you need the CCG. You can ask for a CCG for any items which are not excluded (see below). If, however, you have been awarded or refused a CCG for a particular item, you cannot get a CCG for the same item for 26 weeks from the date of your application.[252]

- CCGs are most often awarded to help people move out of, or stay out of, institutional or residential care (see p120). This could include hospital, residential care and nursing homes, group homes, supported lodgings, sheltered housing, hostels and any other accommodation which provides residents with a substantial care or supervision. If you are moving out of care you need to show that a CCG will help you establish yourself in the community (eg, by helping you set up home). If you live in your own home, you need to show that a CCG will lessen the risk of you going into hospital or residential care – eg, by improving your ability to cope at home and to stay healthy. The type of items you could claim for include furniture and household equipment, moving expenses, clothing and footwear and non-medical items needed because of sickness and disability, including wheelchairs and special beds, mattresses, chairs and equipment to help with everyday living.

- You can also claim a CCG to ease exceptional pressures on you and your family. 'Family' is not defined in the law and could encompass couples (married or not, of any sex[253]), children and adult sons and daughters and other relatives living together. People living on their own, however, are probably excluded under this provision.[254] 'Exceptional pressures' are not defined in the law and could include disability, sickness, depression, bereavement, family breakdown, poor living conditions and child behavioural problems.

Excluded items

You cannot get a CCG for any of the following items:[255]

- the cost of domestic assistance (including home care) or respite care;
- a medical, surgical, optical, aural or dental item. A medical item, however, should not include an everyday item needed because of a medical condition – eg, non-allergic bedding, a special bed or mattress, special shoes, equipment for everyday living and a wheelchair;
- most housing costs including repairs and improvements (other than minor ones), rent, deposits, mortgage payments, residential accommodation charges and council tax and water charges;
- telephone and fuel charges, educational or training needs, work-related expenses, debts to government departments, court fines and fees, needs which a local authority has a statutory duty to meet and most daily living expenses;
- a need which occurs outside the UK.

Amount

You must specify the amount of CCG you need on your application form (see below). There is no legal maximum but the minimum you can be awarded is £30 (unless the CCG is for travel expenses).[256] You should state the actual or estimated cost or each item you need on your application form. The amount you request should be allowed unless it is unreasonable. The Benefits Agency often refers to catalogue prices as a guide to what is reasonable.

Any CCG you are awarded is reduced by the amount of capital you and your partner have in excess of £500 (£1000 if either of you is aged 60 or over).[257]

How to claim

You should apply for a CCG on form SF300 obtainable from your local Benefits Agency office. You should list all the items you need and the actual or estimated cost of each item. You should explain why you need the items, with reference to the purposes for which a CCG can be awarded (see p124), and why your application should be given high priority. A supporting letter from your doctor, social worker or other professional involved in your care may help your case.

Budgeting loans

Budgeting loans (BLs) are interest-free loans paid to help people on IS or income-based JSA, with intermittent expenses. They usually have to be re-paid on a weekly basis by direct deductions from benefit.

Who can claim

You are eligible for a BL if:[258]

- you are in receipt of IS (see p93) or income-based JSA (see p125) when you claim a BL and you and/or your partner have been receiving one of those

benefits throughout the 26 weeks before your claim is determined, apart from any breaks of up to 28 days; *and*
- you must not have too much capital (see p123); *and*
- the BL must be for one or more of the following items:
  - furniture or household equipment;
  - clothing and footwear;
  - rent in advance and/or removal expenses on moving;
  - improvement, maintenance and security of the home;
  - travelling expenses;
  - expenses related to seeking or re-entering work;
- HP and other debts for any of the above.

As with community care grants (CCGs – see p120), there is no legal entitlement to a payment and each district Benefits Agency office is given a fixed annual budget for loans. Unlike CCGs, however, applications are decided in accordance with set criteria, rather then on a discretionary basis (see below).

Repayment of BLs can cause hardship and you should always apply for a CCG rather than a BL if you are eligible (see p120).

Amount

You can request a BL of between £30 and £1,000.[259] Whether you are actually offered a BL and the amount you are offered depends on a number of factors including:[260]
- the length of time you have been receiving benefit;
- the size of your family;
- the amount of any outstanding BLs you have;
- your ability to repay a BL within 78 weeks.

If you are offered a loan, you will be given details of the weekly repayment rate, which can vary from 5 per cent to 25 per cent of your IS applicable amount (excluding housing costs). You will sometimes be given more than one offer of different amounts with different terms.

Any award, however, is reduced by the amount of any capital you or your partner have in excess of £500 (£1,000 if either of you is aged 60 or over).[261]

BLs are normally recovered by direct deductions from your weekly benefit.

How to claim

You should apply for a BL on form SF500 obtainable from your local Benefits Agency. If you are offered a loan, you are given 14 days to return your acceptance.

Crisis loans

Crisis loans (CLs) are paid to people who have no money because of a crisis. Unlike budgeting loans, they are not restricted to people on benefit.

Who can claim

You are eligible for a CL if:[262]

- you are aged 16 or over; *and*
- you have insufficient resources to meet the immediate needs of your self and/or your family; *and*
- you need a CL to prevent serious damage or serious risk to your (or a member of your family's) health and safety following an emergency or disaster; or you need a CL for rent in advance to secure for private accommodation following a stay in care (you must also have been awarded a community care grant – see p120); *and*
- you are not in hospital or a care home (unless your discharge is planned within the next two weeks) and the CL is not for an excluded item (items excluded are the same as for community care grants – see p122 – except that living expenses and fuel costs are not excluded but holidays, TVs and cars are); *and*
- you are likely to be able to repay the loan.

As with community care grants (see p120), there is no legal entitlement to a CL. Payments are discretionary and must take into account the circumstances of each case (including the urgency of the need) and guidance is set out in the *Social Fund Guide*. The *Guide* gives examples of when a CL may be appropriate, including where you have lost money, you are waiting for a benefit claim to be processed, your fuel has been disconnected, or you have suffered an emergency or disaster such as a fire or flood. You can, however, claim in any situation where you have no money.

Amount

You can request a lump sum CL of up to £1,000, or a weekly sum of up to 75 per cent of your IS personal allowance (see p97) plus £20.20 for each child, for living expenses.[263] You will not usually be offered more than you can repay in 78 weeks. You will be given details of the weekly repayment rate which is normally between 5 per cent and 15 per cent of your IS applicable amount excluding housing costs (see p99).

How to claim

You should claim a CL on form SF400 or SF401. It is common for Benefits Agency counter staff to advise potential applicants that they do not qualify. You should always insist on completing an application form and being given a written decision. You will normally be interviewed and you should always fully explain your circumstances and why you need a CL.

Other means-tested benefits

Other means-tested benefits are briefly described below. For more details see CPAG's *Welfare Benefits Handbook*.

Income-based jobseeker's allowance

Income-based jobseeker's allowance (JSA) is paid to people whose income and capital are below set limits. Claimants must be working less than 16 hours a week and not have a partner who is working more than 24 hours a week. They must also satisfy the labour market conditions ie, be capable of work, available for work and actively seeking work and signing on at a local JobCentre. Income-based JSA is calculated in the same way as IS, taking into account the applicable amount and resources of the claimant's family (see p96). People who have paid sufficient NI contribution conditions may be able to claim contribution-based JSA allowance (see p93) instead of, or in addition to, income-based JSA. People who are eligible to claim IS may be better off doing so, to avoid having to satisfy the labour market conditions.

Working families' tax credit

Working families' tax credit (WFTC), which replaced family credit in October 1999, is paid to people with dependent children who are working for at least 16 hours a week and whose earnings and capital are below set levels. The rules and structure are similar to disabled person's tax credit (DPTC – see p115) but you will usually be better off claiming DPTC if you qualify because it is a more generous benefit.

Bonuses
- A back to work bonus of up to £1,000 is payable to some people who cease claiming IS (see p93) or income-based JSA (see p125) as a result of moving from part-time to full time work of at least 16 hours a week.
- A child maintenance bonus of up to £1,000 is payable to people receiving child maintenance who cease claiming IS or income-based JSA as a result of working.
- People who cease claiming IS or income-based JSA can claim extended payments of housing benefit (see p102) and council tax benefit (see p111) for the first four weeks they are working. Lone parents who start working can continue to claim IS for two weeks.

4. **People in hospital**

Your benefit may be reduced after you or your dependants have been in hospital for specified periods. The rules apply to anyone who is being maintained free of charge, while undergoing treatment as an in-patient in a hospital or similar institution (this could include some nursing homes and hospices). This covers all in-patients, apart from fee-paying private patients in NHS or private hospitals.[264]

Separate stays in hospital which are separated by less than 28 days are linked together when calculating how long someone has been an in-patient.[265] This means that your benefit may be reduced immediately, or sooner than normal, if you are re-admitted to hospital within 28 days of a previous stay. You do not count as an in-patient on the day you enter hospital, but you do on the day you are discharged.[266]

You may lose or gain entitlement to different benefits as a result of the hospital rules and you should always seek advice if you are unsure about the situation. It is important that you inform the benefit authorities about any hospital admission or discharge as soon as possible, to avoid any overpayment or underpayment of benefit. In particular, if your IS stops, your HB and CTB will also stop and you may need to make a fresh claim.

If you need to claim benefit on the basis of incapacity for work, the hospital can issue medical certificates. You can arrange for someone to collect your benefit while you are in hospital and if you are unable to manage your affairs another person can act as your appointee (see p226).

See p139 if you need help with fares to hospital. You may also be eligible for a community care grant to cover fares to visit someone in hospital (see p120).

Non-means-tested benefits

Attendance allowance and disability living allowance

If you become entitled to attendance allowance (AA – see p85) or disability living allowance (DLA – see p81) while you are an in-patient, you cannot receive any benefit until the day following your discharge.[267] If you are already entitled to AA or DLA when you become an in-patient, payment stops after you have been in hospital for 28 days (84 days if you are aged under 16).[268] Note the linking rule on p125 if you have been re-admitted to hospital after less than 28 days. Your benefit should be restored when you are discharged from hospital (you should not have to make a fresh claim but should inform the Benefits Agency of your discharge).

You should also note the following special rules:

- You can continue to receive the mobility component of DLA (see p83) while you are an in-patient if you had a Motability agreement (see p83) when you entered hospital (benefit normally continues until the agreement ends).[269] You can also continue to receive the mobility component if you had been receiving it for at least a year in July 1996.[270]
- If you are terminally ill you can continue to receive AA or DLA while you are in a hospice.[271]
- If you enter hospital from residential or nursing care, you are not normally entitled to AA or the care component of DLA. This is because periods spent in special accommodation in which AA and the care component of DLA are not payable (see p356), link with periods spent as an in-patient (unless they

are separated by more than 28 days) precluding re-instatement of benefit when a resident becomes an in-patient.[272] If you have been receiving AA/DLA care component while in an independent care home (eg, because you have been self-funding) it will remain payable for the first 28 days in hospital. Note, however, that in all cases the mobility component of DLA remains payable for at least the first 28 days in hospital (see above).

Invalid care allowance

You remain entitled to invalid care allowance (ICA – see p88) for up to 12 weeks in any period of 26 weeks while you, or the person you are caring for, are an in-patient.[273] Your ICA stops, however, when the person you are caring for loses her/his AA or care component of DLA, which will usually happen after s/he has been an in-patient for 28 days (84 days if s/he is a child) (see above). Any increase of ICA you receive for a spouse is reduced to £13.35 a week after s/he has been an in-patient for six weeks.[274]

Other non-means-tested benefits

The following benefits are reduced after the periods in hospital specified below:
• retirement pension;
• widow's pension and widowed mother's allowance;
• incapacity benefit;
• severe disablement allowance

Other benefits are generally unaffected by stays in hospital but note that:
• you can only continue to receive benefit for a child who has been an in-patient for more than 12 weeks if you are regularly incurring expenditure in respect of her/him;
• you can only continue to claim contribution-based JSA for two weeks while you are an in-patient.

After six weeks

Your basic entitlement to the above benefits is reduced by:
• £26.70 a week if you are a single claimant; *or*
• £13.35 a week if you have one or more dependants

after you have been an in-patient for six weeks, but your benefit will not be reduced to below £13.35 a week.[275]

If your spouse has been an in-patient for more than six weeks, any dependant's increase you are receiving is reduced by £13.35 a week, subject to a minimum payment of £13.35.[276]

After 12 weeks

Any increase you are receiving for a child stops after s/he has been an in-patient for 12 weeks, unless you continue to regularly incur expenditure in respect of her/him.[277]

After 52 weeks

Your basic entitlement to the above benefits is reduced to £13.35 a week after you have been an in-patient for more than 52 weeks.[278] You can be paid less that this if you are unable to act for yourself, your benefit is being paid to the hospital (as your appointee or on your appointee's request) and your doctor certifies that the benefit cannot be used for your comfort or enjoyment.[279]

If you have a dependant, you can opt for the remainder of your normal weekly entitlement, less a further deduction of £26.70, to be paid to her/him (you should be sent a form for this purpose).[280] Any increase you receive for a spouse is reduced to £13.35 after s/he has been an in-patient for 52 weeks.[281]

Entering hospital from residential or nursing care

Special rules apply if you are admitted into hospital from a residential care or nursing home, unless your placement is self-funded. If you are a permanent home resident, the above benefits are reduced to £13.35 (or less if the circumstances set out above in 'after 52 weeks' apply) from the first day you become an in-patient, or, where you reside in an independent care or nursing home, after you have been an in-patient for six weeks. If you are a temporary home resident, your period of residence counts towards the periods of six weeks and 52 weeks, after which your benefit is reduced when you are an in-patient (see above).[282]

Means-tested benefits

Income support

Your income support (IS) applicable amount (see p96), is reduced after you or a member of your family (see p96) have been an in-patient for the periods specified below. Note the linking rule on p125 if you have been re-admitted to hospital after less than 28 days. Special rules apply if you are admitted into hospital from a residential or nursing care home (see Chapter 21).

After four weeks

Your entitlement to a severe disability premium (see p97) ceases when your attendance allowance (AA) or disability living allowance (DLA) care component stops (usually after you have been an in-patient for four weeks – see p126), unless you are a member of a couple and one or both of you are in hospital, in which case you can qualify for the premium at the single person's rate.[283] Your entitlement to a disability, higher pensioner, or disabled child premium (see p97) is not affected by the withdrawal of AA of DLA.[284] You remain entitled to a carer's premium (see p97) for eight weeks after your invalid care allowance stops.[285]

After six weeks

- If you are a single claimant, your IS applicable amount is reduced after you have been an in-patient for six weeks, to £16.70 plus any housing costs (see p99).[286] All premiums are withdrawn. Housing costs remain payable as long as your period of absence from home is unlikely to substantially exceed 52 weeks.[287] Note that you can be treated as a single claimant if you are likely to be away from your family for substantially more than 52 weeks.[288]
- If you are a lone parent, your IS applicable amount is reduced to £16.70 plus child allowances, the family premium and where applicable, the disabled child premium (see p97) and housing costs (see above).[289]
- If you are a member of a couple and one of you has been an in-patient for six weeks, your IS applicable amount is reduced by (not to) £13.35. If both of you have been in hospital for more than six weeks, your applicable amount is reduced to £33.40, plus, if applicable, child allowances, the family premium, the disabled child premium and any housing costs (see above).[290]

After 12 weeks

The IS personal allowance for a child or young person (see p97) is reduced to £13.35 after s/he has been an in-patient for 12 weeks.[291] Child-related premiums remain payable, including the disabled child premium (even after the cessation of DLA).[292]

After 52 weeks

- If you are a single claimant, your IS applicable amount is reduced to £13.35 (or less if the circumstances set out on p128 apply) when you have been an in-patient for 52 weeks.[293] Housing costs can be paid to another person if s/he can be treated as liable to pay them.
- If you are a lone parent or a member of a couple, your IS applicable amount is reduced to £13.35 (or less if the circumstances set out on p128 apply) once your absence from your family is likely to substantially exceed 52 weeks.[294] If your partner remains at home, s/he can claim normal rate IS as a single claimant or lone parent, if s/he is eligible to do so.
- You will lose the IS personal allowance and any premiums paid in respect of a child or young person if s/he is likely to be away for substantially longer than 52 weeks.[295]

Housing benefit and council tax benefit

You can continue to claim housing benefit (HB – see p102) and council tax benefit (CTB – see p111) for up to 52 weeks while you are an in-patient, as long as your absence from home is unlikely to substantially exceed 52 weeks.[296] You should also remain entitled to CTB for as long as your home remains your sole or main residence (see p112).[297]

Subject to the above, you remain entitled to maximum HB (see p104) and CTB (see p113) as long as you are receiving IS or income-based JSA. If your entitlement to IS or income-based JSA stops because of the hospital rules, your HB and CTB will also stop and you must submit fresh claims for them.

If you are not receiving IS or income-based JSA, your HB and CTB applicable amount is reduced in the same way as for IS (see p128) after you or your partner have been an in-patient for more than four or six weeks.[298]

You can continue to claim for members of your family who are in-patients as long as, in the case of HB, they are unlikely to be away for substantially longer than 52 weeks, and in the case of CTB, their absence remains temporary.[299]

Other means-tested benefits

Other means-tested benefits are generally unaffected by stays in hospital. Note, however, that you can only continue to claim income-based JSA (see p125) for two weeks while you are an in-patient (but you may be able to claim IS instead). If your partner is an in-patient, your applicable amount is reduced after s/he has been in hospital for 4, 6 or 52 weeks in line with the rules which apply to IS (see p128).

5. **Increasing your entitlement to benefit – examples**

Many people do not claim all the benefits to which they are entitled. To ensure you do so, you will need to be familiar not only with the conditions relating to any of the benefits or allowances which may be relevant to you and anyone you can claim for, but also with how the different benefits which may apply to you may affect other benefits or allowances which you or someone else may be able to claim. The details set out in this chapter should enable you to identify which benefits and allowances may apply to you. The following are typical examples of circumstances where benefits are commonly underclaimed and where claimants have been able to increase their incomes. For examples of common problems and how to overcome them, see Chapter 11.

Example 1
Monica is 63 years old and owns her own home (for which she no longer pays any mortgage). She receives a basic retirement pension of £66.75 a week, from which she pays £12.75 a week council tax. She has no savings.

Because her income (£66.75) is less than her IS applicable amount of £75, she should be advised to claim IS which will be worth £8.25 a week. She will also be entitled to maximum CTB so that she will not have to pay any of her £12.75 a week council tax. By claiming both IS and CTB she will be able to increase her income by £21 a week. (For more details of how she may also be able to backdate any claims and payments, see Chapter 10.) By claiming IS, she will now be eligible for higher winter payments and community care grants from the social fund (see also Chapter 4 for other sources of financial assistance which may now be available to her).

Example 2

Margaret and Steve are a married couple who live together in their own home (for which they no longer pay any mortgage). They are both aged 70. Their combined income from retirement and occupational pensions is £160 a week, out of which they pay £22 a week council tax. They have no savings. Both Margaret's and Steve's health has been deteriorating recently and they are now being provided with community care services for several hours a day (see Chapter 2) to assist them with their personal care needs.

Because their income (£160) is higher than their IS applicable amount (£116.00) they are not currently entitled to IS, but they are entitled to CTB. If they claimed CTB they would only have to pay £8.68 a week council tax. However, because of the extent of their personal care needs, they should each be advised to claim AA. If they are each awarded AA for their care needs during the day, this will be worth £35.40 a week each and will increase their IS applicable amount to £204.80 (because they will each be entitled to a severe disability premium and they will be entitled to the couple rate of the higher pensioner premium instead of the ordinary pensioner premium). They should therefore be advised to claim IS as well which will be worth an extra £44.80. They will then also be entitled to maximum CTB so that they will no longer have to pay the £8.68 council tax. By claiming AA (worth £70.80) they have become entitled to IS (worth £44.80) and extra CTB (worth £8.68). They have, therefore, increased their income by £124.28 a week. (For details of how they may also be able to backdate any claims and payments, see Chapter 10.) By claiming IS, they will now be eligible for higher winter payments and community care grants from the social fund (see also Chapter 4 for other sources of financial assistance which may now be available to them).

Example 3

Brian and Sheila are a married couple aged 60 and 55 who live together in rented accommodation. Brian has physical disabilities and depends on Sheila to help with his personal care needs throughout the day and night. They each receive an award of long term incapacity benefit of £66.75 a week (totalling £133.50), HB, and CTB, out of which they have to pay £6.97 towards their rent and council tax.

Because of his extensive personal care needs, Brian should be advised to claim DLA. He may expect to be paid the higher rate care component of £52.95 a week. Sheila should, therefore, also be advised to claim ICA. ICA will not be paid to Sheila because it overlaps with her long term IB. However, so long as she is awarded ICA, they will be entitled to a carer's premium worth £13.95 a week. They will then be entitled to IS worth £5.75 a week as well as maximum HB and CTB so that they will no longer have to contribute towards their rent and council tax. By claiming DLA and ICA and IS, they will be able to increase their total weekly income by £65.67 a week. (For details of how they may also be able to backdate any claims and payments, see Chapter 10.) By claiming IS, they will now be eligible for higher winter fuel payments and social fund grants (see also Chapter 4, for other sources of financial assistance which may now be available to them).

Example 4:

Liz is 70 years old and is severely disabled. She lives in rented accommodation for which she gets maximum HB and CTB because her pension is topped up with IS (worth £82.25 a week in total) as well as AA. Her IS does not include a severe disability premium because her son, Ernie, who lives nearby, is receiving ICA for looking after her. Ernie is 45 years old and lives alone. He also depends on IS, and his combined income from ICA and IS is £65.35 a week. Ernie had to give up work some years ago both to look after his mother and because he had become incapable of work due to poor health.

Ernie should be advised to claim incapacity benefit (IB). Although his ICA will then no longer be payable (because this will overlap with his claim for IB) his IS will still include a carer's premium. However, because ICA will no longer be in payment to him, his mother will now be entitled to the severe disability premium. If it is accepted that Ernie has been incapable of work for more than 12 months, Ernie will also be entitled to a disability premium (worth £21.90 a week). By claiming IB, Ernie may manage to increase his income by £21.90 a week, and will increase his mother's income by £39.75 a week. (For details of how they may also be able to backdate any claims and payment, see Chapter 10.)

Notes

1. Which benefits you can claim
1 Reg 4 SS (OB) Regs

2. Non means-tested benefits
2 s122(1) SSCBA 1992
3 s44(1) SSCBA 1992
4 s48A SSCBA 1992
5 ss48B SSCBA 1992
6 s51 SSCBA 1992
7 s78(3) SSCBA 1992; reg 10 SS(WB&RP) Regs
8 Sch 3 para 5 SSCBA 1992
9 s44 and sch 4 SSCBA 1992
10 ss82-85, 86A and 90 SSCBA 1992; SS(Dep) Regs; SSB(PRT) Regs
11 s80, 81 and sch 4 SSCBA 1992
12 ss45, 46, 48A, 48B SSCBA 1992
13 Sch 5 paras 1 and 2 SSCBA 1992
14 ss36(2), 37(4) and 38(3) SSCBA 1992
15 s36 SSCBA 1992
16 s37 SSCBA 1992
17 s38 SSCBA 1992
18 ss 36, 39, 80(5) and sch 4 SSCBA 1992
19 Reg 19(2) SS(C&P) Regs
20 s3 SSAA 1992
21 s30A SSCBA 1992
22 Sch 12, para 1 SSCBA 1992
23 ss30A and 30C SSCBA 1992
24 s171B SSCBA 1992; reg 2 SS (ME) Regs
25 s171C SSCBA 1992
26 s171C SSCBA 1992; Sch to SS (IFW) Regs
27 Reg 25 SS (IFW) Regs
28 Regs 6 and 8 SS (IFW) Regs
29 Reg 6 (2)(g) SS&CS (D&A) Regs
30 Reg 28 SS (IFW) Regs
31 Reg 10 SS (IFW) Regs
32 Regs 10 , 11 SS (IFW) Regs
33 Reg 27 SS (IFW) Regs
34 Reg 13 SS (IFW) Regs
35 Reg 31 SS(IB) T Regs
36 Regs 16 and 17 SS (IFW) Regs
37 Reg 10 SS&CS (D&A) Regs
38 s21 and Sch 3 SSCBA 1992
39 ss30A and 30B and Sch 4 SSCBA 1992
40 s30B(4) SSCBA 1992
41 ss30A and 30B SSCBA 1992
42 s30B(3) SSCBA 1992
43 s86A and Sch 4 SSCBA 1992; SS (IB-ID) Regs
44 ss 80-81 and Sch 4 SCBA 1992; SS(IB-ID) Regs.
45 SS IB (TP) Regs
46 s68 SSCBA 1992
47 Reg 8 SS (SDA) Regs
48 Reg 6 SS (SDA) Regs
49 Reg 10 SS (SDA) Regs
50 s68(6) SSCBA 1992; Sch 2 SS (GB) Regs.
51 s68 and Sch 4 SSCBA 1992
52 s69 SSCBA 1992; Reg 10A SS(SDA) Regs
53 ss 71-73 and 75 SSCBA 1992; Reg 2 SS (DLA) Regs
54 s74 SSCBA 1992
55 s72 SSCBA 1992
56 s72(6) SSCBA 1992
57 *R v NI Commissioner ex parte Sec. Of State for Social Services* [1981], reported as an appendix to R(A) 2/80; *Mallinson v Sec of State for Social Security* [1994], reported as an appendix to R(A) 3/94
58 *R v NI Commissioner ex parte Sec of State for Social Services* (see above); CA/281/1989
59 CDLA/58/1993
60 *R v NI Commissioner ex parte Sec of State for Social Services* (see above)
61 See note 50
62 *Moran v Sec of State for Social Services*, reported as an appendix to R(A) 1/88
63 R(A) 2/75
64 R(A) 3/86; *Mallinson v Sec of State for Social Services* (see above)
65 *Sec of State for Social Security v Fairey (aka Halliday)* (HL), 21 May 1997
66 CDLA/85/1994
67 s73(8) SSCBA 1992
68 s73(1) and (2) SSCBA 1992
69 Reg 12(1)(a) SS (DLA) Regs
70 CM/98/1989
71 Reg 12(4) SS (DLA) Regs
72 CM/208/1989

73 R(M) 1/81
74 R(M) 1/83
75 CDLA/42/1994; CDLA/14307/1996
76 s73(1) SSCBA 1992
77 s73(4) SSCBA 1992
78 s66(2)(a) SSCBA 1992
79 ss72(5) and 73(12) SSCBA 1992
80 Reg 2(4) SS (DLA) Regs
81 s1(3) SSAA 1992
82 Reg 4 SS (DLA) Regs
83 Reg 6(8) SS (C&P) Regs
84 s54(1) SSAA 1992
85 ss64 -66 SSCBA 1992; reg 2 SS (AA) Regs
86 s64 SSCBA 1992
87 s66 SSCBA 1992
88 Reg 2(3) SS (AA) Regs
89 s65(3) and Sch 4 SSCBA 1992
90 Reg 6(8) SS (C&P) Regs
91 s54(1) SSAA 1992
92 s70 SSCBA 1992; regs 5, 8 and 9 SS (ICA) Regs; regs 10 and 13 SS (CE) Regs
93 Reg 4 SS (ICA) Regs
94 Reg 4(2) SS (ICA) Regs
95 R(G) 3/91
96 Reg 4(1A) SS (ICA) Regs
97 s70(7) SSCBA 1992
98 Regs 9, 10, 13 and Sch 3 SS(CE) Regs
99 s90 and Sch 4 SSCBA 1992; SS (Dep) Regs
100 Reg 6(21) and (22) SS (C&P) Regs
101 ss94, 108 and 109 SSCBA 1992
102 ss103 and 108 SSCBA 1992
103 Sch 7 paras 11 and 12 SSCBA 1992
104 Sch 7 para 13 SSCBA 1992
105 R(I) 22/59; CI/257/1949; CI/159/1950
106 *Fenton v Thorley* [1903] AC 443 (HC)
107 *Moore v Manchester Liners Ltd* [1910] AC 498 (HL)
108 *R v Industrial injuries Commissioner ex parte AEU* [1966], reported as an appendix to R(I) 4/66
109 s99 SSCBA 1992; R(I) 1/88;R(I) 12/75; R(I) 4/70; R(I) 7/85
110 s2(1) SSCBA 1992
111 ss108 and 109 SSCBA 1992; Sch 1 S(IIPD) Regs
112 *Jones v Sec of State for Social Services* [1972] reported as an appendix to R(I) 3/69
113 Reg 11(8) and Sch 2, SS (GB) Regs
114 Reg 11 SS (GB) Regs

115 Sch 6 SSCBA 1992
116 Sch 4 SSCBA 1992
117 s 104 and Sch 4 SSCBA 1992; Reg 19 SS (GB) Regs

3. **Means-tested benefits**
118 s105 SSCBA 1992
119 Sch 7 para 11(10) SSCBA 1992
120 Sch 7 para 13 SSCBA 1992
121 s124 SSCBA 1992
122 Reg 4ZA and Sch 1B IS Regs
123 Reg 5 IS Regs
124 Reg 6 IS Regs
125 Regs 4ZA (3), 13 (2)(b) and Sch 1B paras 10 and 12 IS Regs
126 s137(1) SSCBA 1992;
127 Regs 14-16 and para 9 Sch 7 IS Regs;
128 s124 (4) SSCBA 1992
129 Sch 2, Part 1, IS Regs
130 Sch 2, para 5 IS Regs
131 Sch 2, Part II, IS Regs
132 Sch 2, paras 9, 9A and 15 IS Regs
133 Sch 2, paras 10, 12 and 15 IS Regs
134 Sch 2 paras 11, 12 and 15 IS Regs
135 Sch 2, paras 13 and 15 and regs 2(1) and 3 IS Regs
136 Reg 3(10), (4) and (5) IS Regs
137 Reg 3 and Sch 3 para 13(3) IS Regs
138 Sch 2, paras 14 and 15 IS Regs
139 Sch 2, paras 14ZA and 15 IS Regs
140 Sch 3 IS Regs
141 Sch 3 para 3(1) IS Regs
142 Sch 3 para 3(10) IS Regs
143 Sch 3 para 3(8) and (9) IS Regs
144 Sch 3 para 3(11) IS Regs
145 Sch 3 para 3 (5) IS Regs; CIS 719/1994
146 *R v Penwith DC ex parte Burt* [1988] 22 HLR 292, QBD
147 Sch 3 para 3(6) 15 Regs
148 Sch 3 para 3(7) IS Regs
149 s130 SSCBA 1992; HB Regs
150 Reg 10 HB Regs
151 *R v Rugby BC HBRB ex parte Harrison* (1994) 28 HLR; *R v Poole BC ex parte Ross* (1995) 28 HLR; *R v Warrington BC ex parte Williams* (1997)
152 Reg 6(1)(c) HB Regs
153 s134(2) SSCBA 1992; reg 7(1) HB Regs
154 Reg 10(5) HB Regs
155 s130(1)SSCBA Reg 5 HB Regs
156 Reg 7A HB Regs
157 Reg 48A HB Regs
158 Reg 48A (2) HB Regs

159 Regs 7(1)(k) and 8 HB Regs
160 Regs 8(2) and 10(2) HB Regs
161 Regs 7(1)(a) and (1A) HB Regs
162 Reg 7(1)(b) HB Regs
163 Reg 2(1) HB Regs
164 Regs 3(4) and 7(1)(b) HB Regs
165 Reg 7(1)(c) HB Regs
166 Reg 7(1)(d) HB Regs
167 Reg 7(1)(h) HB Regs
168 Reg 7(1) (e) – (g) HB Regs
169 Reg 7(1)(l) HB Regs
170 s137 SSCBA 1992; regs 13 – 15 HB
     Regs
171 s130(3)(a) SSCBA 1992; reg 61 HB
     Regs
172 s130(3)(b) SSCBA 1992; reg 61 HB
     Regs
173 Reg 16 and Sch 2 HB Regs
174 Reg 3(3) HB Regs
175 Regs 19 – 45 HB Regs
176 Reg 51 HB Regs
177 Sch 1 Part II, HB Regs
178 Sch 1 paras 4 and 7 HB Regs
179 Reg 10(3)(a) and (6) HB Regs
180 Sch 1, para 1A HB Regs
181 Sch 1 paras 1(a) – (e) HB Regs
182 Reg 10(3) HB Regs
183 Reg 10(1)(e) HB Regs
184 Sch 1 para 3 HB Regs
185 Sch 1 para 1(a)(iii) HB Regs
186 Sch 1 para 1(a)(ii) HB Regs
187 Sch 1 para 1(b) HB Regs
188 Sch 1 para 1(a)(iv) HB Regs
189 Sch 1 para 1(a)(iv) HB Regs
190 Sch 1 para 1 (c) HB Regs; para A4.75
     GM
191 Sch 1 para 1(f)(i) HB Regs
192 *R v Sutton LBC HBRB ex parte Harrison*
     23 July 1997, QBD, now upheld by
     the Court of Appeal on 15 July 1998
193 Sch 1 para 1(f) (ii) HB Regs; paras
     A4.77-79 GM
194 Sch 1 para 1(f)(iii) HB Regs
195 Sch 1 para 7 HB Regs
196 Sch 1 paras 1(f) and 7 HB Regs
197 See HB/CTB A37/97
198 HB (General) Amendment (No.3)
     Regs 1999, SI 1999 No. 2734; HB/
     CTB A47/99
199 Reg 12A and Sch 1A HB Regs; reg 10
     HB (Amd.) Regs
200 Regs 10(6B) and 11 HB Regs
201 Reg 12A HB Regs
202 Reg 11 HB Regs

203 Reg 12A (1)(c) HB Regs
204 Reg 3 HB Regs
205 Regs 3 and 63 HB Regs
206 Reg 63 HB Regs
207 Reg 61 HB Regs
208 Reg 66 HB Regs
209 Regs 93 and 94 HB Regs
210 s131 SSCBA 1992; Regs 4A and 40
     CTB Regs
211 s131(6) SSCBA 1992
212 ss6(5) and 99(1) LGFA 1992
213 s131(3) SSCBa 1992; reg 4c CTB regs
214 The Council Tax (Exempt Dwellings)
     Order 1992
215 ss13 and 80 LGFA 1992; The Council
     Tax (Reductions for Disabilities) Regs
     1992
216 The Council Tax (Reductions for
     Disabilities Amdendment) Regs 1999,
     SI No. 1999/1004
217 ss11 and 79 LGFA 1992
218 s137 SSCBA 1992; regs 5 – 7 CTB
     Regs
219 s131 SSCBA 1992; regs 51-53 CTB
     Regs
220 Regs 8 – 37 and Sch 1 CTB Regs
221 Reg 51(3) CTB Regs
222 Reg 51(2A) CTB Regs
223 Reg 51(5) CTB Regs
224 Regs 54 and Sch 2 CTB Regs
225 Reg 3 CTB Regs
226 Reg 52(6) – (8) CTB Regs
227 Reg 52 CTB Regs

4. People in hospital

228 Reg 52 CB Regs
229 TC(MA) Regs 1999
230 Reg 7 SFM&FE Regs
231 Reg 7(1)(e) SFM&FE Regs
232 Reg 3(1) SFM&FE Regs
233 Reg 7(5) SFM&FE Regs
234 Reg 3(1) SFM&FE Regs
235 Reg 7(1), (3) and (4) SFM&FE Regs
236 Reg 7(6)(a) SFM&FE Regs
237 Reg 7A SFM&FE Regs
238 Reg 9 SFM&FE Regs
239 Reg 8(1)(a) SFM&FE Regs
240 s78(4) SSAA 1992
241 Reg 8(1) SFM&FE Regs
242 Sch 4 para 9 SS(C&P) Regs
243 Reg 5(1) SFM&FE Regs
244 Reg 5(2) SFM&FE Regs
245 Reg 9(1) SFM&FE Regs
246 Regs 1A and 2 SFCWP Regs
247 SFWFP Regs

248 Opinion of Advocate General Case C-382/98, 23.9.99
249 SF Dir 25
250 SF Dir 4
251 s140 SSCBA 1992
252 s140(4)(a) SSCBA 1992: SF Dir 7
253 This now appears to have been confirmed in *Fitzpatrick (A.P.) v Sterling Housing Association Ltd*, HL 28 October 1999
254 *R v Sec. Of State ex parte Healey*, The Times, 22 April 1991
255 SF Dirs 23 and 29
256 SF Dir 28
257 SF Dir 27
258 SF Dirs 2, 8 and 9
259 SF Dir 10
260 SF Dirs 50 – 53
261 SF Dir 9
262 SF Sirs 3, 14-16, 22 and 23
263 SF Dirs 18, 20 and 21
264 Reg 2(2) SS(HIP) Regs
265 Reg 21(2) IS Regs; reg 18(3) HB Regs; Reg 10(3) CTB Regs; reg 17(4) SS (HIP) Regs; reg 8(2) SS(AA) Regs; Regs 10(5)(a) and 12B(3) SS(DLA) Regs
266 Reg 2(2A) SS(HIP) Regs; reg 6(2A) SS(AA) Regs; regs 8(2A) and 12(2A) SS(DLA) Regs
267 Reg 8(3) SS(AA) Regs; regs 10(3) and 12B(2) SS(DLA) Regs
268 Regs 6 and 8(1) SS(AA) Regs; regs 8, 10(2), 12A and 12B(1) SS(DLA) Regs
269 Regs 12B(7) and (8) SS(DLA) Regs
270 Reg 12B(3) – (5) SS(DLA) Regs
271 Reg 8(4) SS(AA) Regs; regs 10(6) and 12B(9A) SS(DLA) Regs
272 Reg 8(2) SS(AA) Regs; reg 10(5) SS(DLA) Regs
273 Reg 4(2) SS(ICA) Regs
274 Regs 9 and 11 SS(HIP) Regs
275 Reg 5 SS(HIP) Regs
276 Regs 9 and 11 SS(HIP) Regs
277 Reg 13 SS(HIP) Regs
278 Reg 6(2) SS(HIP) Regs
279 Reg 16 SS(HIP) Regs
280 Regs 6, 10, 11 and 12 SS(HIP) Regs
281 Reg 11(1)(b) SS(HIP) Regs
282 Regs 17(2) and (3) SS(HIP) Regs
283 Sch 2 paras 13(3A) and 15(5) IS Regs
284 Sch 2 paras 12(1)(c)(ii) and 14(3) IS egs
285 Sch 2 para 14ZA(3) IS Regs
286 Sch 7 para 1(a) IS Regs
287 Sch 3 para 3(11) and (12) IS Regs
288 Reg 16(2)(b) IS Regs
289 Sch 7 para 1(3) IS Regs
290 Sch 7 para 1(c) and Sch 2 para 12(1)(c)(ii) IS Regs
291 Sch 7 para 3 IS Regs
292 Sch 2 para 14(6) IS Regs
293 Sch 7 para 2 IS Regs
294 Reg 16(2)(b) and Sch 7 para 2(b) IS Regs
295 Reg 16(2)(b) and (5)(b) IS Regs
296 Reg 5(8B)(c)(ii) and (8C) HB Regs; Regs 4C(4)(c)(ii) and 5 CTB Regs
297 s131(3)(a) SSCBA 1992
298 Reg 18 and Sch 2 paras 12(1)(a)(iii), 13(3A), 14(b), 14ZA(3) and 15(5) HB Regs; reg 10 and Sch 1 paras 13(1)(a)(iii), 14(3A), 15(b), 16(3) and 19(6) CTB Regs
299 Reg 15(2)(b) HB Regs; reg 7(1) CTB Regs

Chapter 4

Other sources of financial assistance

This chapter explains what other financial assistance you may be able to apply for, apart from social security benefits and help from social services. It covers:

1. Health benefits (p137)
2. Transport concessions for disabled people (p141)
3. Special funds for sick and disabled people (p143)
4. Housing grants (p147)
5. Housing grants in Scotland (p150)
6. Charities (p152)

For information about legal advice and assistance under the legal aid scheme see Appendix 4.

1. Health benefits

This section deals with the following areas of provision under the National Health Service (NHS):

- prescriptions;
- dental treatment and dentures;
- sight tests;
- glasses;
- wigs and fabric supports;
- fares to hospital;
- the qualifying benefit and low income scheme;
- applications for help with health care costs;
- health care equipment.

Although the NHS generally provides free health care, there are charges for some items and services. You will be exempt from these charges:

- if you receive a qualifying benefit or qualify for the low income scheme (see p139); *or*

- (except for sight tests and glasses) if you are a permanent resident in a care home and social services are assisting you with the costs of your accommodation; *or*
- (unless otherwise stated) because you are under 16 or under 18 and in full-time education; *or*
- because of your age or specific health needs as detailed under each of the schemes below.[1]

Prescriptions

You qualify for free prescriptions if:
- you are aged 60 or over;[2] *or*
- you suffer from:
  - a continuing physical disability which prevents you leaving your home except with the help of another person;
  - epilepsy, requiring continuous anti-convulsive therapy;
  - a permanent fistula, including a caecostomy, ileostomy, laryngostomy or colostomy, needing continuous surgical dressing or an appliance; *or*
- you suffer from, and require specific substitution therapy for, diabetes mellitus, myxoedema, hypoparathyroidism, diabetes insipidus and other forms of hypopituitarism, forms of hypoadrenalism (including Addison's disease), or myasthenia gravis; *or*
- you are a war disablement pensioner and you need the prescription for your war disability.

Exemptions also apply to people who are pregnant or who have a child under the age of one.

Dental treatment and dentures

You qualify for free NHS dental treatment (including check-ups) and appliances (including dentures) only if you receive a qualifying benefit or if your income is low enough or if social services are assisting you with the costs of your accommodation as a permanent resident in a care home (unless you are pregnant or you have a child under the age of one).

Sight tests

You qualify for a free NHS sight test if:
- you are aged 60 or over; *or*
- you are registered blind or partially sighted; *or*
- you have been prescribed complex lenses; *or*
- you suffer from diabetes or glaucoma; *or*

- you are aged 40 or over and are the parent, brother, sister or child of someone suffering from glaucoma; *or*
- you are a patient of the Hospital Eye Service.

Glasses

If you qualify for free glasses you are entitled to a voucher which you can use to buy or repair glasses or contact lenses if:
- you require glasses or contact lenses for the first time; *or*
- your new prescription differs from your old one; *or*
- your old glasses have worn out through fair wear and tear; *or*
- you are a Hospital Eye Service patient needing frequent changes of glasses or lenses; *or*
- you have been prescribed complex lenses; *or*
- as a result of an illness you have lost or damaged your glasses or lenses and the cost is not covered by insurance and you have been prescribed complex lenses.

Wigs and fabric supports

You qualify for free wigs and fabric supports if you are a hospital in-patient when the wig or fabric support is supplied.

Fares to hospital

You qualify for help with your fares to hospital if you are attending an NHS hospital or a disablement services centre for treatment or services only if you receive a qualifying benefit or if social services are assisting with the costs of your accommodation as a permanent resident in a care home or your income is low enough (unless you are a patient at a sexually transmitted disease clinic more than 15 miles from your home).

You are entitled to help with the cost of travelling by the cheapest means of transport available. This usually means normal class public transport. If you have to go by car or taxi, you should be paid your petrol costs or taxi fare. The travel expenses of a companion can also be met if you need to be accompanied for a medical reason.

If you are receiving income support (IS) or Jobseeker's allowance (JSA) you may also be eligible for help from the social fund with the costs of visiting a close relative or partner (see Chapter 3).

The qualifying benefit and low income scheme

You will automatically qualify for full assistance with the costs of any of the above health benefits if:
- you (or your partner) receive IS or JSA. The same also applies to working families and disabled person's tax credits, provided less than £70 of the

maximum tax credit has been withdrawn (see p116), and to family credit and disability working allowance (which have now been replaced by tax credits); or
- you are a war disablement pensioner and you need the health benefit because of your war disability; or
- (except sight tests and glasses) you are a permanent resident in a care home and social services are assisting you with the costs of your accommodation.

You may also be entitled to full or partial remission of any charges on the grounds of low income if you are not already exempt on other grounds. To qualify for help under the low income scheme you must have less than £8,000 in capital, or less than £16,000 if you are permanently resident in a care home. A calculation is then carried out to compare your income with your requirements and any excess income will affect your entitlement to a remission of charges.

Income

Your income is calculated in the same way as for IS (see Chapter 6) except that:
- your income is normally only taken into account in the week in which it is paid;
- regular maintenance payments count as weekly income and irregular payments are averaged over the 13 weeks prior to your claim;
- insurance policy payments for housing costs not met by IS count as income but payments for unsecured loans for repairs and improvements (including premiums) are ignored.

Requirements

Your requirements are the same as your IS applicable amount (see p96) except that:
- the higher pensioner premium is allowed if you or your partner are 60 or over and the severe disability premium is allowed even if you are jointly liable for your housing costs with a close relative; and
- your housing costs include interest and capital payments on all loans secured on your home, any loans to adapt your home for the needs of a disabled person, any council tax liabilities (less council tax benefit), and any rent (less housing benefit).

Excess income

Your excess income is the difference between your income and your requirements.
The amount of help you can claim for hospital fares is reduced by the amount of your excess income.

The cost of a sight test is reduced to the amount of your excess income.

The value of a voucher for glasses or lenses is reduced by twice your excess income.

Charges for dental treatment and for wigs and fabric supports which are higher than three times your excess income are remitted.

You cannot get partial remission of charges for prescriptions (but see below for pre-payment certificates).

Applications for help with health care costs

If you are exempt because of age or receipt of a qualifying benefit, you need only complete the declaration on the back of the prescription form, or complete a form provided by your dentist, optician or hospital receptionist before you receive treatment. For free treatment for war pensioners contact the War Pensions Agency.

To apply for remission of charges on the grounds of low income, you need to complete form HC1, available form your doctor, dentist, optician, hospital or the Benefits Agency. If you qualify for free services you will be sent a certificate HC2; for partial remission you will be sent certificate HC3. Certificates are normally valid for six months, or 12 months if you are 60 or over or entitled to a disability premium or living permanently in a care home. In the latter case a special short form application HC1(RC) is available.

Refunds may be obtained if you apply within three months (or longer if you have good reasons) on forms available from your chemist, optician, dentist, hospital or the Benefits Agency.

Pre-payment certificates for prescriptions are available and will save you money if you need more than five prescriptions in four months or 14 prescriptions in a year. Application forms can be obtained from the Benefits Agency, post office or chemist (and refunds can be made if, within a month of paying, you qualify for free prescriptions or you die).

Health care equipment

Health care equipment such as special footwear, leg appliances, wigs, surgical supports, wheelchairs, commodes, incontinence pads, hearing aids and low vision aids can be provided by health authorities, hospitals and GPs, either free of charge or on prescription. Equipment for daily living can also be provided by social services but may be subject to a charge (see Chapter 2).

2. Transport concessions for disabled people

In addition to any help with travel costs which you may be entitled to from social services (see Chapter 2) or from the social fund (see Chapter 3) or from the NHS (see p139), you may also be entitled to:

- Motability scheme;
- road tax exemption;
- orange badge parking concessions;
- disabled person's railcard concessions.

Motability

Motability is a registered charity incorporated by Royal Charter to assist people with disabilities with the hire purchase or hire and running costs of a car.

You may only be entitled to assistance from Motability if you receive the higher rate mobility component of disability living allowance (or war pensioner's mobility supplement) (see p83). Motability can assist you if this has been awarded to you for life, or if it has been awarded for a period which will last at least another two years (to buy a used car), or three years (to hire a car), or four years (to buy a new car). Motability can arrange for the Disability Benefits Unit to pay all or part of your disability living allowance direct to them so that they can arrange for concessionary rates for the hire or hire purchase, adaptation, insurance and service costs (as appropriate) of a suitable vehicle for your use (or for the use by another person for your benefit). You may be expected to make a down payment on the cost of an unusually expensive car, and higher contributions may be necessary if you drive more than 12,000 miles a year. Motability may also be able to help with the costs of driving lessons.

For information, advice and assistance, contact: Motability, Goodman House, Station Approach, Harlow, Essex CM20 2ET (tel: 01279 635666).

Road tax exemption

If you get the higher rate mobility component of disability living allowance (or war pensioner's mobility supplement) you are also entitled to exemption from road tax (vehicle excise duty) for one car which will apply so long as it is being used solely by you or for your benefit. Applications for exemption certificates (which can then be used for applying for a tax exempt disc from the Vehicle Licensing Agency) are available from the Disability Benefits Unit or War Pensions Agency responsible for paying your benefit. Road tax exemption cannot be backdated even if there is a delay in processing your claim for benefit.

Road tax exemption is also still available for cars used by passengers who have been getting attendance allowance or the care component of disability living allowance since before 12 April 1993, provided they had already been granted exemption by that date.

Orange badge parking concessions

The orange badge scheme[3] provides parking concessions to allow people with severe walking difficulties and people who are blind (or people who are driving them) to park (either in specially reserved parking bays for badge holders or in certain other restricted parking areas) near shops, public buildings and other places, usually for extended periods and without charge. The scheme applies throughout England, Wales and Scotland except in four London areas (the City of London, Westminster, Kensington and Chelsea, and parts of Camden).

You are entitled to an orange badge if you are over two years old and you:

- receive the higher rate mobility component of disability living allowance (or war pensioner's mobility supplement); *or*
- are registered blind; *or*
- have a 'permanent and substantial disability which causes inability to walk or very considerable difficulty in walking'; *or*
- drive regularly and have a severe disability in both arms so that you cannot turn a steering wheel by hand (even if the wheel is fitted with a turning knob).

Orange badges are normally administered by social services departments in local authorities (who have a discretion to charge up to £2 to issue a badge). The orange badge is expected to be replaced by a new blue badge, which will be phased in throughout the European Community from January 2000.

Disabled person's railcard concessions

You are entitled to a disabled person's railcard if you:

- receive attendance allowance; *or*
- receive the middle or higher rate care component (or higher rate mobility component or war pensioner's mobility supplement) of disability living allowance; or
- receive severe disablement allowance; *or*
- receive 80 per cent or more war pension; or
- are registered as visually impaired or are deaf; *or*
- have recurrent attacks of epilepsy.

The railcard entitles you to one third off the cost of most train journeys. For details, contact your local station which may also provide details of other fare concessions offered by train operators and about assistance with access and travel arrangements

3. **Special funds for sick and disabled people**

The Independent Living Funds

There are two Independent Living Funds which may make cash payments to you so you can employ carers to help you live independently in your own home. These are government-funded but independent and discretionary trust funds managed by a Board of Trustees. A legally binding trust deed sets out the scope of the schemes. Awards are discretionary, but the trustees must follow basic eligibility criteria and guidelines.[4]

The Independent Living (Extension) Fund has taken over from the original Fund which was set up in 1988 as an interim measure until the implementation of community care legislation and a review of social security benefits for people with disabilities. It was wound up in 1993 and no new applications are accepted. You can only get help if you were being assisted under the original arrangements. These were relatively generous, and often enabled people to buy care without any involvement from social services before the new community care arrangements were introduced.

The Independent Living (1993) Fund applies to all new applications for assistance and works in partnership with social services to devise 'joint care packages' combining services and/or direct payments from social services (see Chapter 2) with cash payments from the Fund.

To be eligible for help from the Independent Living (1993) Fund you must:

- be so severely disabled that you need help with personal care or household duties to maintain an independent life in the community; *and*
- be living alone or with people who are unable to fully meet your care needs. No payments will be made in respect of paying a partner or close relative who lives with you but payment may be made to those who do not. In such cases the carer may even also be able to claim invalid care allowance (see p87) for looking after you even if this means that the contribution you may be expected to make may be reduced if you are no longer entitled to the severe disability premium (see below); *and*
- be at least 16 and under 66 years old; and
- be receiving the higher rate care component of disability living allowance (see p81); *and*
- be receiving IS or JSA (or have an income at or about that level after you have contributed to your own care costs – see below); *and*
- have less than £8,000 in savings (which are calculated in the same way as for IS (see Chapter 7) and therefore include the savings of your partner); *and*
- be receiving (or it is planned that you will receive) services costing at least £200 a week, paid for by social services, and which will cost no more than £500 a week in total – ie, counting a maximum payment of £300 from the Fund. The cost to social services for providing home care, day centre care, supervision, regular respite care and meals on wheels, for example, *less* any charge you pay to them for it, will count towards the £200, but capital or running costs of any equipment, social work salaries, services provided exclusively by health authorities, and childcare costs, for example, will not count; *and*
- have care needs that are generally stable and will be met by the joint care package for the following six months.

This last condition means that some people who are terminally ill may not qualify. The requirement that you must be in receipt of disability living allowance (DLA) may cause practical problems if there is any delay in processing your claim as no retrospective awards are ever paid and social services may be reluctant to arrange care packages costing over £200. It may also cause practical problems if your award is terminated or reduced. Although the Fund will continue to make their payments provided you are seeking a review of or appealing against the decision to stop or reduce your benefit until any appeal has run its course, you will still be expected to pay your contribution to the care package based on the award of DLA you will no longer have (see below).

If you meet all of these eligibility criteria, you will still be expected to make a contribution towards the cost of your care. Contributions are also expected if you are receiving help from the Independent Living (Extension) Fund. This will be half of your DLA care component plus all of your severe disability premium if it is payable with any IS/JSA you receive (see p97). If you do not get IS/JSA you will be expected to contribute all of your income in excess of the amount you would get if you did qualify (excluding the severe disability premium). Excess income calculations are based on IS rates, except that most housing costs (including all mortgage payments and endowments or rent, and council tax and water rates liabilities), child support maintenance payments, and a £30 disregard on earnings, are usually taken into account. The Independent Living Fund will also usually refuse to become involved if a substantial sum is held in a trust fund for you.

If you are paying charges to social services for the care they are providing, this may also be taken into account in new awards, but will not always be taken into account in revised awards (see below). For a new application this means that if social services are expecting you to contribute all or part of your award of DLA and/or severe disability premium, the Fund may offset this from any contribution it would otherwise expect from you. In practice this could mean that any charge you are asked to pay to social services may simply be picked up by the Fund. Special attention will need to be given to charges applied to new applicants to the 1993 Fund, as these may either reduce the value of services provided by social services to less than £200 or increase the contribution expected from the Fund to more than £300, so that in either case the conditions will not be met.

Applications to the 1993 Fund can only be made through social services. The Fund will then arrange for one of its own social workers to discuss your care needs with you and negotiate an appropriate joint care package (and provide advice and assistance with meeting the duties you will have as an employer of your carers).

If there is a significant change in your circumstances the Fund will reassess, and may increase, your award if appropriate and if there are sufficient funds in its budget. The Fund will, not, however, increase its own contribution if the change is due to any reduction in care provided by social services or to a new or increased charge payable to them for their services. If your award is under the Extension Fund, it may contact social services any extra services you now need which they should provide. If the Fund agrees to pay any extra, this will be subject to a total limit of £560.

If your award is under the 1993 Fund it will always attempt to renegotiate a care package with social services to see who should take on responsibility for meeting any of your additional needs. Provided you have been receiving assistance for a reasonable period (usually six months), the 1993 Fund's contribution will not be discontinued (and there appears to be no limit to how much it may be increased to, budgets permitting) even if social services considers it necessary to increase their contribution to the extent that the total cost of the care package then exceeds £500.

If any services provided by social services in respect of your increased needs are subject to a charge, the Fund may offset this charge from any contribution you would otherwise be expected to make.

Awards will be suspended if you go into hospital or a care home, but will be reinstated if you return home within 26 weeks.

Complaints or appeals may be made to the Director of the Funds and may be considered by a subcommittee of the Board of Trustees. For details contact your local social services department or the Independent Living Fund, PO Box 183, Nottingham NG8 3RD (tel: 0115 942 8191/2).

The Macfarlane and Eileen Trusts

The Macfarlane Trust, the Macfarlane (Special Payments) Trust, and the Macfarlane (Special Payments) (No. 2) Trust make payments to haemophiliacs.

The Macfarlane Trust also administers the Eileen Trust which helps people infected with HIV through NHS blood transfusions or transplants.

The Fund was set up in 1992 for haemophiliacs who contract HIV through blood or tissue transfusions. For further information, contact the Macfarlane Trust, PO Box 627, London SW1H OQG (tel: 0171 233 0342).

The Family Fund

The Family Fund gives grants and other help to families with children who have severe disabilities. It commonly helps with holidays, furniture, equipment and transport needs.

For information, contact the Family Fund, PO Box 50, York YO1 1UY (tel: 01904 621115).

4. **Housing grants**[5]

Housing renovation grants

Housing renovation grants are discretionary and subject to a means test, but may be available for the improvement or repair of a dwelling (or for the provision of dwellings by conversion of a house or other building).

They are available only to owners (or certain leaseholders) of properties at least 10 years old which they must normally have occupied for at least the last three years.

Renovation grants may be awarded to:

- make a property fit for human habitation (ie, so it is structurally stable, free from serious disrepair and damp, has adequate provision for lighting, heating, water supply, drainage, and ventilation, and has a toilet, washbasin, bath or shower, and facilities for cooking, including a sink);
- bring a property up to a reasonable standard of repair or improve services (such as fuel and water) or amenities (such as a bath or toilet);
- improve thermal insulation;
- provide heating facilities;
- improve the internal arrangements (such as staircases); *or*
- provide adequate fire precautions.

The means-test is similar to that which applies to claims for housing benefit (HB) and council tax benefit (CTB) (see Chapters 6 and 7 and p102 and p111) except that:

- the resources of the applicant and anyone else who is both entitled to apply and lives or intends to live in the property are considered;
- there are no non-dependant deductions;
- the applicable amount is increased by £40;
- there is no maximum capital limit and the first £5,000 is disregarded (with tariff income applying on capital above this);
- there is a system of stepped tapers on excess income which is used to calculate how much you would be able to repay on a notional loan to pay for the work over a period of 10 years.

Grants may have to be repaid if the property is sold within five years of any work being completed (unless the applicant has died).

For further details and application forms, contact your local housing department.

Disabled facilities grants

Means-tested disabled facilities grants are available for the provision of facilities for a disabled person in a dwelling or a common part of a building (eg, a staircase) containing one or more flats.

They are available to home owners or tenants (or landlord of a disabled tenant), who is disabled, ie:
- your sight, hearing or speech is substantially impaired; *or*
- you have a mental disorder or impairment; *or*
- you are physically substantially disabled by illness, injury, or impairment present since birth, or otherwise; *or*
- you are registered (or registrable) as disabled with social services.

Mandatory grants (up to a maximum of £20,000 in England or £24,000 in Wales) can be awarded for:
- facilitating disabled access to a dwelling room for use as the principal family room, bedroom, toilet, bath or shower;
- making a dwelling safe;
- facilitating a disabled occupant's use of a source of power, light or heat, or food preparation facilities;
- improving or providing a suitable heating system; or
- facilitating access and movement around the home to enable the disabled occupant to care for someone dependent on them who also lives there.

Discretionary grants may also be awarded for adaptations which make the property more suitable for the accommodation, welfare or employment of the disabled occupant.

The means-test is similar to that which applies to renovation grants (see p147) except that only the resources of the person who is disabled (and her/his partner) are considered.

Applications should be made to your local housing department, which must then consult with social services. In practice, people are commonly referred first to social services who then arrange for an occupational therapy assessment. Applications should be determined within six months. If approved, the work must normally be carried out within one year. Housing departments have a discretion to approve a grant but stipulate that it will not be paid for up to a year after the application was made, and may revise their decision if your circumstances change before the works are completed.

Home repair assistance

Home repair assistance is a discretionary grant to help meet the cost of smaller scale repairs, improvements and adaptations (up to a maximum of £2,000 per application or £4,000 for the same dwelling in three years).

Such grants are only available if:
- you receive IS/JSA/HB/CTB (or family credit or disability working allowance or one of the tax credits which have replaced them), or you are (or the application is to facilitate the care of someone who is) aged 60 or over or

disabled (as for disabled facilities grants, above) or infirm (which is not defined); *and*

- you are at least 18 years old; *and*
- the dwelling is your only or main residence (unless you are applying on behalf of someone who is at least 60 years of age or disabled or infirm); *and*
- you are a home owner or private tenant or have the right to exclusive occupation of the property for, normally, at least five years, and you are entitled to carry out the works.

Home repair assistance is also available to some occupiers of houseboats and mobile homes.

For details and application forms contact your local housing department.

Home energy efficiency scheme

The home energy efficiency scheme (HEES) is administered by the Energy Action Grants Agency and offers grants to owners and tenants (including council tenants) who receive IS/JSA/HB/CTB (or family credit or disability working allowance or one of the tax credits which have replaced them) or disability living allowance or attendance allowance (or constant attendance or war pensioners mobility supplement).

If you do not get one of these benefits, you will still qualify for up to 25 per cent of the full grant if you or your partner are at least 60 years old.

Grants of up to £315 (or £160 for materials if you want to carry out the work yourself) are available for draught-proofing doors and windows, loft insulation, cavity wall insulation, improvements to heating system controls, and energy advice (which can include the provision of two low energy light bulbs and a hot water tank jacket). The maximum £315 grant will be increased to £700 from April 2000.

The HEES has recently been reviewed and a 'New HEES Plus' scheme is expected to be introduced from April 2000. This will provide grants of up to £2,000 for insulation and central heating in main living areas for people aged 60 or over who receive one of the means-tested benefits referred to above (although grants will have to be repaid by those who move house). Beneficiaries of the New HEES Plus will also be offered a home security assessment (see below).

For details and application forms contact the Energy Action Grants Agency, PO Box 1NG, Newcastle upon Tyne NE99 2RP (freephone 0800 072 0150).

Other housing grants

Houses in multiple occupation grants (for landlords for repairs or improvements to certain properties), common parts grants (for repairs or improvements to the common parts of a building – eg, containing flats with a roof) and group repair schemes (for external works to a group of properties, such as a block or a terrace) may also be available from your local housing department.

From summer 2000, if you are entitled to a New HEES Plus grant (see above) you will also be entitled to a home security assessment and free window and door locks and similar measures.[6]

---

5. Housing grants in Scotland

Improvement and repair grants

In Scotland, grants are available to owners and tenants to help meet the cost of improvement and repair work to houses in the private sector. Almost all grants are awarded at the discretion of the local councils. As a general rule, grants are automatically available only when a council has served a statutory notice, such as a repairs notice or an improvement order, or if your house is in an area which has been declared a Housing Action Area for Improvement.

Local authorities also decide the total amount of money which will be available for grant assistance. Their budgets are limited and they can only give grants up to the budget they have set for the purpose. The level of grant and the maximum amount which can be paid are set by law.

Grants are mandatory when standard amenities are required and the expense limits for each standard amenity are:

- fixed bath or shower   £450
- hot and cold water supply at a fixed bath or shower   £570
- wash-hand basin   £170
- hot and cold water supply at a wash-hand basin   £305
- sink   £450
- hot and cold water supply at a sink   £385
- toilet   £680

Total   £3,010

Standard amenity grants are awarded at 50 per cent of whatever costs are approved by the council. Discretionary grants can be awarded for work to both the internal and external fabric of a house which is necessary to maintain the useful life of the property eg, repairs to the roof or replacing rotten window frames.

In general, grants are awarded at 50 per cent of approved costs, but the level can be increased to 75 per cent or 90 per cent in certain cases. To be eligible for grant assistance, your house should normally be more than ten years old and be in council tax band A, B, C, D or E.

The Scottish Executive intends to reform the present system to target grants on houses in the worst condition, and on those people in greatest financial need. Some local authorities already take an applicant's resources into consideration when making a decision about awarding grant. For further information, contact your local council housing department.

Improvement grants for people with disabilities

In Scotland, if you are registered disabled, or could be registered disabled, you have a right to an assessment of your needs by the social work department, including your needs for 'adaptations to your home, or equipment for your use for your greater safety, comfort or convenience'.[7] Following assessment, the social department should either provide what is needed or provide assistance, including financial assistance to help with the cost of the adaptation. The housing department may offer a discretionary improvement grant towards the costs of the works.[8] The grant may cover:

- alteration or enlargement; *or*
- making the house suitable for your accommodation, welfare or employment.

The housing department can pay up to 75 per cent of the approved costs of works, within prescribed limits. Mandatory grants are available to all households for the provision of standard amenities (see, improvement and repairs grants). Even if the house already has one of these amenities, a disabled person may still be entitled to a grant for another if this is essential to her/his needs eg, a further toilet on the ground floor.

Financial assistance from the social work department is separate from and can be paid in addition to any improvement grant for adaptation, eg, to meet the 25 per cent (or more) of the cost not met by the grant.[9]

For further details contact your local council housing and social work departments.

The Warm Deal

In Scotland, the Warm Deal replaces the former Home Energy Efficiency Scheme (HEES) and is administered by the Energy Action Grants Agency (EAGA), freephone 0800 181667. The grant covers a package of energy efficiency measures, all or some of which may be offered, according to the energy needs of the home. Grants may be offered to owners and tenants (including council tenants) who receive IS/JSA/HB/CTB (or family credit or disability working allowance or one of the tax credits which have replaced them), or disability living allowance, or attendance allowance (or constant attendance or war pensioners mobility supplement). The maximum grant is £500. Those over 60, but not in receipt of any of the benefits listed above, may qualify for a reduced grant of £78.75, or 25 per cent of the cost of the work, whichever is the lower. Those who received a HEES grant in the past may still qualify for a grant for further works, within certain limits.

Other housing grants

In Scotland, discretionary grants can also be available for replacing lead plumbing or reducing exposure to radon gas, or for mutual repairs to common parts of a building. Mandatory grants may be available in certain circumstances to provide fire escapes in houses in multiple occupation. Contact your local housing department for further information.

6. Charities

There are hundreds of local and national charities that provide a wide range of help to people in need. Your local social services may know of appropriate charities which may be able to assist you, or you can consult publications such as the *Guide to grants for Individuals in Need* or the *Charities Digest* in your local library.

Notes

1. Health benefits
1 NHS(TERC) Regs 1988; NHS(CDA) Regs 1980; NHS (DC) Regs 1989; NHS (GOS) Regs 1986; NHS (OCP) Regs 1977; NHSA 1977
2 *R v Secretary of State for Health ex parte Cyril Richardson,* House of Lords Case C-137/94

2. Transport concessions for disabled people
3 DP(BMV) Regs 1982

3. Special funds for sick and disabled people
4 Independent Living (Extension) Fund Guidance Notes and Independent Living (1993) Fund Guidance Notes

4. Housing grants
5 HGCRA 1996; the Housing (FEP) Order 1996; HRA Regs 1996; the Disabled Facilities Grants and Home Repair Assistance (Maximum Amounts) Order 1996; The Housing Renewal Grants (Services and Charges) Order 1996; HRG Regs 1996; HRG(PF&P) Regs 1996
6 Home Office Press Release 305/9, 30.9.99

5. Housing grants in Scotland
7 s2 CSDPA 1970
8 H(S)A 1987 Part X111
9 Scottish Office Circular SDD 40/1985. Provision of Aids Equipment and House Adaptations for Disabled People Living at Home

Chapter 5
· ·
Supported housing

This chapter explains the different types of accommodation which may be considered as alternatives to residential or nursing care homes and for which special rules may apply. It covers types of accommodation which may or may not fall within the definition of 'supported accommodation' in the housing benefit scheme (see pp106) and includes:

1. Sheltered and very sheltered housing (p154)
2. Unregistered care homes and hostels (p156)
3. Adult Placement Schemes (p156)
4. Abbeyfield Homes (p158)
5. Less dependent residents in local authority care homes (p159)
6. Registered care homes where housing benefit is payable (p161)
7. Cluster homes (p162)
8. Temporary stays in supported housing (p163)

Many people encounter difficulties in trying to live independently in their own homes, yet their personal care needs may not be so great that residential or nursing care would be a desirable, appropriate or available option. There are many different types of supported accommodation schemes which aim to meet their needs. Some offer accommodation which has been specially adapted or designed to suit particular physical needs. Others offer services with the support of wardens or other care staff and additional facilities, which may sometimes be supplemented by community care services arranged by social services (see Chapter 2). Some offer so much care and support that it can be difficult to distinguish them from care homes.

Most of these different supported housing schemes do not have to be registered as care homes. Residents may claim social security benefits in much the same way as if they were living in ordinary accommodation. There will often be no need for social services to be involved in making any arrangements for residents to live there. This means there will be no question of social services being seen as having responsibility for, or recovering any contribution towards, the cost of the accommodation. In other cases, although social services may be involved in arranging the accommodation, special arrangements sometimes apply.

There may be financial advantages to residents and social services if someone lives in supported housing rather than a care home. This is because those living in supported housing rather than care homes can usually claim more social security benefits, and these can be used to meet the costs of the accommodation and services. Housing benefit (HB) in particular may be effectively used to pay for relatively expensive accommodation and extensive support services (see p104) which can be comparable to those provided in care homes. A resident may then have more money for personal or other expenses than if s/he was in a care home. Also, the benefits paid to meet the accommodation and support costs may reduce the expense that would otherwise fall on social services.

The arrangements currently available for paying for the costs of supported accommodation have been the subject of government review and are in the process of being revised.

1. Sheltered and very sheltered housing

The term sheltered housing (or very sheltered housing, depending on the level of support provided) is commonly used to refer to groups of flats usually supported by a warden and mainly intended for occupation by older people. Sheltered housing schemes are usually provided by local authority housing departments or housing associations and tend to be graded according to the level of independence of the resident in the following categories:[1]

- category 1, containing specially designed units of accommodation for the relatively active elderly, where communal facilities and a warden are optional;
- category 1.5, offering warden support but no communal facilities;
- category 2, designed for the less active elderly resident and offering communal facilities (eg, common rooms, laundry rooms and guest rooms) and warden support, as well as alarms for alerting the warden;
- category 2.5, more often referred to as 'very sheltered' or 'extra care' schemes, are designed for frail elderly people and offer more enhanced care and facilities than in category 2.

Much of the supported accommodation for people who are under pensionable age tends to be referred to instead as hostels.

The terms 'sheltered' and 'very sheltered' housing have no particular significance in themselves for social security or community care purposes, but are commonly used to distinguish between the types of accommodation provided in local authority or registered care homes where different rules on benefits claims (see Chapter 21) and social services responsibilities (see Chapters 2, 12 and 23) generally apply.

If you live in sheltered or very sheltered housing you will be able to claim social security benefits in the same way as if you were living in ordinary accommodation or your own home (see Chapter 3). For example, you could claim all appropriate income support (IS) personal allowances and premiums, attendance allowance (AA) or any care component (and mobility component) of disability living allowance (DLA) for your own needs, and housing benefit (HB) to meet eligible housing costs (for the accommodation and for certain services which may include those provided by the warden). If you have personal care needs which the housing scheme cannot provide, additional community care services may be provided, although you may be charged for them (see Chapter 2).

Sheltered housing schemes will, therefore, usually be more financially attractive to both residents and social services than local authority or registered care homes. There is also greater security of tenure in sheltered schemes (where residents will usually be tenants) than in care homes (where residents will usually only have a licence to occupy). As sheltered housing is not covered by the registration requirements for care homes[2] (see p269), it is not subject to the same standards of inspection and monitoring, and may therefore not offer the same degree of accountability, although it may offer greater personal freedom than in the regulated environment of a registered home.

The level of support in some very sheltered housing schemes may be as great as, if not greater than, that provided in some registered care homes. The distinction in treatment for social security purposes depends on whether the accommodation needs to be registered as a care home – ie, whether it is an establishment which is considered by the social services registration and inspection unit to provide both board and personal care (or, in Scotland, registration is linked to the provision of 'care and support whether or not it is combined with the board') (see Chapter 12).

Some sheltered housing schemes have managed to avoid the registration requirements simply because board (or, in Scotland, support) is not provided, or else because personal care is not provided as a condition of occupation of the accommodation – eg, because it is paid for separately and residents have a genuine choice as to whether or not to receive it. Whether or not the link between the provision of the accommodation and personal care is sufficient to require registration will depend on the full nature and extent of the individual arrangements in each establishment. This will include consideration of the extent of the interdependence between the accommodation and personal care services and the choice available to residents, whether personal care is provided by the landlord or by another agency on her/his behalf or whether the resident has made her/his own separate arrangements (either privately or through the provision of community care services). If you are considering sheltered housing you should check with the landlord or seek independent advice to see what arrangements will apply.

2. **Unregistered care homes and hostels**

Some care homes and hostels do not have to be registered as care homes (see p268) eg, because they do not provide the necessary degree of board or personal care. This also includes some homes set up by Royal Charter or Act of Parliament such as Salvation Army homes which are nevertheless treated as care homes by the Benefits Agency (so that residents may still be able to claim the IS residential allowance) (see p352).

A wide variety of hostels offer support for those with a broad range of different needs (eg, for those with mental health difficulties or drug/alcohol dependencies) and the extent of the support available varies widely from hostel to hostel. Residents of unregistered care homes and hostels are normally licensees rather than tenants.

If you are resident in an unregistered care home or hostel, you can claim benefits in the same way as if you were living in ordinary accommodation or your own home (see Chapter 3), including IS personal allowances and premiums and AA or DLA. You can also claim HB to meet eligible housing costs (which may include some of your care costs – see p104), although you will not be able to claim IS residential allowance. If you live in a Royal Charter or Salvation Army home you cannot claim HB[3] but you may be able to claim the IS residential allowance. Additional community care services may be provided to meet personal care needs not provided in your accommodation, although you may be charged for them (see Chapter 2).

3. **Adult placement schemes**

'Adult placement schemes' are arrangements where (usually) social services find suitable carers to look after adults with personal care needs in the carer(s)' own home.

The National Association of Adult Placement Services defines the arrangements as[4] 'the provision of accommodation for vulnerable adults in the homes of specially recruited people living in the community who are approved for this purpose by an official agency. The carers undertake to integrate such service users into their household and provide appropriate help, for an agreed fee, whilst the agency continues to ensure that both the carer and the service user placed receive support and assistance'.

Placements may be arranged on a long-term basis, or for short-term breaks, or for regular (sometimes even non-residential) befriending purposes. Such accommodation arrangements have the advantage of offering a home environment in the community and a greater degree of individual care and attention, which will have been considered more appropriate for a person's needs than a local authority or registered care home. Such arrangements are most commonly used to accommodate adults under pensionable age who have severe physical or learning disabilities, but older and less dependent adults sometimes also opt, for or are placed in, such schemes.

Since April 1993 most adult placements in England and Wales have fallen within the scope of the Registered Homes Act 1984 and have been required to register as small care homes (see Chapter 12). Some adult placements have escaped the registration requirements because they do not provide the required degree of personal care or board – eg, because residents pay for their meals not as an inclusive charge, but on a pay-as-you-eat basis. In Scotland, it is much less common for adult placements to be registered.

The term 'adult placement' has no particular significance in itself for social security or community care purposes. The extent to which social security benefits may be relied on by those in adult placement schemes depends instead on whether the accommodation is registered as a care home or not, and how long the arrangement has lasted. It may also depend on the extent to which social services have been involved in the arrangements for the placement – eg, sometimes social services formally place adults with carers because they have a statutory duty to do so (see Chapter 12), yet sometimes they merely introduce the adult and the carer who then make their own independent arrangements.

If you have been resident in an adult placement since 31 March 1993 you *may* have preserved rights so that you will be entitled to higher rates of IS (and AA/DLA but not HB) as explained in Chapter 22. Although it was not possible for small homes to be registered before April 1993, certain residents of unregistered homes receiving particularly high levels of care were entitled to a residential care home rate of IS before April 1993 which has continued. You may also have preserved rights if before April 1993 you were living in a larger registered care home and have since moved into an adult placement which has been required to register since April 1993.

If you do not have preserved rights you *may* nevertheless be entitled to transitional HB if it was payable in respect of your placement before it was required to register and will continue to be payable, together with ordinary rates of IS and AA/DLA as appropriate, as explained on p9.

If your placement has been arranged since 1 April 1993, you will not normally have preserved rights, and if the accommodation is registered as a care home you will not normally be entitled to HB. However, you *may* instead be entitled to IS residential allowance (see Chapter 21). If this is insufficient to meet the costs of your care, social services may be responsible for paying for your accommodation for which you may have to make a contribution on the basis explained in Chapters 12 and 23.

Placements in unregistered adult placements since April 1993 should be treated in the same way as for unregistered care homes (see above).

If social services are not making any payment towards the cost of your accommodation (even if they are paying towards the cost of any care you need) or if the accommodation is not registered (or if you were entitled before it was registered), you may also be entitled to AA/DLA (see p356). You may also be provided with community care services in respect of personal care needs which are not met by your carer(s), although you may be charged for them (see Chapter 2).

4. **Abbeyfield Homes**

Special arrangements apply to residents of homes provided by the Abbeyfield Society because they are considered by the government to offer supported accommodation of a type which exemplifies good practice in community care.

Most Abbeyfield Homes are not considered to provide board (or, in Scotland, support) or personal care and so are not required to be registered as care homes (see p269). However, a small number are registered and some are registered as nursing care homes.

Residents of Abbeyfield Homes usually have their own room, although they may share communal facilities and meals, and are generally more independent than those who need residential care. Residents are often moved into care homes when they become more dependent, and consequently the majority of residents in Abbeyfield Homes have only been resident since April 1993. Such residents are treated in the same way as if they were in sheltered accommodation (see p154), except that residents in Abbeyfield Homes are treated as licensees rather than tenants[5]), and may therefore claim social security benefits as if they were in ordinary accommodation or in their own homes (see Chapter 3), which may include all appropriate IS allowances and premiums, AA/DLA and HB for any eligible housing costs (see Chapter 3). Residents may also be provided with community care services, however, may be charged for them (see Chapter 2).

Residents of Abbeyfield Homes who have been resident since before 1 April 1993, however, are considered to have preserved rights

(see Chapter 22) so that IS is paid as if they are in a registered care home whether it is registered or not. However, there may be significant disadvantages in having preserved rights (see Chapter 22). Unlike residents with preserved rights in care homes who can only lose their preserved rights if they leave residential or nursing care, Abbeyfield residents may lose their preserved rights without leaving the home. If you are an Abbeyfield resident with preserved rights you will lose those rights if:[6]

- you still live in an Abbeyfield Home; *and*
- it is not a registered home; *and*
- you require personal care, including assistance with bodily functions; *and*

- the personal care you require is not provided by Abbeyfield; *and*
- you contract with another person or body to provide that care.

'Contract' will in practice usually, but not necessarily, mean 'pay', although it is not clear to what extent this condition may be met simply by paying charges for community care services (see Chapter 2), as both the charges and services are arranged under statutory provisions rather than by way of a 'contract'. 'Personal care' is not clearly defined, although the context would suggest that it refers to the broad meaning of the term used in the law relating to registration requirements (see Chapter 12) rather than, for example, the specific meaning given to the term used in the conditions of entitlement to AA/DLA (see Chapter 3).

Your preserved rights will, however, be re-acquired as soon as any of the conditions above no longer apply.

If you lose your preserved rights in this way, you may then claim benefits in the normal way as if you had only been resident since April 1993 (see above) – ie, including ordinary rates of IS, AA/DLA and HB, as appropriate. This may usually (but not necessarily) mean that you will have more money to pay for your accommodation and care and for your own personal expenditure than if you retained your preserved rights.

For further details contact (for England and Wales) the Abbeyfield Society, Abbeyfield House, 53 Victoria Street, St. Albans, Hertfordshire AL1 3UW (01727 857536); or (for Scotland) Abbeyfield (Scotland), 15 West Martland Street, Edinburgh EH12 5EA (0131 225 7801).

5. **Less dependent residents in local authority care homes**

Before April 1993, local authority social services departments in England and Wales had powers to arrange for the provision of accommodation not only under the National Assistance Act 1948 but also under the National Health Service Act 1977. The 1977 Act was used to provide accommodation mainly for people who were able to live more independently than those accommodated under the 1948 Act, but who nevertheless required some degree of care and support. These were mostly (but not always) people under pensionable age. There were powers, but not duties, to ask for a reasonable charge for such accommodation which meant that residents were usually left with more money for their personal use than the personal expenses allowance (see Chapter 15) available to those accommodated under the 1948 Act. Although the 1977 Act did not apply in Scotland, there were powers to vary the personal expenses allowance to achieve the same effect. This arrangement existed so that less dependent residents could be encouraged to live as independently as possible, perhaps with a view to eventually living completely independently in the community, by allowing them to have more responsibility over how their money was spent on – eg, on food, household or other living expenses or travel costs.

Since 1 April 1993, arrangements by social services in England and Wales for the placement of adults in care homes are now made under the National Assistance Act 1948 and under this Act a charge must be made for the accommodation (see Chapter 12 and note the exceptions which apply to certain aftercare services for those recovering from mental health problems on p261). It is still recognised, however, that the normal charging rules would not be appropriate for less dependent residents because they will usually need to be left with more than the standard personal expenses allowance if they are to live as independently as possible. In Scotland, social work departments have since 1993 had a discretion not to charge less dependent residents as well as vary the personal expenses allowance.[7]

Special arrangements therefore apply to less dependent residents. A less dependent resident is a person who lives in:[8]

- independent accommodation which is not required to be registered as a care home; *or*
- a local authority home which does not provide board (eg, in a cluster or group home or hostel – see p162). 'Board' means at least some cooked or prepared meals, cooked or prepared by someone other than the resident (or a member of her/his family) and eaten in the accommodation, where the cost of meals is included in the standard rate fixed for the accommodation. This means that residents who pay for their food in a cafeteria or pay-as-you-eat arrangement should be classed as less dependent.

If you are a less dependent resident:

- you will be entitled to the normal rates of IS personal allowances and premiums payable to those who live independently in the community (see Chapter 3), and neither the residential allowance nor the applicable amount normally payable to residents in local authority care homes (see Chapter 21) will apply;
- you will be entitled to claim HB towards your eligible housing costs (see Chapter 3). Although you are not normally entitled to HB if you live in a residential home owned or managed by a local authority this exclusion will only apply if you pay an inclusive charge for accommodation and meals[9] (except that, even if meals are not included, you will still not be entitled to HB if you were living in such a home on 31 March 1993[10]). Note, however, that HB is only payable if you are liable for the costs of occupying your accommodation, and although there is clearly a policy intention that you should be able to claim HB as a less dependent resident in local authority

residential accommodation, it has been argued that such an arrangement may be in breach of the Local Authorities (Goods and Services) Act 1970 which prohibits local authorities in England and Wales from selling a service (ie, the provision of your accommodation) to a non-public body (ie, you) which would be the very arrangement necessary to enable you to qualify for HB[11];

- for both IS and HB, the higher capital limits (£10,000 and £16,000 – see Chapter 7) for those living permanently in care homes will apply;
- special provisions will apply to enable social services to continue to treat you differently where they consider it reasonable to do so[12] by disregarding income or capital;
- normally taken into account (see Chapters 13 and 14) and disregarding the rules on the treatment of liable relatives (see Chapter 17). Factors to be taken into account will include:[13]
  - your commitments – ie, the extent to which you may be incurring costs directly for necessities such as food, fuel and clothing;
  - the degree of your independence – ie, the extent to which you should be encouraged to take on expenditure commitments;
  - whether you need a greater incentive to become more independent eg, the extent to which you may be encouraged to take on paid employment if most or all of your earnings are disregarded.

Note, however, you will not be entitled to AA or any care component of DLA if you are living in a local authority care home even if you are a less dependent resident (so that you will still not be entitled to certain premiums such as the severe disability premium) – see Chapter 21.

6. **Registered care homes where housing benefit is payable**

Most residents of registered care homes have been excluded from entitlement to HB since 14 January 1991.[14] Prior to that date, however, there were no specific rules excluding residents from entitlement to HB, although most people claimed IS to meet the costs of their home and now have preserved rights (see Chapter 22) if they have lived there continuously since then, or else rely on IS and social services assistance (see Chapters 12, 21 and 23) if they have left but since returned. However, some residents may not have been entitled to IS (eg, because they had savings in excess of £8,000) but could still claim HB (because their savings were less than £16,000).

Transitional arrangements allow for entitlement to HB to continue in the following circumstances:

- if you were entitled to HB in respect of the costs of a particular registered care home on 29 October 1990[15] and you continue to live in *any* registered care home;
- if you were entitled to HB on 31 March 1993 and you were either:
  - in remunerative work; *or*
  - paying a commercial rent to a non-resident close relative; *or*
  - living in an unregistered home with less than four residents (in England and Wales) (a small home which may not have been required to register until April 1993 – see Chapter 12)

then you remain eligible for HB as long as you do not break your claim and you continue to live in the *same* home (even if it is a small home which since April 1993 has been required to register), disregarding temporary absences of up to 13 or 52 weeks.[16]

Note that these rules on transitional HB apply separately to the transitional HB scheme for people in supported accommodation (see p107).

---

7. Cluster homes

Apart from the exceptions for the transitional arrangements (see above), the general exclusion from entitlement to HB applies to the whole of any registered accommodation. Certain parts of some registered care homes may, however, be exempt from the registration requirements – eg, because board (or, in Scotland, support) and personal care are not provided there. This may be because certain units of accommodation attached to the home are sometimes used for less dependent residents (or for staff). Sometimes these are self-contained units or bungalows in the grounds of the core home and are often referred to as 'cluster' homes. Similarly, some self-contained units may be clustered around the grounds of a core local authority care home or even in the grounds of a hospital. Units are often used to accommodate a number of residents together for mutual support and to encourage independent living, and these are often referred to as 'group' homes. There is no restriction on entitlement to HB in such clustered accommodation[17] where residents may also claim the usual rates of IS (personal allowances and premiums but not the residential allowance) and may also be provided with additional community care services as appropriate. AA/DLA may also be payable, although you will not be entitled to AA or any care component of DLA if you are living in local authority accommodation which has been provided by social services (see Chapters 12 and 21).[18]

8. **Temporary stays in supported housing**

If you depend on IS or HB for help with the mortgage or rent you pay for the home you normally live in and you need to stay in supported housing on a temporary basis (eg, for a period of respite for you and/or your carer or as part of a programme of treatment for recovering alcohol/drug addicts), the housing costs on your own home will normally only continue to paid for up to 13 weeks (see p99), or 52 weeks if your temporary accommodation is a care home (see Chapter 21 p351), for each period of temporary absence from your own home.

You will also not be able to claim IS or HB for the housing costs of your temporary accommodation while you are receiving IS or HB for the costs of your own home (but see Chapter 21 p8, if your temporary accommodation is a care home).

If you are away from your home for more than 13 (or 52) weeks, you will permanently lose any entitlement you have to transitional HB for your normal home (see p159), or preserved rights (see above and Chapter 22), and (unless you or your partner are aged 60 or over) there may be a waiting period before you can start to be paid housing costs with your IS when you return (see p99).

If you are unable to pay for the costs of any temporary accommodation, social services may arrange to pay for it if they consider that you need it (see Chapter 12). Although they may then make a financial assessment to see whether you should contribute towards the costs, they will make allowances for any costs you still have to make to maintain your own home. However, they will not be able to pay for any costs on your own home (eg, because you do not qualify for IS housing costs or HB because your temporary absence from it is for more than 13/52 weeks) if you do not have sufficient income of your own to pay for them (see Chapters 21 and 23).

It may, therefore, be impossible to pay for the costs of prolonged temporary stays in supported housing without accruing debts on your own home. The only alternatives would be to arrange for a series of temporary stays (even if you only return to your own home for one weekend or day every 13 weeks), or for community care services to meet your needs as far as possible in your own home instead (see Chapter 2), or to give up your own home and move into supported housing or a care home on a permanent basis.

Notes

1. **Sheltered and very sheltered housing**
   1 The categories appear to be derived from a Ministry of Health and Local Government Circular No. 82/69 which was cancelled in 1980 but continues to be referred to in design standards for new schemes in England and Wales.

2. **Unregistered care homes and hostels**
   2 England/Wales: RHA 1984; Scotland: SW(S)A 1968
   3 Reg 7(1)(e) and (3) HB Regs

3. **Adult placement schemes**
   4 'Information on the funding of adult placements' – *National Association of Adult Placement Services* 1997

4. **Abbeyfield Homes**
   5 *Abbeyfield (Harpenden) Society Ltd v Woods* [1968] 1 All ER 352, CA
   6 Reg 19 (1ZR) IS Regs

5. **Less dependent residents in local authority care homes**
   7 England/Wales:CRAG 2.001 – 2.011; Scotland: ss13B and 15 SW(S)A 1968 and s7 MH(S)A 1984 and SWSG 2.001-2.006
   8 Reg 2 NA (AoR) Regs 1992; reg 8 HB Regs
   9 Reg 8(2)(b) HB Regs
   10 Reg 8(2ZA) and (2ZB) HB Regs
   11 See *Community Care News,* issue no. 1, February 1999, Rowe & Maw
   12 Reg 5 NA (AoR) Regs 1992
   13 Reg 5 NA (AoR) Regs 1992; CRAG 2.010

6. **Registered care homes where housing benefit is payable**
   14 Reg 7(1)(e) and (3) HB Regs
   15 Reg 7(2)(c) and (d) HB Regs
   16 Reg 7(4)-(12) HB Regs

7. **Cluster homes**
   17 GM A4.30-36
   18 CDLA 13479/96

Part 3

• •

General provisions for social security benefits in the community and in care homes

Whether you are living at home in the community or in a care home, there are many common rules which apply to most social security benefits you may be entitled to.

This Part explains the common rules which apply to the treatment of any income (see Chapter 6) or capital and property (see Chapter 7) you (or your partner) may have if you (or your partner) are claiming any of the means-tested benefits, ie income support (IS), income-based jobseeker's allowance (JSA), housing benefit (HB) and/or council tax benefit (CTB) (for details of the rules in Chapter 3 which apply to claims for disability working allowance, family credit and tax credits, see CPAG's *Welfare Benefits Handbook*). It also highlights the rules on income, capital and property which are different for people who live at home in the community and people who live in care homes.

This Part also covers the rules which may affect the liable relatives (see Chapter 8) of those who claim IS/income-based JSA, and the special rules which apply to special groups of people seeking to claim IS, income-based JSA, HB and/or CTB (see Chapter 9).

This Part also covers how all (means-tested and non-means-tested) social security benefits are administered (see Chapter 10) and some of the common problems encountered in trying to claim them (see Chapter 11).

Certain social security benefits which may be paid when you are living at home in the community may not be paid at all if you are living in a care home, or the amount of benefit payable may be quite different. For the main rules which apply to social security benefits payable to those who live in care homes, see Chapter 21.

Chapter 6

Income – social security benefits

This chapter explains how your income affects your entitlement to income support, income-based jobseeker's allowance, housing benefit and council tax benefit. It covers:

1. General rules about income (p168)
2. Income other than earnings (p169)
3. Earnings from employment and self-employment (p179)
4. Notional income (p182)

Your entitlement to income support (IS) (see p93), income-based jobseeker's allowance (JSA) (see p125), housing benefit (HB) (see p102) and council tax benefit (CTB) (see p111), and the amount of benefit you receive, depends on how much income you have. Some of your income may be completely ignored, or partially ignored, or counted in full. Some income may be treated as capital (see p195), and some capital may be treated as income (see p174). The rules for working out your income are very similar for IS, income-based JSA, HB and CTB, and are similar whether you are living at home in the community or living in a care home. Where there are differences, these are indicated.

For how income affects claims for tax credits (formerly family credit and disability working allowance) – (see pp115 and 125), and for how income affects claims for IS/income-based JSA if you are, or have recently been, involved in a trade dispute, see CPAG's *Welfare Benefits Handbook*.

For the treatment and effect of certain forms of earnings-related income on claims for: contribution-based JSA; invalid care allowance; incapacity benefit and severe disablement allowance; increases of those benefits and retirement pension; maternity allowance; widowed mother's allowance; and industrial injuries benefit unemployability supplement in respect of child and adult dependants (see Chapter 3).

There are many similarities, and some significant differences, between the way your income is treated for benefit purposes and the way it is treated by social services if they are assisting you with the costs of your care home. For details see Chapter 13.

1. General rules about income

This section explains the rules about whose income counts when working out your entitlement to IS/income-based JSA/HB/CTB, how the income of your partner is treated, how income is converted into weekly amounts to calculate your entitlement to those weekly benefits, and the special rules on the periods covered by income in claims for IS and income-based JSA.

Whose income counts

If you are a member of a couple (see p96) your partner's income is added to yours and calculated in the same way as if it were yours.[1] Note that if you are living in a care home (unless you are only in the home on a temporary basis) you will not usually be treated as living in the same household as your partner, and your partner's income will therefore be ignored in calculating your entitlement to IS/income-based JSA/HB/CTB (but see Chapter 8 for the rules on liable relatives and IS/income-based JSA).

Special rules apply to the treatment of income of a dependent child (see CPAG's *Welfare Benefits Handbook*).

Converting income into a weekly amount

IS, income-based JSA, HB and CTB are all calculated on a weekly basis. Therefore, your income is converted into a weekly amount to determine your entitlement to benefit. For IS/income-based JSA, this amount is attributed to a forward period and affects the benefit payable for that period. For HB/CTB, an appropriate past period is used where possible to assess your normal weekly income, and this figure is used to calculate benefit. There are special rules on the treatment of fluctuating income (especially from earnings) to convert it into an average weekly amount (see CPAG's *Welfare Benefits Handbook*).

For IS/income-based JSA it is sometimes necessary to calculate income for part weeks. This applies when other income covers part of the week for which IS/income-based JSA is paid – eg, when an award of incapacity benefit or severe disablement allowance is paid from a different day from the day on which your IS/income-based JSA starts. In such circumstances, a daily rate is calculated and only the amount paid for the days covered by IS/income-based JSA is taken into account.[2]

The period covered by income

For HB/CTB, a past period is normally looked at to assess what your current normal weekly income is. Earnings of employees are usually averaged out over the previous five weeks if you are paid weekly, or two months if you are paid monthly. However, a different period can be used if this would give a fairer reflection of what your earnings would be over the period of your claim.[3]

Earnings from self-employment are averaged out over an appropriate period (usually based on the last year's trading accounts) of up to a year.[4]

For IS/income-based JSA there are special rules for deciding the length of the period for which and the date from which payments of income count. These rules are designed to give a clearer indication of how you are expected to make use of any earnings or other income you receive for each week of your claim for IS/income-based JSA. For further details see CPAG's *Welfare Benefits Handbook*.

2. **Income other than earnings**

Most forms of income are taken into account for each of the means-tested benefits (IS/income-based JSA/HB/CTB), although some rules about how income is treated are different for different benefits. Different rules apply to the treatment of:

- other social security benefits;
- charitable and voluntary payments;
- income from capital;
- income from tenants and lodgers; *and*
- miscellaneous income.

All income is taken into account only after deducting any tax due on it.[5] For HB/CTB, any changes in tax rates may be ignored for up to 30 weeks.[6] If income is paid in another currency, any bank charges for converting the payment into sterling are also deducted.[7]

Other social security benefits

When calculating your entitlement to IS/income-based JSA/HB/CTB, any other social security benefits paid to you (or your partner) are taken into account. Some are counted in full, some are fully ignored, and some are partially disregarded.

Benefits which count in full

- Contribution-based JSA;
- incapacity benefit;
- severe disablement allowance;
- invalid care allowance;
- retirement pensions;
- widows' benefits (including industrial death benefit, but note that the widow's payment counts not as income but as capital – see p198);
- industrial injuries benefits (except constant attendance allowance and exceptionally severe disablement allowance which are fully disregarded);

- maternity allowance;
- child benefit;
- child's special allowance and war orphan's pension;
- for IS/income-based JSA only, guardian's allowance;
- family credit or working families tax credit (WFTC), disability working allowance or disabled person's tax credit (DTPC), and earnings top-up;
- for IS/income-based JSA only, statutory sick pay (SSP) and statutory maternity pay, less any tax, Class 1 National Insurance (NI) contributions and half of any pension contributions (for HB/CTB, SSP and statutory maternity pay are treated as earnings and you may therefore benefit from an earnings disregard – see p181).

For further details of these benefits, see Chapter 3.

Problems may arise where the Benefits Agency tries to take into account a benefit you are not receiving (eg, invalid care allowance) because it has been delayed or suspended or is not payable because it overlaps (see p69) with another benefit you receive. You should insist on being paid your full benefit and the Benefits Agency should instead deduct the difference from arrears of the delayed benefit only when it is eventually paid.[8]

For IS/income-based JSA/HB/CTB, arrears of any means-tested benefit and any of those disability benefits which are disregarded as income (see below) should be treated as capital and ignored for 52 weeks (see p198).[9] This rule only applies to arrears of benefit you actually receive, so only the amount paid to you after the Benefits Agency has deducted any amount because another benefit is delayed should be counted.

Benefits which are ignored completely

- Attendance allowance (AA) or any care component of disability living allowance (DLA) (or constant attendance allowance, exceptionally severe disablement allowance or severe disablement occupational allowance paid because of an injury at work or a war injury), unless, for IS/income-based JSA, you are a person with preserved rights because you have been living in a care home since before 31 March 1993 (see Chapter 22) (or unless you are accommodated under the Polish Resettlement Act), in which case it is taken into account in full (up to the amount of the highest rate of AA – ie £52.95 a week);[10]
- any mobility component of DLA[11] (or mobility supplement under the War Pensions Scheme);[12]
- any extra-statutory payment made to you to compensate for non-payment of IS/income-based JSA or AA or DLA (or mobility allowance or mobility supplement);[13]
- pensioner's Christmas bonus (see p93);[14]

- social fund payments (see p117)[15] (which are also disregarded as capital indefinitely[16] – see p199);
- certain special war widows' payments,[17] including any special or supplementary payments (currently £56.45) to pre-1973 war widows;[18]
- resettlement benefit paid to certain patients who are discharged from hospital and who had been in hospital for more than a year before 11 April 1988;[19]
- any increase of incapacity benefit, maternity allowance, widowed mother's allowance, retirement pension, industrial injuries benefit unemployability supplement, invalid care allowance or a service pension paid for adult or child dependants who are not members of your family;[20]
- any payment in consequence of a reduction in liability for council tax (or, formerly, community charge);[21]
- for HB/CTB only, guardian's allowance.[22]

There are also special rules to ensure that payments of IS/income-based JSA/HB/CTB (and certain transitional and extra-statutory payments to compensate for any loss of these benefits) are disregarded in calculating entitlement to IS/income-based JSA/HB/CTB.[23] There are special rules for HB/CTB claimants who are awarded IS/income-based JSA which ensures that their income does not have to be separately assessed by the local authority. For the treatment of payments of arrears of benefits (see p199).

Benefits which are partially ignored

The first £10 of any award of any of the following benefits is ignored:
- war disablement pension (including any tax-free service invaliding pension or 'service attributable pension';[24]
- war widow's pension;
- widow's pension payable to widows of members of the Royal Navy, Army or Royal Air Force who were disabled or died in consequence of service in the armed forces;
- an extra-statutory payment made instead of the above pensions;
- similar payments made by another country;
- a pension from Germany or Austria paid to the victims of Nazi persecution.[25]

Only £10 in all can be ignored, even if you have more than one payment which attracts a £10 disregard.[26] However, the £10 disregard allowed on these war pensions is additional to the total disregard of any mobility supplement or AA (ie, constant attendance allowance, exceptionally severe disablement allowance and severe disablement occupational allowance) paid as part of a war disablement pension. The £10 disregard may, however, overlap with other disregards on student loans (see p178) and charitable or voluntary payments (see below), when a combined maximum of £20 is allowed.

Local authorities are given a limited discretion to increase the £10 disregard on war disablement, war widows' pensions and the pension payable to widows of members of the Royal Navy, Army or Royal Air Force, when assessing income for HB and CTB.[27] Some local authorities disregard the full amount of these pensions and some do not increase the disregard at all, so you should check your own local authority's policy on this issue.

Charitable and voluntary payments

Charitable payments are payments made under a charitable trust (although it does not have to be registered or administered by a registered charity) for the promotion of a public benefit (eg, the relief of poverty, or the advancement of education or religion, or other purposes which benefit a significant group of people) at the discretion of the trustees. Voluntary payments are payments which have a benevolent purpose and are given without anything being given in return (although the person making the payment may sometimes come under an obligation to do so). Voluntary payments are similar to charitable payments but they will not be made from charitable trusts and they will usually be paid for the benefit of an individual. Payments made by central government cannot be classed as charitable or voluntary, but payments made by local authorities can be.[28]

Most charitable or voluntary payments which are made *irregularly* and are intended to be made irregularly are treated as capital and are unlikely to affect your claim unless they take your capital above the capital limit.[29]

Charitable or voluntary payments made, or due to be made, *regularly* are completely ignored if they are intended, and used, for anything *except* food, ordinary clothing or footwear, household fuel, council tax, water rates and rent (less any non-dependant deductions) for which HB is payable. For IS/ income-based JSA only, they are also ignored if they are for housing costs met by IS/income-based JSA, or residential or nursing care home accommodation charges for people with preserved rights (see Chapter 22) met by IS/income-based JSA or by a local authority. Where you do not have a preserved right and the local authority has placed you in a residential or nursing care home that is more expensive than normal for a person of your needs because you preferred that home, a charitable or voluntary payment towards the *extra* cost is ignored for IS/income-based JSA.[30]

If not ignored altogether, charitable or voluntary payments have a £20 disregard, although that may overlap with other disregards for certain war pensions (see p171) or student loans (see p178) when a combined maximum of £20 is allowed.[31] Note that this is a weekly disregard so payments spread over different or successive benefit weeks attract a £20 disregard for each.

For HB and CTB it has been decided that discretionary grants to Canadian war veterans or their widows settled in the UK should also be treated as voluntary payments and attract a £20 disregard.[32] It is arguable that this should also apply to IS/income-based JSA and to any other discretionary grants paid to any other overseas war veterans (or their widows) who are settled in the UK.

Any payments from a former partner or the parent of your child, whether voluntary or not, are treated as maintenance payments (see p178).

Concessionary coal that is provided free by British Coal to a former employee or widow is classed as income in kind and ignored for all benefits.[33] Cash in lieu of coal is not a voluntary payment[34] but counts in full as income, or as earnings if paid to a current employee.[35]

See also payments made to someone else on your behalf (p184) and payments disregarded as miscellaneous income (p175).

Charitable payments from the Macfarlane and similar trusts

Any payments, including payments in kind, from the Macfarlane Trust, the Fund, the Eileen Trust or either of the Independent Living Funds (see p143) are disregarded in full.[36] There are also special rules allowing for the disregard of certain payments by you, or on your behalf, for the benefit of yourself or certain relatives and members of your family, out of money which originally came from these sources.[37]

Income from capital

In general, actual income generated from capital (eg, interest on savings) is ignored as income[38] but counts as capital[39] from the date you are due to receive it. However, income derived from the following categories of disregarded capital (see p195) is treated as income:[40]

- your home;
- your former home if you are estranged or divorced;
- property which you have acquired for occupation as your home but which you have not yet been able to move into;
- property which you intend to occupy as your home but which needs essential repairs or alterations;
- property occupied wholly or partly by a partner or relative or any member of your family who is 60 or over or incapacitated;
- property occupied by your former partner, but not if you are estranged or divorced (unless, for HB/CTB only, s/he is a lone parent);
- property for sale;
- property which you are taking legal steps to obtain to occupy as your home;
- your business assets;
- a trust of personal injury compensation.

Income from any of the above categories (other than your current home, business assets or a personal injuries trust) is ignored up to the amount of the total mortgage repayments (ie, capital and interest, and any payments that are a condition of the mortgage such as insurance or an endowment policy),[41] council tax and water rates paid in respect of the property for the same period over which the income is received.[42] This might apply, for example, to any rent you receive from letting your home while you are in a care home (but see p175 for the treatment of rent from other properties).

Tariff income from capital over £3,000[43]

Capital over £3,000 is considered to have an assumed income from it, called tariff income. You are assumed to have an income of £1 for every £250, or part of £250, by which your capital exceeds £3,000 but does not exceed £8,000 (for IS/income-based JSA) or £16,000 (for HB/CTB).

Note, however, that for IS/income-based JSA/HB, if you are in a care home, tariff income applies only between £10,000 and £16,000.

You should report any increases or decreases in any capital over £3,000 as soon as possible otherwise you may have to repay any overpaid benefit (see p245) from failing to report any increases, or there may be restrictions on how far back any underpaid benefit may be repaid to you (see Chapter 10) if you do not report any decreases in time.

Capital which counts as income

The following count as income:
- instalments of capital outstanding either when your benefit claim is decided or when you are first due to be paid benefit, whichever is earlier, or at the date of any subsequent review,[44] if they would bring you over whichever capital limit is applicable. Any balance outstanding over the capital limit counts as income by spreading it over the number of weeks between each instalment;[45]
- any payment from an annuity[46] (but see p175 for when this is disregarded);
- certain lump sum payments from liable relatives (see Chapter 8).

In addition, there are special rules on career development loans from the Employment Service and educational maintenance grants if you leave a course early. For details see CPAG's *Welfare Benefits Handbook*.

Capital which is counted as income cannot also be treated as producing a tariff income.[47]

For HB/CTB, withdrawals from a capital sum are sometimes treated as income, including loans to cover extra expenses for a particular period – eg, for a period of respite care.[48] You should, however, argue that unless it is paid in instalments it should be treated as capital.[49] Any payments of capital, or any irregular withdrawals from a capital sum which are clearly for one-off items and not regular living expenses, should be treated as capital. Furthermore, if no withdrawals are in fact made, the sum should be treated as capital.[50]

Income from tenants and lodgers

Lettings without board

If you let room(s) in your home to tenants, sub-tenants, or licensees under a formal contractual arrangement, £4 of the weekly charge for each tenant, sub-tenant, licensee (and her/his family) is ignored. An extra £9.25 is ignored if the charge covers heating costs.[51] The balance counts as income.

If someone shares your home under an informal arrangement, any payment made by them to you for their living and accommodation costs is ignored,[52] but a non-dependant deduction may be made from any HB/CTB or housing costs paid with IS/income-based JSA (see Chapter 3).

Boarders

If you have a boarder(s) on a commercial basis and the boarder or any member of her/his family is not a close relative of yours, the first £20 of the weekly charge is ignored and half of any balance remaining is then taken into account as your income.[53] For HB/CTB, there is no specific reference in the rules to non-commercial arrangements or close relatives, but the rules on contrived tenancies could possibly apply (see p103). The £20 disregard applies for each boarder you have, but the charge must normally include at least some meals.[54]

Note: Whether you let part of your home to tenants or lodgers, with or without board, any income left after applying the above disregards may be considered to be intended to be used to meet any housing costs of your own which are not met by IS/income-based JSA/HB, and may therefore also be offset accordingly.[55]

If the person for whom you are providing board has been placed with you on a temporary basis under community care arrangements, all payments you receive are disregarded (see p177).[56]

Tenants in other properties

If you have a freehold interest in a property other than your own home and you let it out, the rent is treated as capital.[57] This rule also applies if you have a leasehold interest in another property which you are sub-letting. There is disagreement between commissioners as to whether it is the gross rent which should be taken into account, or only the sum left after deducting expenses.[58]

Miscellaneous income

Income which counts in full

- Any occupational pension or income from a personal pension or retirement annuity contract apart from any discretionary payment from a hardship fund). However, for IS/income-based JSA, half of any such payments will be disregarded if you are in a care home and have 'preserved rights' (see

Chapter 22) and an amount equal to at least half of your pension payments are being paid by you for the maintenance of your spouse.[59] This disregard applies only if it is in respect of a spouse (and not an unmarried partner), and will not apply if less than half of your pension payments are being used for her/his maintenance. It will apply even if the share of the pension is not being paid directly to your spouse – eg, if it is being paid to a building society to pay her/his mortgage. However, if your spouse is reliant on a means-tested benefit the share of your pension will be treated as a maintenance payment (see p178) when her/his own claim(s) for benefit is assessed, and you should check, or seek advice, to make sure that s/he will not be worse off if you arrange to make the payments for her/him.

- Payments from an annuity, *except that* in the case of 'home income plans' income from the annuity equal to the interest payable on the loan with which the annuity was bought is ignored if the following conditions are met:
  – you used at least 90 per cent of the loan made to you to buy the annuity; *and*
  – the annuity will end when you and your partner die; *and*
  – you or your partner are responsible for paying the interest on the loan; *and*
  – you, or both your partner and yourself, were at least 65 at the time the loan was made; *and*
  – the loan is secured on a property which you or your partner owns or has an interest in, and the property on which the loan is secured is your home, or that of your partner.

If the interest on the loan is payable after income tax has been deducted, it is an amount equal to the net interest payment that is disregarded, otherwise it is the gross amount of the interest payment.[60]

Income which is fully disregarded

Payments for care home costs

- For IS/income-based JSA, any payments made by social services to a care home in respect of the costs of the accommodation which they have arranged for you.[61] Note that, due to an unintentional oversight, this particular disregard was drafted ambiguously between April 1994 and April 1998 and such payments may have not have been disregarded in some cases. It is clearly contrary to policy intention for such payments to be taken into account, and you should seek advice if this has happened to you.
- For IS/income-based JSA, if your accommodation in a care home has been arranged by social services and you do not have preserved rights, any charitable or voluntary payments (see p172) to make up the difference between the actual charge for the home and the maximum fee which would

normally be met by social services for a person with your particular needs provided that it was your choice to move into the more expensive home.[62]
- For IS/income-based JSA, if you live in a care home and have preserved rights, any payment you receive which is intended to be used and is used to meet that part of your accommodation charge which is above the maximum payable by IS.[63]
- For IS/income-based JSA, if your accommodation in a care home has not been arranged by social services and you do not have preserved rights, payments towards the costs of the care home up to the amount of the difference between your applicable amount less your personal expenses allowance (see Chapter 21) and the weekly charge for the home.[64]

Payments by local authorities
- Certain payments from social services for the costs of your accommodation in a care home (see above).
- Any payments made under the Community Care (Direct Payments) Act 1996 (or under s12B of the Social Work (Scotland) Act 1968)[65] – see p46.
- Any payment you receive for looking after a person temporarily in your care if it is paid under community care arrangements by a local authority. This disregard also applies if the payment is made instead by a health authority, voluntary organisation or by the person being looked after.[66]
- Certain payments from social services to assist children in need.[67]
- Educational maintenance allowances to assist children staying on at school beyond school-leaving age.[68]

Loan insurance payments
For IS/income-based JSA, payments you receive under a mortgage protection policy which you took out, and which you use, to pay housing costs which are not included in your IS/income-based JSA[69] (see p99). However, if the amount you receive exceeds the total of the following, the excess counts as your income:
- interest on a qualifying loan which is not met by the Benefits Agency;
- capital repayments on a qualifying loan; *and*
- premiums on the policy in question and building insurance policy.

For HB/CTB, payments you receive under an insurance policy you took out to insure against the risk of being unable to maintain payments on a loan secured on your home. However, anything you get above the total of the following counts as your income:
- the amount you use to maintain your payments; *and*
- any premium you pay for the policy; *and*

- any premium for an insurance policy which you had to take out to insure against loss or damage to your home.[70]
- any payments you receive under an insurance policy you took out to insure against the risk of being unable to maintain hire purchase or similar payments or other loan payments – eg, credit card debts. However, anything you get above the amount you use to make your payments and the premium for the policy counts as your income.[71]

Payments by the Employment Service

Certain payments made by the Employment Service to assist people with the expense of obtaining or retaining employment (eg, expenses payments under the New Deal programme), other than training allowances which count in full as income, may be disregarded (for details see CPAG's *Welfare Benefits Handbook*).

Other payments

For IS/income-based JSA, as long as you have not already used insurance payments for the same purpose, any money you receive which is intended to be used and is used to make:[72]

- capital and interest payments which do not qualify as housing costs;
- payments of premiums on a building insurance policy or on an insurance policy which you took out against the risk of not being able to make the payments on a loan secured on your home;
- any rent that is not covered by HB (see p108);
- any payment to cover expenses if you are working as a volunteer;[73]
- payments in kind[74] which may include food, fuel, cigarettes[75]clothing, holidays, gifts, accommodation, or transport[76] (but see p000 for the treatment of payments in kind by employers and see p000 for the rules on notional income);
- any payments, other than for loss of earnings or of a benefit, made to jurors or witnesses for attending at court;[77]
- Victoria Cross or George Cross payments or similar awards;[78]
- income paid outside the UK which cannot be transferred here;[79]
- fares to hospital;[80]
- payments by the Home Office to assist prison visits;[81]
- income tax refunds, which are instead treated as capital;[82]

Income which is partially disregarded

There are special rules on the treatment of:
- fostering allowances, adoption allowances and residence order allowances paid by social services (see CPAG's *Welfare Benefits Handbook*);
- grants and loans paid to students (see CPAG's *Welfare Benefits Handbook*);

- maintenance payments (or child support maintenance) which you and/or your partner receive for yourself/selves (and/or any children in your family). Most maintenance payments count in full while you are claiming IS/income-based JSA/HB/CTB (although up to £15 of maintenance may be disregarded for HB/CTB if there is a child in your family).[83] If you *pay* maintenance, your payments are not disregarded when calculating your income, unless you are in a care home and the payments are for the maintenance of your spouse and amount to at least half of certain pension payments you receive. For further details on the treatment of maintenance payments see Chapter 8. For details of child support maintenance payments see CPAG's *Child Support Handbook* and *Welfare Benefits Handbook*.

3. Earnings from employment and self-employment

This section explains how your (or your partner's) earnings from employment or self-employment are treated for IS/income-based JSA/HB/CTB. Different rules apply to the calculation of earnings from employment and earnings from self-employment. Only net earnings are counted as income.

The following rules do not apply to the earnings of childminders. Childminders are treated as self-employed but their net profit is deemed to be one third of their earnings less income tax, NI contributions and half of certain pension contributions; the rest of their earnings are completely ignored.[84]

Calculating net earnings from employment

Both gross and net earnings need to be calculated. 'Gross' earnings means the amount received from your employer less deductions for expenses 'wholly, necessarily and exclusively' incurred by you in order to carry out the duties of your employment – eg, deductions could be made for expenditure on tools or work equipment, special clothing or uniform, or the costs of running a car.[85]

'Net' earnings means your gross earnings less deductions for income tax, Class 1 NI contributions and half of contributions made to a personal or occupational pension scheme.[86]

What counts as earnings

Earnings means 'any remuneration or profit derived from . . . employment'. As well as wages, this includes:[87]

- bonus or commission (including tips);
- holiday pay;
- payments made by your employer for expenses which are *not* 'wholly, exclusively and necessarily' incurred in carrying out your job (including

travel expenses to and from work and payments to you for looking after members of your family);
- a retainer fee or a guarantee payment;
- for HB/CTB, any sick pay or maternity pay (for IS/income-based JSA this is treated as income other than earnings);
- non-cash vouchers (except to the extent that they are exempt from liability for NI contributions);
- certain compensation payments in respect of your employment (for further details see CPAG's *Welfare Benefits Handbook*).

The following are examples of payments *not* counted as earnings:[88]
- payments in kind (other than non-cash vouchers – see above). But see p182 for the rules on notional income, including the value of any accommodation provided as part of your job;
- an advance of earnings or a loan from your employer (which counts instead as capital);
- payments towards expenses which are 'wholly, exclusively and necessarily' incurred – eg, travelling expenses in the course of your work. Such disregards may apply in addition to any allowances deducted in assessing gross earnings;
- occupational pension (which counts in full as income other than earnings).

There are special rules on the treatment of expenses paid to local councillors, earnings payable abroad, and payments from the Employment Service for participating in a New Deal programme.

There are also special rules on the treatment of certain payments when you leave a job – eg, holiday pay, pay in lieu of notice and other compensation payments (see CPAG's *Welfare Benefits Handbook*).

Calculating net earnings from self-employment

Your net profit over the period before you claim must be worked out. Net profit consists of all your earnings from self-employment minus:[89]
- any reasonable expenses (see below); *and*
- income tax and NI contributions; *and*
- half of any premium paid in respect of a personal pension scheme or a retirement annuity contract which is eligible for tax relief.

Reasonable expenses

Expenses which may be offset from earnings from self-employment must be reasonable and 'wholly, necessarily and exclusively' incurred for the purposes of your business.[90] Similar considerations apply as those which apply to the assessment of gross earnings from employment (see p179).

Reasonable expenses include repayments of capital on loans for replacing equipment and machinery or repairing business assets, and interest on certain loans for business purposes, but do not include any capital repayments on loans for business purposes, capital expenditure or expansion costs, most depreciation costs, entertainment expenses, losses incurred before the current assessment period or, for HB/CTB only, debts (other than proven bad debts), although the expenses of recovering debts may be deducted.

Disregarded earnings

Some of your net earnings from employment or self-employment are disregarded and do not affect your benefit. The amount of the disregard depends on your circumstances. There are three levels of earnings disregard and the highest one which applies to your circumstances will be allowed. An additional disregard applies to some claimants who work 30 hours or more a week. Certain childcare costs may also be offset from earnings.

£25 disregard
Lone parents claiming HB or CTB have £25 of their earnings ignored.[91] This does not apply to anyone claiming IS or income-based JSA.

£15 disregard
£15 of your earnings is disregarded if:
- for IS/income-based JSA, you are a lone parent;[92]
- you (or your partner) qualifies for the disability premium (see p97). For IS/ income-based JSA, you are treated as qualifying for the premium if you would do so but for being in hospital or a care home;[93]
- you (or your partner) qualifies for the higher pensioner premium (see p97) (or, for IS/income-based JSA, would do so but for being in hospital or a care home), *and*
 – you were entitled to the £15 disregard because you qualified for the disability premium immediately before you (or your partner) became 60 (or, for HB/ CTB, would have done but for the fact that the higher pensioner premium was payable instead) *and*
 – you have been in continuous employment since then. Breaks in employment of up to eight weeks are ignored, and for IS/income-based JSA this is increased to 12 weeks if you stopped getting IS/income-based JSA because you or your partner started full-time work, and breaks when you were not entitled to IS/ income-based JSA because you or your partner went on a government training scheme are ignored);[94]
- you have a partner, one of you is under 60, and your benefit would include a disability premium but for the fact that one of you qualifies for (or, for IS/ income-based JSA, would do but for being in hospital or a care home) the

higher pensioner premium or the enhanced rate of pensioner premium instead;[95]

- you have a partner, one of you is aged 75-79 and the other over 60, and immediately before that person became 60 either of you were entitled to the £15 disregard because of qualifying, or being treated as qualifying, for an enhanced pensioner premium (see above) and either of you have been continuously employed since then (disregarding any breaks as above);[96]
- you, or your partner, qualifies for a carer's premium.[97]
- you are an auxiliary coastguard, part-time fire fighter or lifeboat crew member, or in the Territorial Army.[98]

Basic £10 or £5 disregard

If you do not qualify for a £25 or £15 disregard, £5 of your earnings is disregarded if your are single, or £10 if you have a partner (whether or not you are both working).[99]

Additional full-time work disregard

For HB/CTB, an additional disregard of £11.05 is allowed if you (or your partner):[100]

- receive family credit, disability working allowance, or one of the tax credits (see pp115- 125) which, in either case, includes the £11.05 credit for working full time (30 hours or more a week); or
- work 30 hours or more a week and your HB/CTB includes the family premium, disability premium or higher premium (although if the partner in respect of whom the disability or higher pensioner premium is awarded works 16 hours or more, this will still apply provided her/his partner also works at least 30 hours).

Childcare costs disregard

For HB/CTB, certain childcare costs can be deducted from earnings to provide an additional disregard of up to £70 in respect of one child or £105 in respect of two or more children[101] (for details see CPAG's *Welfare Benefits Handbook*).

4. Notional income

For all means-tested benefits you may, in certain circumstances, be treated as having income even if you do not possess it or if you have used it up. This only applies to income which is available to you (or your family) for your own benefit.[102]

Deprivation of income in order to claim or increase benefit[103]

If you deliberately get rid of income in order to claim or increase your benefit, you are treated as though you are still in receipt of the income. The same considerations apply to deprivation of income as apply to deprivation of capital (see p203). This rule can only apply if the purpose of the deprivation is to gain benefit for yourself (or your family). It should not apply if, for example, you stop claiming invalid care allowance solely so that another person (who is not a member of your family) can become entitled to the severe disability premium[104] (see p97). However, if you do not claim a benefit which would clearly be paid if you did, it may be argued that you have failed to apply for income (see below).

A deliberate decision to 'de-retire' and give up your retirement pension (in the expectation of achieving an overall increase in benefit in the future) can come within this deprivation rule.[105]

Failing to apply for income[106]

If you fail to apply for income to which you are entitled without having to fulfil further conditions, you are deemed to have received it from the date you could have obtained it.

This does *not* include income from:

- a discretionary trust; *or*
- a trust set up from money paid as a result of a personal injury; *or*
- funds administered by a court as a result of a personal injury or the death of a parent of someone under 18; *or*
- where you are under 60, a personal pension scheme or retirement annuity. However, if you are 60 or over you are treated as receiving income in certain circumstances if you fail to purchase an annuity with the money available from such funds; *or*
- an Employment Service Rehabilitation Allowance.[107]

For IS/income-based JSA only, failure to apply for a tax credit does not count as failing to apply for income and you should argue that the same applies to HB/CTB.

For other income or benefits it must still be certain that they would be paid upon application. It may therefore be difficult to establish that there is 'no doubt' that, for example, invalid care allowance would be paid to a carer who does not wish to claim it because of the effect on another person's severe disability premium (see p97).

Income due to you which has not been paid[108]

For IS/income-based JSA only, you may be treated as possessing any income owing to you (provided that the income is due to *you*, or your family, and would be *for your own benefit*). Examples could be wages legally due but not paid, or an occupational pension payment that is due but has not been received (although that cannot apply where the reason for non-payment of an amount of occupational pension is due to insufficient funds in the pension scheme). This rule does not apply if any social security benefit, or a benefit from a European Economic Area, or a government training allowance or pension under the Job Release Scheme, has been delayed. Nor does it apply in the case of money due to you from a discretionary trust, or a trust set up from money paid as a result of a personal injury.

If you are treated as having income due to you which has not been paid, an urgent cases payment should be considered (see CPAG's *Welfare Benefits Handbook*).

Unpaid wages[109]

For IS/income-based JSA only, if you have wages due to you, but you do not yet know the exact amount or you have no proof of what they will be, you are treated as having a wage similar to that normally paid for that type of work in that area.

Income payments made to someone else on your behalf[110]

For all means-tested benefits, if money is paid to someone on your behalf (eg, the landlord for your rent) this can count as notional income. This rule applies in the same way as the rule on notional capital (see p205).

Income payments paid to you for someone else[111]

If you or a member of your family get a payment for somebody not in your family (eg, for a relative living with you), it counts as your income if you keep any of it yourself or spend it on yourself or your family. This does not apply if it is a payment from the Macfarlane Trust, the Fund, the Eileen Trust or either of the Independent Living Funds, or in the form of concessionary coal from British Coal.

Cheap or unpaid labour[112]

If you are helping another person or an organisation by doing work of a kind which would normally command a wage, or a higher wage, you are deemed to receive a wage similar to that normally paid for that kind of job in that area. This rule does not apply if *either*:

- you can show that the person cannot, in fact, afford to pay, or pay more; *or*
- you work for a charitable or voluntary organisation, or as a volunteer (or on a government work or training scheme);

and it is accepted that it is reasonable for you to give your services free of charge.

Even if you are caring for a sick or disabled relative or another person, it may be considered reasonable for her/him to pay you from her/his benefits, unless you can bring yourself within these exceptions.[113] It may, for example, be more reasonable for a close relative to provide services free of charge out of a sense of family duty, particularly if a charge would otherwise break up a relationship. Whether it is reasonable to provide care free of charge depends on the basis on which the arrangement is made, the expectations of the family members concerned, the housing arrangements and the reasons (if appropriate) why a carer gave up any paid work. The risk of a carer losing entitlement to invalid care allowance if a charge were made should also be considered as should the likelihood that a relative being looked after would no longer be able to contribute to the household expenses. If there is no realistic alternative to the carer providing services free to a relative who simply will not pay, this would also make it reasonable not to charge.[114] It may also be worth arguing that carers should not charge because they will otherwise lose their statutory right to an assessment of their needs by social services (see Chapter 2).

Sometimes it may be reasonable to do a job for free out of a sense of community duty, particularly if the job would otherwise have remained undone, and there would be no financial profit to an employer.[115]

Notes

1. General rules about income
1 **IS/HB/CTB** s136(1) SSCBA 1992
  JSA s13(2) JSA 1995
2 **IS** Reg 32(2)-(4) IS Regs;
  JSA Reg 97(2)-(4) JSA Regs
3 **HB** Reg 22(1) HB Regs
  CTB Reg 14(1) CTB Regs
4 **HB** Regs 23(1) and 25(2) HB Regs
  CTB Regs 15(1) and 17(2) CTB Regs

2. Income other than earnings
5 **IS** Reg 40 and Sch 9 para 1 IS Regs;
  JSA Reg 103(1) and (2) and Sch 7 para 1 JSA Regs;
  HB Reg 33 and Sch 4 para 1 HB Regs;
  CTB Reg 24 and Sch 4 para 1 CTB Regs;
6 **HB** Reg 26 HB Regs
  CTB Reg 18 CTB Regs

7 **IS** Sch 9 para 24 IS Regs
  JSA Sch 7 para 25 JSA Regs
  HB Sch 4 para 32 HB Regs
  CTB Sch 4 para 33 CTB Regs
8 s74(S) SSAA 1992
9 **IS** Sch 10 para 7 IS Regs
  JSA Sch 8 para 12(b) JSA Regs
  HB Sch 5 para 8 HB Regs
  CTB Sch 5 para 8 CTB Regs
10 **IS** Sch 9 para 9 IS Regs
  JSA Sch 7 para 10 JSA Regs
  HB Sch paras 5 and 8 HB Regs
  CTB Sch 4 paras 5 and 8 CTB Regs
11 **IS** Sch 9 para 6 IS Regs
  JSA Sch 7 para 7 JSA Regs
  HB Sch 4 para 5 HB Regs
  CTB Sch 4 para 5 CTB Regs

12 **IS** Sch 9 para 8 IS Regs
JSA Sch 7 para 9 JSA Regs
HB Sch 4 para 7 HB Regs
CTB Sch 4 para 7 CTB Regs
13 **IS** Sch 9 paras 7 and 8 IS Regs
JSA Sch 7 paras 8 and 9 JSA Regs
HB Sch 4 paras 6 and 7 HB Regs
CTB Sch 4 paras 6 and 7 CTB Regs
14 **IS** Sch 9 para 33 IS Regs
JSA Sch 7 para 35 JSA Regs
HB Sch 4 para 31 HB Regs
CTB Sch 4 para 32 CTB Regs
15 **IS** Sch 9 para 31 IS Regs
JSA Sch 7 para 33 and Sch 8 para 23
JSA Regs
HB Sch 4 para 30 HB Regs
CTB Sch 4 para 31 CTB Regs
16 **IS** Sch 10 para 18 IS Regs
JSA Sch 8 para 23 JSA Regs
HB Sch 5 para 19 HB Regs
CTB Sch 5 para 19 CTB Regs
17 **IS** Sch 9 para 47 IS Regs
JSA Sch 7 para 46 JSA Regs
HB Sch 4 para 43 HB Regs
CTB Sch 4 para 42 CTB Regs
18 **IS** Sch 9 paras 54-56 IS Regs
JSA Sch 7 paras 53-55 JSA Regs
HB Sch 4 paras 53-55 HB Regs
CTB Sch 4 paras 52-54 CTB Regs
19 **IS** Sch 9 para 38 IS Regs
JSA Sch 7 para 40 JSA Regs
HB Sch 4 para 37 HB Regs
CTB Sch 4 para 39 CTB Regs
20 **IS** Sch 9 para 53 IS Regs
JSA Sch 7 para 52 JSA Regs
HB Sch 4 para 52 HB Regs
CTB Sch 4 para 51 CTB Regs
21 **IS** Sch 9 para 46 IS Regs
JSA Sch 7 para 45 JSA Regs
HB Sch 4 para 41 HB Regs
CTB Sch 4 para 41 CTB Regs
22 **HB** Sch 4 para 50 HB Regs
CTB Sch 4 para 49 CTB Regs
23 **IS** Sch 9 paras 5, 40-42, 45 and 52 IS
Regs
JSA Sch 7 paras 6, 42, 44 and 51 JSA
Regs
HB Sch 4 paras 4, 35, 36, 40, 48 and
51 HB Regs
CTB Sch 4 paras 4, 36-38, 47 and 50
CTB Regs
24 CIS/276/1998

25 **IS** Sch 9 para 16 IS Regs
JSA Sch 7 para 17 JSA Regs
HB Sch 4 para 14 HB Regs
CTB Sch 4 para 14 CTB Regs
26 **IS** Sch 9 para 36 IS Regs
JSA Sch 7 para 38 JSA Regs
HB Sch 4 para 33 HB Regs
CTB Sch 4 para 34 CTB Regs
27 ss134(8) and 139(6) SSAA 1992; regs
7 and 8 IRBS (Amdt 2) Regs
28 R(IS) 4/94; *R v Donaster MBC ex parte
Boulton* [1992] 25 HLR 195; CIS/
12175/1996; paras 33490 – 33495
AOG
29 **IS** Reg 48(9) IS Regs
JSA Reg 110(9) JSA Regs
30 **IS** Sch 9 paras 15 and 15A IS Regs
JSA Sch 7 paras 15 and 16 JSA Regs
HB Sch 4 para 13 HB Regs
CTB Sch 4 para 13 CTB Regs
31 **IS** Sch 9 paras 15(4) and 36 IS Regs
JSA Sch 7 paras 15(4) and 38 JSA Regs
HB Sch 4 paras 13(4) and 33 HB Regs
CTB Sch 4 paras 13(4) and 34 CTB
Regs
32 HB/CTB Circular A17/97
33 **IS** Sch 9 para 21 IS Regs
JSA Sch 7 para 15 JSA Regs
HB Sch 4 para 21 HB Regs
CTB Sch 4 para 22 CTB Regs
34 *R v Doncaster MBC ex parte Boulton*
[1992] 25 HLR 195; R(IS) 4/94
35 **IS** para 31047 AOG
JSA para 33496 AOG
HB/CTB para C3.90 GM
36 **IS** Reg 48(10)(c) and Sch 10 para 22
IS Regs
JSA Sch 7 para 41(1) JSA Regs
HB Sch 4 para 34 HB Regs
CTB Sch 4 para 35 CTB Regs
37 **IS** Sch 9 para 39 IS Regs
JSA Sch 7 para 41(2) JSA Regs
HB Sch 4 para 34 HB Regs
CTB Sch 4 para 35 CTB Regs
38 **IS** Sch 9 para 22(1) IS Regs
JSA Sch 7 para 23(2) JSA Regs
HB Sch 4 para 15(1) HB Regs
CTB Sch 4 para 15(1) CTB Regs
39 **IS** Reg 48(4) IS Regs
JSA Reg 110(4) JSA Regs
HB Reg 40(4) HB Regs
CTB Reg 31(4) CTB Regs

40 **IS** Sch 9 para 22(1) IS Regs
JSA Sch 7 para 23(2) JSA Regs
HB Sch 4 para 15(1) HB Regs
CTB Sch 4 para 15(1) CTB Regs
41 CFC/13/1993
42 **IS** Sch 9 para 22(2) IS Regs
JSA Sch 7 para 23(2) and (3) JSA Regs
HB Sch 4 para 15(2) HB Regs
CTB Sch 4 para 15(2) CTB Regs
43 **IS** Reg 53 IS Regs
JSA Reg 116 JSA Regs
HB Reg 45 HB Regs
CTB Reg 37 CTB Regs
44 **IS** Reg 41(1) IS Regs
JSA Reg 104(1) JSA Regs
HB Reg 34(1) HB Regs
CTB Reg 25(1) CTB Regs
45 **IS** Reg 29(2)(a) IS Regs
JSA Reg 94(2)(a) JSA Regs
HB Reg 25 HB Regs
CTB Reg 17 CTB Regs
46 **IS** Reg 41(2) IS Regs
JSA Reg 104(2) JSA Regs
HB Reg 34(2) HB Regs
CTB Reg 25(2) CTB Regs
47 **IS** Sch 10 para 20 IS Regs
JSA Sch 8 para 25 JSA Regs
HB Sch 5 para 21 HB Regs
CTB Sch 5 para 21 CTB Regs
48 *R v SBC ex parte Singer* [1973] 1 All ER
931; *R v Oxford County Council ex
parte Jack* [1984] 17 HLR 419; *R v West
Dorset DC ex parte Poupard* [1988] 20
HLR 295; para C3.118 GM
49 paras C2.09(xix) and 3.118 GM
50 *R v West Dorset DC ex parte Poupard*
[1988] 20 HLR 295
51 **IS** Sch 9 para 19 IS Regs
JSA Sch 7 para 20 JSA Regs
HB Sch 4 para 20 HB Regs
CTB Sch 4 para 20 CTB Regs
52 **IS** Sch 9 para 18 IS Regs
JSA Sch 7 para 19 JSA Regs
HB Sch 4 para 19 HB Regs
CTB Sch 4 para 19 CTB Regs
53 **IS** Sch 9 para 20 IS Regs
JSA Sch 7 para 19 JSA Regs
HB Sch 4 para 19 HB Regs
CTB Sch 4 para 19 CTB Regs

54 Definition of 'board and lodging
accommodation'
IS Reg 2(1) IS Regs
JSA Reg 1(3) JSA Regs
HB Sch 4 para 42(2) HB Regs
CTB Sch 4 para 21(2) CTB Regs
55 CIS/13059/1996
56 **IS** Sch 9 para 58 IS Regs
JSA Sch 7 para 56 JSA Regs
HB Sch 4 para 67 HB Regs
CTB Sch 4 para 62 CTB Regs
57 *CAO v Palfrey and Others, The Times*,
17 February 1995
IS Reg 48(4) IS Regs
JSA Reg 110 (4) JSA Regs
HB Reg 40(4) HB Regs
CTB Reg 31(4) CTB Regs
58 CIS/25/1989; CIS/563/1991; CIS/85/
1992 (Palfrey)
59 **IS** Reg 40(4) and Sch 9 para 15B IS
Regs
JSA Regs 103(6) and 98(2)(e) JSA
Regs
HB Reg 33(4) HB Regs
CTB Reg 24(5) CTB Regs
All Definition of 'occupational
pension' in reg 2(1) of each of those
regs
60 **IS** Reg 41(2) and Sch 9 para 17 IS
Regs
JSA Reg 104(2) and Sch 7 para 18 JSA
Regs
HB Reg 34(2) and Sch 4 para 16 HB
Regs
CTB Reg 25(2) and Sch 4 para 16 CTB
Regs
61 **IS** Reg 42(7) and Sch 9 para 64 IS
Regs
JSA Reg 105(11) and Sch 7 para ? JSA
Regs
62 **IS** Sch 9 para 15A IS Regs
JSA Sch 7 para 16 JSA Regs
63 **IS** Sch 9 para 30(1)(e) IS Regs
JSA Sch 7 para 31(1)(e) JSA Regs
64 **IS** Sch 9 para 30A IS Regs
JSA Sch 7 para 32 JSA Regs
65 **IS** Sch 9 para 58 IS Regs
JSA Sch 7 para 56 JSA Regs
HB Sch 4 para 67 HB Regs
CTB Sch 4 para 62 CTB Regs
66 **IS** Sch 9 para 27 IS Regs
JSA Sch 7 para 28 JSA Regs
HB Sch 4 para 25 HB Regs
CTB Sch 4 para 26 CTB Regs

67 **IS** Sch 9 para 28 IS Regs
JSA Sch 7 para 29 JSA Regs
HB Sch 4 para 26 HB Regs
CTB Sch 4 para 27 CTB Regs
68 **IS** Sch 9 para 11 IS Regs
JSA Sch 7 para 12 JSA Regs
HB Sch 4 para 10 HB Regs
CTB Sch 4 para 10 CTB Regs
69 **IS** Sch 9 para 29 IS Regs; para 33240
AOG
JSA Sch 7 para 30 JSA Regs
70 **HB** Sch 4 para 28 HB Regs
CTB Sch 4 para 29 CTB Regs
71 **IS** Sch 9 para 30ZA IS Regs
JSA Sch 7 para 31A JSA Regs
72 **IS** Sch 9 para 30 IS Regs
JSA Sch 7 para 31 JSA Regs
73 **IS** Sch 9 para 2 IS Regs
JSA Sch 7 para 2 JSA Regs
HB Sch 4 para 2 HB Regs
CTB Sch4 para2 CTB Regs
74 **IS** Sch 9 para 21 IS Regs
JSA Sch 7 para 22 JSA Regs
HB Sch 4 para 21 HB Regs
CTB Sch 4 para 22 CTB Regs
75 Para C3.73(xiii) GM
76 See para 63596 on related provisions
for child benefits
77 **IS** Sch 9 para 43 IS Regs
JSA Sch 7 para 43 JSA Regs
HB Sch 4 para 38 HB Regs
CTB Sch4 para 40 CTB Regs
78 **IS** Sch 9 para 10 IS Regs
JSA Sch 7 para 11 JSA Regs
HB Sch 4 para 9 HB Regs
CTB Sch 4 para 9 CTB Regs
79 **IS** Sch 9 para 23 IS Regs
JSA Sch 7 para 24 JSA Regs
HB Sch 4 para 22 HB Regs
CTB Sch 4 para 23 CTB Regs
80 **IS** Sch 9 para 48 IS Regs
JSA Sch 7 para 47 JSA Regs
HB Sch 4 para 44 HB Regs
CTB Sch 4 para 43 CTB Regs
81 **IS** Sch 9 para 50 IS Regs
JSA Sch 7 para 49 JSA Regs
HB Sch 4 para 46 HB Regs
CTB Sch 4 para 45 CTB Regs

82 **IS** Reg 48(2) IS Regs
JSA Reg 110(2) JSA Regs
HB Reg 40(2) HB Regs
CTB Reg 31(2) CTB Regs
83 **HB** Sch 4 paras 13(3) and 47 HB Regs
CTB Sch 4 paras 13(3) and 46 CTB
Regs

3. Earnings from employment and self-employment

84 **IS** Reg 38(9) IS Regs
JSA Reg 101(10) JSA Regs
HB Reg 31(9) HB Regs
CTB Reg 22(9) CTB Regs
85 *Parsons v Hogg* [1985] 2 All ER 897,
CA, appendix to R(FIS) 4/85; R(FC) 1/
90
86 **IS** Reg 36(3) IS Regs
JSA Reg 99(1) and (4) JSA Regs
HB Reg 29(3) HB Regs
CTB Reg 20(3) CTB Regs
87 **IS** Regs 35, 40(4) and 48(3) IS Regs
JSA Regs 98, 103 and 110 JSA Regs
HB Regs 28(1) and 40(3) HB Regs
CTB Regs 19(1) and 31(3) CTB Regs
88 **IS** Regs 35(2) and 48(5) and Sch 9
para 21 IS Regs
JSA Regs 98(2) and 110(5) and Sch 7
para 22 JSA Regs
HB Regs 28(2) and 40(5) and Sch 4
para 21 HB Regs
CTB Regs 19(2) and 31(5) and Sch 4
para 22 CTB Regs
89 **IS** Reg 38(3) IS Regs
JSA Reg 101(4) JSA Regs
HB Reg 31(3) HB Regs
CTB Reg 22(3) CTB Regs
90 **IS** Reg 38 IS Regs
JSA Reg 101 JSA regs
HB Reg 31 HB Regs
CTB Reg 22 CTB Regs
91 **HB** Sch 3 para 4 HB Regs
CTB Sch 3 para 4 CTB Regs
92 **IS** Sch 8 para 5 IS Regs
JSA Sch 6 para 6 JSA Regs
93 **IS** Sch 8 para 4(2) IS Regs
JSA Sch 6 para 5 JSA Regs
HB Sch 3 para 3(2) HB Regs
CTB Sch 3 para 3(2) CTB Regs
94 **IS** Sch 8 paras 4(4) and (7) IS Regs
JSA Sch 6 paras 5 and 21 and reg
87(7) JSA Regs
HB Sch 3 para 3(4) HB Regs
CTB Sch 3 para 3(4) CTB Regs

95 **IS** Sch 8 para 4(3) and (5) IS Regs
JSA Sch 6 para 5(3) and (5) JSA Regs
HB Sch 3 para 3(3) and (5) HB Regs
CTB Sch 3 para 3(3) and (5) CTB Regs

96 **IS** Sch 8 para 4(6) IS Regs
JSA Sch 6 para 5(6) JSA Regs
HB Sch 3 para 3(6) HB Regs
CTB Sch 3 para 3(6) CTB Regs

97 **IS** Sch 8 paras 6A and 6B IS Regs
JSA Sch 6 paras 7 and 8 JSA Regs
HB Sch 3 paras 4A and 4B HB Regs
CTB Sch 3 paras 4A and 4B CTB Regs

98 **IS** Sch 8 para 7 IS Regs
JSA Sch 6 paras 9 and 10 JSA Regs
HB Sch 3 para 6 HB Regs
CTB Sch 3 para 6 CTB Regs

99 **IS** Sch 8 paras 6 and 9 IS Regs
JSA Sch 6 paras 11 and 12 JSA Regs
HB Sch 3 paras 5 and 8 HB Regs
CTB Sch 4 paras 5 and 8 CTB Regs

100 **HB** Sch 3 para 16 HB Regs
CTB Sch 3 para 16 CTB Regs

101 **HB** Reg 21A HB Regs
CTB Reg 13A CTB Regs

4. Notional income

102 CIS/15052/1996, para 11

103 **IS** Reg 42(1) IS Regs
JSA Reg 105(1) JSA Regs
HB Reg 35(1) HB Regs
CTB Reg 26(1) CTB Regs

104 Paras 33608-16 AOG; CIS/15052/1996

105 CSIS/57/1992

106 **IS** Reg 42(2) IS Regs
JSA Reg 105(2) JSA Regs
HB Reg 35(2) HB Regs
CTB Reg 26(2) CTB Regs

107 **IS** Reg 42(2A) IS Regs
JSA Reg 105(3) JSA Regs
HB Reg 35(2A) HB Regs
CTB Reg 26(2A) CTB Regs

108 **IS** Reg 42(3) IS Regs
JSA Reg 105(6) JSA Regs

109 **IS** Reg 42(5) IS Regs
JSA Reg 105(12) JSA Regs

110 **IS** Reg 42(4)(a)(ii), (4A) and (9) IS Regs
JSA Reg 105(10)(a)(ii) JSA Regs
HB Reg 35(3)(a) and (8) HB Regs
CTB Reg 26(3)(a) and (8) CTB Regs

111 **IS** Reg 42(4)(b) IS Regs
JSA Reg 105(10)(b) JSA Regs
HB Reg 35(3)(b) HB Regs
CTB Reg 26(3)(b) CTB Regs

112 CIS/191/1991
IS Reg 42(6) IS Regs
JSA Reg 105(13) JSA Regs
HB Reg 35(5) HB Regs
CTB Reg 26(5) CTB Regs

113 *Sharrock v CAO* (CA) 26 March 1991;
CIS/93/1991

114 CIS/93/1991; CIS/422/1992; CIS/701/1994

115 CIS/147/1993

7

Chapter 7

Capital and property – social security benefits

This chapter explains how capital and property affect entitlement to income support, income-based jobseeker's allowance, housing benefit and council tax benefit. It covers:
1. The capital limit (p191)
2. Whose capital counts (p191)
3. What counts as capital (p192)
4. Disregarded capital (p195)
5. How capital is valued (p200)
6. Notional capital (p202)

Your entitlement to income support (IS – see p93), income-based jobseeker's allowance (JSA – see p125), housing benefit (HB – see p102) and council tax benefit (CTB – see p111), and the amount of benefit you receive, depends on the value of any property and other capital assets you have. Some of your capital and property may be completely ignored, or partially ignored, or counted in full. Some capital may be treated as income (see p174) and some income may be treated as capital (see p195). You may also be treated as having some capital or property which you do not actually have (see p202). The rules on the treatment of your capital and property are very similar for IS, income-based JSA, HB and CTB. They are also similar whether you are living in your own home or in a care home, although there are some significant differences. Where there are differences, these are indicated.

For the treatment of capital and property on claims for tax credits (formerly family credit and disability working allowance – see pp115 and 125) see CPAG's *Welfare Benefits Handbook*.

There are no rules on the treatment of capital and property for non-means-tested benefits (see p70) as they are not affected capital assets.

There are many similarities but also some very significant differences, between the way property and capital is treated for benefit purposes and the way it is treated by social services if they are assisting you with the costs of your care home. For details see Chapter 14.

1. **The capital limit**

Different capital limits apply depending on whether you are living at home or whether you are living permanently in a care home.

If you live at home you are not entitled to IS/income-based JSA if you have capital worth over £8,000, and you are not entitled to HB/CTB if you have capital over £16,000.[1] For IS/income-based JSA/HB/CTB, capital worth up to £3,000 is completely ignored, but if you have between £3,000.01 and £8,000 (IS/income-based JSA) or £16,000 (HB/CTB), you may still be entitled to benefit but some income from your capital is assumed.[2] That is known as tariff income (see p174).

For IS/income-based JSA, higher limits apply if you live permanently in:[3]

- a residential care or a nursing home and in either case you are given board and personal care because of old age, disablement, past or present dependence on alcohol or drugs, or past or present mental disorder; *or*
- a local authority care home whether board is provided or not; *or*
- an Abbeyfield Society home (see p156); *or*
- a home provided under the Polish Resettlement Act in which you are receiving personal care because of old age, disablement, past or present dependence on alcohol or drugs, past or present mental disorder, or a terminal illness.

You are treated as living permanently in one of these homes in spite of periods of absence of up to 13 weeks (or up to 52 weeks if you are over pensionable age or, in some cases, you were getting supplementary benefit as a residential care home boarder before 27 July 1987).

For HB, the higher limits apply if you live in a care home for which HB is payable[4] (see Chapter 5).

If the higher limits apply, capital worth up to £10,000 is completely ignored, and tariff income starts to apply on capital between £10,000.01 and £16,000. The upper limit, above which benefit is no longer payable at all, is £16,000 for IS/income-based JSA as well as HB.

2. **Whose capital counts**

Your partner's capital is added to yours and calculated in the same way as if it were yours.[5] Note that if you are living in a care home, unless you are only in the home on a temporary basis, you will not usually be treated as living in the same household as a partner (see p96) and your partner's capital will therefore be ignored.

Special rules apply to the treatment of any capital of a dependent child (see CPAG's *Welfare Benefits Handbook*).

3. **What counts as capital**

The term 'capital' is not defined. In general, it means lump sum or one-off payments rather than a series of payments.[6] It includes savings, property and redundancy payments. Capital payments can normally be distinguished from income because they are not payable in respect of any specified period or periods, and they do not form nor are intended to form part of a regular series of payments[7] (although capital can be paid by instalments). However, some capital is treated as income (see p174), and some income is treated as capital (see p173).

Savings

Your savings (eg, cash you have at home or in a bank or building society, premium bonds, stocks and shares and unit trusts) generally count as capital.

Your savings from past earnings can only be treated as capital when all relevant debts, including tax liabilities, have been deducted.[8] Savings from other past income (including social security benefits) will also be treated as capital (although payments of arrears of certain benefits may be disregarded for certain periods – see p198). There is no provision for disregarding money put aside to pay bills.[9] If you have savings close to the capital limit it may be best to pay bills (eg, gas, electricity, telephone) as soon as possible or by standing order etc, to prevent your capital going over the limit.

Fixed-term investments

Capital held in fixed-term investments counts. However, if it is presently unobtainable it may have little or no value (but see p201 for jointly held capital). If you can sell your interest, or raise a loan through a reputable bank using the asset as security, or otherwise convert the investment into a realisable form, its value counts. If it takes time to produce evidence about the nature and value of the investment, you may be able to get an interim payment of HB,[10] or a crisis loan from the social fund (see p117).

Property and land

Any property or land which you own counts as capital, although many types of property are disregarded (see p195).

Loans

A loan usually counts as money you possess. However, you should not be treated as having any capital from:
- a loan granted on condition that you only use the interest but do not touch the capital because the capital element has never been at your disposal;[11]

- money paid to you to be used for a particular purpose on condition that the money must be returned if not used in that way;[12]
- a property you have bought on behalf of someone else who is paying the mortgage;[13]
- money you are holding in a bank account on behalf of someone else and which has to be returned to them at a future date.[14]

For HB/CTB, some loans might be treated as income even if it is paid as a lump sum (see p174).

Trusts

A trust is a way of owning an asset. In theory, the asset is split into two notional parts: the legal title owned by the trustee, and the beneficial interest owned by the beneficiary. A trustee can never have use of the asset, only the responsibility of looking after it. An adult beneficiary, on the other hand, can ask for the asset at any time. Anything can be held on trust – eg, money, houses or shares.

Beneficiaries of trusts

If you are the adult beneficiary of:
- a *non-discretionary trust*, you can obtain the asset from the trustee at any time and therefore effectively own it, so it counts as your capital;
- a *discretionary trust*, the asset itself does not normally count as your capital because you cannot demand payments (of either income or capital) which are only made at the discretion of the trustee within the terms of the trust;
- a trust which gives you the *right to receive payments in the future* (eg, on reaching the age of 25), this right has a present capital value, unless it is disregarded (see p198);
- a *life interest* (or, in Scotland, a liferent) only in an asset (ie, you have the right to enjoy the asset in your life time but the asset will pass on to someone else when you die), the value of your interest is disregarded,[15] but not the income itself if you get any.

If the beneficiary is under 18, even with a non-discretionary trust s/he has no right to payment until s/he is 18 (or later if that is what the trust stipulates). Her/his interest may nevertheless have a present value.[16]

Trustees

If you hold an asset as a trustee, it is not part of your capital. You are only a trustee either if someone gives you an asset on the express condition that you hold it for someone else (or use it for their benefit), or if you have expressed the clearest intention that your own asset is for someone else's benefit, and renounced its use for yourself[17] (assets other than money may need to be transferred in a particular way to the trust).

It is not enough to only *intend* to give someone an asset. However, in the case of property and land, proprietary estoppel may apply. This means that if you lead someone to believe that you are transferring your interest in some property to them, but fail to do so (eg, it is never properly conveyed), and they act on the belief that they have ownership (eg, they improve or repair it, or take on a mortgage), it would then be unfair on them were they to lose out if you insisted that you were still the owner.[18] In this case, you can argue the capital asset has been transferred to them, and you are like a trustee. Thus you can insist that it is not your capital asset, but theirs, when claiming benefit.

If money (or another asset) is given to you to be used for a special purpose, it may be possible to argue that it should not count as your capital. This is called a purpose trust.[19]

Trust funds from personal injury compensation

The value of any trust fund is ignored if it has been set up out of money paid because of a personal injury (either to you or a member of your family). Personal injuries compensation held by the Court of Protection (because the injured person in incapable of managing her/his own affairs) and administered by that Court and/or the Public Trustee is treated in the same way (as are 'infant funds in court' in respect of injuries to minors or the death of a parent).[20] It is not necessary for the trust to be set up by a formal deed so long as the beneficiary has no direct access to the funds.

'Personal injury' includes not only accidental and criminal injuries, but also any disease and injury suffered as a result of a disease.

Note that the notional income and capital rules (see pp182 and 202) cannot apply to personal injury compensation paid into trusts (or court funds) even if some time has passed before they are paid in. However, if there is no trust, or until one can be set up, the whole of the compensation counts as capital, even if the money is held by your solicitor.[21]

Payments from trust funds

Any payments made to you from trust funds or court funds (see above) may count in full as income or capital, depending on the nature of the payment.[22] However, trustees may have a discretion to:

- allow such funds to be used to purchase items that would normally be disregarded as capital, such as personal possessions (see p199) – eg, a wheelchair, car, or new furniture; *or*
- to arrange payments that would normally be disregarded as income – eg, ineligible housing costs (see p99).

Similarly, they may have discretion to clear debts or pay for a holiday, leisure items or educational or medical needs. See p172 for the treatment of voluntary payments and pp184 and 206 for the treatment of payments made to third parties.

Income treated as capital

Certain payments which appear to be income are nevertheless treated as capital. These are:[23]

- income from capital (eg, interest on a building society account) and income from rents on properties let to tenants (see p175). However, income from disregarded property listed on p195 (eg, a home you are trying to sell or which is occupied by elderly relatives) and income from business assets or personal injury trusts counts as income not capital;
- irregular one-off charitable payments;
- an advance of earnings or loan from your employer;
- holiday pay which is not payable until more than four weeks after your job ends or is interrupted;
- income tax refunds;
- certain lump sum payments to part-time firefighters or lifeboat crew members or auxiliary coastguards or members of the Territorial Army;
- for IS/income-based JSA, a discharge grant on release from prison.

Any income treated as capital is disregarded as income.[24]

4. **Disregarded capital**

Your home

If you own the home you normally live in, its value is ignored. This also applies if you are living away from your home temporarily – eg, because you are in a care home. Your home includes any garage, garden, outbuildings and land, together with any premises that you do not occupy as your home but which it is impractical or unreasonable to sell separately – eg, croft land. If you own more than one property only the value of the one normally occupied is disregarded under this rule.[25]

Even if you do not live in it, the value of the property can be disregarded during temporary absences and in the following circumstances:[26]

- **If you have left your former home following a marriage or relationship breakdown**, the value of the property is ignored for six months from the date you left, or longer if any of the steps below are taken. For HB/CTB, if it is occupied by your former partner who is a lone parent, its value is ignored as long as s/he lives there.

- **If you have sought legal advice or have started legal proceedings in order to occupy property** as your home, its value is ignored for six months from the date you first took either of these steps, or longer if it is reasonable.

- **If you are taking reasonable steps to dispose of any property**, its value is ignored for six months from the date you *first* took such steps, or longer if it is reasonable. This may include a period before you claimed benefit.[27] 'Property' here may include land on its own, even if there are no buildings on it.[28] The test for what constitutes 'reasonable steps' is an objective one. Putting the property in the hands of an estate agent or getting in touch with a prospective purchaser should count,[29] but any period when the house is advertised at an unrealistic sale price should not.[30] If you need longer to dispose of the property, the disregard can continue for years if it is reasonable – eg, where a husband or wife attempts to realise their share in a former matrimonial home but the court orders that it should not be sold (eg, until a child reaches a certain age).

- **If you sell your home** and intend to use the money from the sale to buy another home, the capital is ignored for six months from the date of sale, or longer if it is reasonable. This also applies even if you do not actually own the home but, for a price, you surrender your tenancy rights to a landlord.[31] You do not need to have decided within the six months to buy a *particular* property. It is sufficient if you intend to use the proceeds to buy *some* other home, although your intention must involve more than a mere hope or aspiration. There must be an element of certainty which may be shown by evidence of a practical commitment to another purchase, although this need not involve any binding obligation.[32] If you intend to use only part of the proceeds of the sale to buy another home, only that part is disregarded even if, for example, you have put the rest of the money aside to renovate your new home.[33]

- **If you have acquired a house or flat for occupation** as your home but have not yet moved in, its value is ignored if you intend to live there within six months. The value can be ignored for longer if it is reasonable.

- **If your home is damaged or you lose it altogether**, any payment, including compensation, which you intend to use for its repair, or for acquiring another home, is ignored for six months, or longer if it is reasonable.

- **If you have taken out a loan or been given money for the express purpose of essential repairs and improvements** to your home, it is ignored for six months, or longer if it is reasonable. If it is a condition of the loan that the loan must be returned if the improvements are not carried out, you should argue that it should be ignored altogether.

- **If you have deposited money with a housing association as a condition of occupying your home**, this is ignored indefinitely. If money deposited for this purpose is now to be used to buy another home, this is ignored for six months, or longer if reasonable, in order to allow you to complete the purchase.

- **Grants made to local authority tenants to buy a home or do repairs/ alterations** to it can also be ignored for six months, or longer if reasonable, to allow completion of the purchase of the repairs/alterations.

When considering whether to increase the period of any disregard, all the circumstances should be considered, especially your (and your family's) personal circumstances, any efforts made by you to use or dispose of the home[34] (if relevant) and the general state of the market (if relevant). In practice, periods of around 18 months are not considered unusual.

It is possible for property to be ignored under more than one of the above disregards in succession.[35]

Some income generated from property which is disregarded is ignored (see p175).

For the treatment of jointly owned property see p201.

For the different rules on the treatment of unoccupied properties in financial assessments by social services, see Chapter 14.

The home of a partner or relative

The value of a house is also ignored if it is occupied wholly or partly as their home by:[36]

- your partner, or a relative of yours, or any member of your family, provided that (in either case) s/he is aged 60 or over or is incapacitated; *or*
- your former partner from whom you are not estranged or divorced; *or*
- for HB/CTB only, your former partner from whom you are estranged or divorced if s/he is a lone parent.

'Partner' means your husband or wife or person with whom you are (or, in the case of a former partner, have been) living together as husband and wife.[37]

'Incapacitated' is not defined. Guidance suggests that it refers to someone who is getting or would get an incapacity or disability benefit,[38] but you should argue for a broader interpretation, if necessary.

'Relative' includes: a parent, son, daughter, step-parent/son/daughter, or parent/son/daughter-in-law; brother or sister; or a partner of any of these people; or a grandparent or grandchild, uncle, aunt, nephew or niece.[39] It also includes half-brothers and sisters and adopted children.[40]

For the treatment of jointly owned property see p201.

For the different rules on the treatment of occupied properties in financial assessments by social services see Chapter 14.

Future interests in property

A future interest in most kinds of property is ignored.[41] A future interest is one which will only revert to you, or become yours for the first time, when some future event occurs. An example of a future interest is where someone else has a life interest (see p193) in a fund and you are only entitled after that person has died.

However, this does not include a freehold or leasehold interest in property which has been let by you to tenants. If you did not let the property to the tenant (eg, because the tenancy was entered into before you bought the property), then your interest in the property should be ignored as a future interest in the normal way. It has been suggested that if you grant someone an 'irrevocable licence' to occupy property, your interest in that property is a future one and should be ignored.[42]

The right to receive a payment in the future

If you know you will receive a payment in the future, you could sell your right to that payment at any time so it has a market value and therefore counts as capital. The value of this is ignored, however, where it is a right to receive:[43]

- income under a life interest (or, in Scotland, a liferent);
- any earnings or income which are ignored because they are frozen abroad;
- any outstanding instalments where capital is being paid by instalments;
- an occupational or personal pension;
- any rent if your are not the freeholder or leaseholder;
- any payment under an annuity;
- any payment under a trust fund that is disregarded (see p193).

As soon as any of these payments are actually received, they may count in full as income (see p173).

Social security and other state benefits

Arrears of certain social security benefits are ignored for 52 weeks after they have been paid.[44] These are IS/income-based JSA/HB/CTB, attendance allowance, disability living allowance, industrial injuries benefit mobility supplement, and tax credits (as well as the benefits these replaced – ie, supplementary benefit, mobility allowance, family income supplement, family credit and disability working allowance), or concessionary payments made instead of these, and certain war widows' payments.

Refunds on council tax (or, formerly, community charge) liabilities, fares to hospital and payments to assist prison visits are also ignored for 52 weeks.[45]

Social fund payments are ignored indefinitely.[46]

Miscellaneous disregarded capital

- All **personal possessions**, including items such as jewellery, furniture or a car, are ignored unless you have bought them in order to be able to claim or get more benefit,[47] in which case the sale value, rather than the purchase price, is counted as actual capital, and the difference is treated as notional capital[48] (see p202). Compensation for damage to, or the loss of, any personal possessions, which is to be used for their repair or replacement is ignored for six months, or longer if reasonable.[49]
- If you are self-employed, your **business assets** are ignored for as long as you continue to work in that business. If you stop working in the business, you are allowed a reasonable time to sell the assets without their value affecting your benefit. It is sometimes difficult to distinguish between personal and business assets. The test is whether the assets are 'part of the fund employed and risked in the business'.[50]Letting out a single house to tenants does not constitute a business.[51]
- **Tax rebates** for the tax relief on interest on a mortgage or loan obtained for buying your home or carrying out repairs or improvements are ignored.[52]
- The value of a fund held under a **personal pension scheme or retirement annuity contract** is ignored.[53]
- The surrender value of any **life assurance or endowment policy or annuity** is ignored. This applies even if the life assurance aspect of a policy is not the sole or even the main aspect[54] (although the other features of any policy may still be considered under the actual or notional income and capital rules – see pp182 and 202). Any payments under the annuity count as income (but see p175 for when these are ignored).
- **Payments by social services for children in need**[55] **are ignored.**
- **Charitable payments** in kind are ignored,[56] as are all payments from the Macfarlane Trust, the Fund, the Eileen Trust and either of the Independent Living Funds[57] (see p143) and certain payments from money which originally came from them (the rules are the same as for income – see p173).
- **Payments to jurors and witnesses** for attending court are ignored, except for payments for loss of earnings or benefit.[58]
- There are special rules on the treatment of **payments by the Employment Service** – eg, under the New Deal programme (see CPAG's *Welfare Benefits Handbook*).
- **Payments in other currencies** are taken into account after disregarding bank charges or commission payable on conversion to sterling.[59]
- Victoria or George Cross payments are ignored.[60]

Capital treated as income

Some payments which appear to be capital are nevertheless treated instead as income (see p174). Any payments treated as income are ignored as capital.[61]

5. **How capital is valued**

All your capital (except for national savings certificates, shares, unit trusts and overseas assets – see below) is valued at its current market or surrender value, less expenses involved in the sale and any debts secured on it.

The **market value** means the amount of money you could raise by selling it or raising a loan against it.[62] The test is the price that would be paid by a willing buyer to a willing seller on a particular date[63]. So if an asset is difficult, or impossible, to realise, its market value should be heavily discounted, or even nil.[64]

In the case of a house, an estate agent's figure for a quick sale is a more appropriate valuation that the district valuer's figure for a sale within three months.[65]

It is not uncommon for an unrealistic assessment to be made of the value of your capital. If you disagree with any decision you should consider challenging it.

If there would be **expenses** involved in selling your capital, 10 per cent is deducted from its value for the cost of sale.[66] This applies until it is actually sold, when the net proceeds, after the actual expenses incurred (subject to the notional capital rules), will count in full.

Deductions are made from the gross value of your capital for any **mortgage or debt secured on the capital**.[67] Where a single mortgage is secured on a house and land and the value of the house is disregarded for benefit purposes, the whole of the mortgage can be deducted when calculating the value of the land.[68]

Unsecured debts (eg, tax liabilities) cannot be offset against the value of your capital,[69] but your capital may be reduced once you have paid off your debts (subject to the notional capital rules).

For the valuation of jointly owned property see p201.

National savings certificates, shares, unit trusts and overseas assets

These are valued in the following way:
- **National savings certificates** are attributed with the value they would have had if purchased on the last day of issue before the 1 July before your claim is decided or benefit awarded (whichever is the earlier), or any subsequent review.[70]
- **Shares** are valued at their current market value (based on a quarter of the difference between the bid price and offer price) less 10 per cent for the cost of sale and after deducting any lien held by brokers for sums owed in the cost of acquisition and commission.[71]

- **Unit trusts** are valued on the basis of the bid price quoted in newspapers (no deduction is allowed for the cost of sale because this is already included in the bid price).[72]
- **Overseas assets**[73] are valued (less 10 per cent if there are expenses for the sale, and any debts secured on the assets) at their current market or surrender value in that country, unless (because of exchange controls or other prohibitions) you are not allowed to transfer the full value to this country, in which case you are treated as having capital equal to what a willing buyer in this country would give for those assets, which may be very little or nothing. If the capital is realised in another currency, charges for conversion into sterling are also deducted.[74]

Capital that is jointly owned with someone else

If you jointly own any capital asset you are treated as owning an equal share of the asset with all other owners. This applies regardless of the actual proportion of your real share in the asset.[75] For example, if you actually own 30 per cent of an asset and your brother owns the other 70 per cent, each of you are treated as owning a 50 per cent share. Similarly, if you actually own 90 per cent of an asset and one other person owns the other 10 per cent, you are treated as owning only 50 per cent and the value of the extra 40 per cent you actually own does not count as your capital.

The value of any deemed share should be calculated in the same way as your actual capital. However, it is only the value of your deemed share looked at in isolation which counts, and this will usually be worth rather less than the same proportion of the value of the whole asset. If the asset is a house, for example, the value of any deemed share, even if it is larger than your actual share, may be very small or even worthless, particularly if the house is occupied and the other owner(s) are unwilling to buy your share or sell their share(s) and there is a possibility that the sale of the property cannot be forced. This is because even a willing buyer could not be expected to pay much for an asset s/he would have difficulty making use of or selling on to someone else.[76] Valuations often fail to take into account official guidance on a range of factors relevant to the assessment of jointly owned properties,[77] and you may need to challenge any decision (see Chapter 10) based on an inadequate valuation.

The rules do not apply to assets which are not really jointly owned. In the case of savings held in a joint bank account with a separated spouse, there is a presumption that both parties have joint beneficial ownership of the whole account. But if there is clear evidence that part of the sum belongs to one party alone, and the joint account has merely been used for convenience, that part will count as if it is in her/his sole ownership.[78] Many couples use joint accounts only for convenience, and it is often only on separation (eg, because one partner needs residential or nursing care) that they will take steps to separate how much belongs to each. The way in which a couple apportions their savings between themselves (see also p202 for the treatment of assets when couples separate) could affect how much benefit each may be entitled to.

If, because you jointly own an asset, you are treated as owning an asset of greater value than it is actually worth to you, you should consider selling your share if possible because as soon as it is sold only the actual proceeds of your actual share should be treated as your capital. Unless you sell it for less than it is actually worth, the notional capital rules (see below) should not apply. Even if you or any other co-owner(s) sell only part of your (or their) share(s), the deemed value of your asset will reduce as the number of co-owners increases. In the meantime, you may be able to apply for a crisis loan from the social fund (see p123).

Treatment of assets when partners separate

When partners separate, assets such as their former home or a building society account may be in joint or sole names. For example, if a building society account is in joint names, under the rule about jointly owned capital, you and your former partner are treated as having a 50 per cent share each. But if your former partner is claiming sole ownership of the account, DSS guidance suggests that your interest in the account should count as having a nil value until the question of ownership is settled.[79] If your former partner puts a stop on the account, in effect freezing it, the account should be disregarded until its ownership is resolved.

On the other hand, a former partner may have a right to some or all of an asset that is in your sole name – eg, s/he may have deposited most of the money in a building society account in your name. If this is established, then the partner in whose name the account is held may well, depending on the circumstances, be treated as not entitled to the whole of the account but as holding part of it as trustee for her/his former partner.[80] In that event, the rule about jointly owned capital may have the effect of treating you as owning half of the amount in the account. However, the point made in the DSS guidance referred to above should logically apply equally here, so you should not be treated as owning half the capital (or indeed any of it) unless or until it is established that you do own at least some share of it, and the value of your interest can be assessed.

6. **Notional capital**

In certain circumstances you are treated as having capital which you do not in fact possess. This is called notional capital.[81] There is a similar rule for notional income (see p182).

You will be treated as having notional capital if:

- you deliberately deprive yourself of capital in order to claim or increase benefit (see p203);
- you fail to apply for capital which is available to you (see p205);
- someone else makes a payment of capital to a third party on your behalf (see p205);
- you receive a payment of capital on behalf of a third party and, instead of handing it on, you use or keep the capital (see p206); *and*
- you are a sole trader or a partner in a limited company (see p206).

Notional capital counts in the same way as capital you actually possess, except that, in cases of deprivation of capital, a diminishing notional capital rule may be applied so that the value of the notional capital you are treated as having will be considered to reduce over time (see p205).

Deprivation of capital in order to claim or increase benefit

If you deliberately get rid of capital in order to claim or increase your benefit, you are treated as still possessing it.[82] This could apply if, at the time of using up your money, you know that you may qualify for benefit (or more benefit) as a result, or qualify more quickly, but it should not apply if you do not know, and could not reasonably be expected to know about the effect of using up your capital[83] or if you have been using your money at a rate which is reasonable in the circumstances.

Even if you do know about the capital limits, it still has to be shown that you intended to obtain, retain or increase your benefit.[84] For example, it has been held that a claimant who, facing repossession of his home, transferred ownership to his daughter (who, he feared, would otherwise be made homeless), in spite of having been warned by Benefits Agency staff that he would be disqualified from benefit if he did so, did not dispose of the property with any intention of gaining benefit.[85]

The longer the period that has elapsed since the disposal of the capital, the less likely it is that it was for the purpose of obtaining benefit,[86] but there is no set safe period after which it may be said that benefit can be claimed without the need for further enquiry.[87]

A person who uses up her/his resources may have more than one motive for doing so. Even where qualifying for benefit as a result is only a subsidiary motive, and the predominant motive is something quite different (eg, ensuring your home is in good condition by spending capital to do necessary repairs or improvements), you may still be counted as having intentionally deprived yourself of capital.[88]

If you pay off a debt which you are required by law to repay immediately, the deprivation rule should not apply.[89] Even if you pay off a debt which you do not have to immediately, it must still be shown that you did so with the intention of gaining benefit.[90]

In practice, arguing successfully that you have not deprived yourself of capital to gain benefit may boil down to whether you can show that you would have spent the money in the way you did regardless of the effect on your benefit entitlement. Where this is unclear, the burden of proof lies with the adjudicating authority. In one case a man lost over £60,000 speculating on the stock market. Due to his wife's serious illness, which affected his own health and judgement, he did not act to avoid losses when the stock market crashed. It was held that it had not been proved that there had been an intentional deprivation.[91]

For IS/income-based JSA, you can only be affected by this rule if the capital in question is actual capital.[92] So if you are counted as owning half a bank account under the rule about jointly held capital (see p201), but your real share is only a quarter, you cannot be affected by any deprivation of the other quarter. It is even arguable that the deprivation rule should not apply to the quarter which you actually own.[93] There is no such express rule spelt out in HB/CTB law, but you should argue that the same principle applies.

If a person acting on your behalf as your attorney has misspent your money for her/his own benefit, the amount spent cannot be notional capital (because the disposal will have been unlawful) or actual capital (because you no longer have it), but your right to recover the money may still have an actual capital value.[94]

If you are treated as possessing notional capital, it is calculated in the same way as if it were actual capital[95] and the same disregards will apply (although conflicting case law suggests that you may not be able to rely on the disregard which applies when steps are being taken to sell a property even if the new owner is trying to sell it[96]), although the diminishing notional capital rule (see p205) may reduce its value over time.

Other points on deprivation of capital

- Any deprivation must be found to have been for the purposes of claiming or increasing your entitlement to that benefit.[97]
- Deprivation for the purposes of claiming one benefit cannot be said to be deprivation for the purposes of claiming another. For example, a deprivation for supplementary benefit purposes could not count as deprivation for IS,[98] because IS did not exist at the time of the original deprivation. The only exception is that a deprivation to gain IS may apply to income-based JSA (but not *vice versa*). Where a deprivation has been found for the purposes of IS it does not necessarily follow that there has also been any intention to gain HB or CTB. Similarly, a deprivation for the purposes of reducing your liability to social services for any contribution to the costs of a care home (see Chapter 14) may not necessarily mean there has been any intention to

gain IS, and *vice versa*. Sometimes, however, it is possible that a deprivation may have been made with more than one purpose in mind.

- Each adjudicating authority must reach its own decision on each benefit.
- Even deprivation decisions on HB must be made independently of decisions for CTB.[99] This may result in different conclusions being drawn on any disposal for each benefit, and even where intent is found in two different benefits, there may be different views about the amount of capital that has been deliberately disposed of.[100] The only exception is that if the deprivation rule has been applied to a claim for HB/CTB, and you then submit a successful claim for IS, the notional capital decision on HB/CTB should be put in abeyance for as long as IS remains in payment.[101] Social services must also apply their deprivation rule independently of any decision on IS/income-based JSA/HB/CTB, and *vice versa*.

The diminishing notional capital rule

There are complicated rules for working out how your notional capital should be treated as spent, so that its value is deemed to have diminished over time.[102] Broadly, the rules aim to provide for your notional capital to be gradually reduced by the weekly amount of any means-tested benefit you would have been entitled to but for the notional capital rule. For details see CPAG's *Welfare Benefits Handbook*.

Failing to apply for capital[103]

Under this rule you are treated as having capital you could get if you applied for it – eg, where money is held in court which would be released on application or an unclaimed premium bond win. This does not apply if you fail to apply to capital from:

- a discretionary trust; *or*
- a trust (or court fund) set up from money paid as a result of a personal injury; *or*
- a personal pension scheme or retirement annuity contract; *or*
- a loan which you could only get if you gave your home or other disregarded capital as security.

Capital payments made to a third party on your behalf

If someone else pays an amount to a third party (eg, the electricity board or a building society) for you (or a member of your family), this may count as your capital.[104] It counts if the payment is to cover certain of your (or your family's) normal living expenses – ie, food, household fuel, council tax, ordinary clothing or footwear, rent for which HB is payable (less non-dependant deductions), water charges or, for IS/income-based JSA only, housing costs met by IS/income-based JSA or the costs of your care home if you have preserved rights.

Payments for other kinds of expenses (eg, care home charges above the IS/income-based JSA limit or mortgage capital repayments) are disregarded.

For IS/income-based JSA, payments derived from certain social security benefits (including war disablement pensions and war widows' pensions) which are paid to a third party count as belonging to you (or a member of your family) if you (or a member of your family) are entitled to that benefit.[105]

For IS/income-based JSA, there are different rules if you could be liable to pay maintenance as a liable relative.

Capital payments paid to you for a third party[106]

If you (or a member of your family) get a payment for someone not in your family (eg, a relative who does not have a bank account) it only counts as yours if it is kept or used by you.

Companies run by sole traders or a few partners

There are special rules on the treatment of the assets of sole traders or small partnerships (see CPAG's *Welfare Benefits Handbook*).

Notes

1. The capital limit
1 **IS** reg 45 IS Regs;
   JSA reg 107 JSA Regs;
   HB reg 37 HB Regs;
   CTB reg 28 CTB Regs
2 **IS** reg 53 IS Regs;
   JSA reg 116 JSA Regs;
   HB reg 45 HB Regs;
   CTB reg 37 CTB Regs
3 **IS** regs 45 and 53(1A), (1B), (1C) and (4) IS Regs;
   JSA regs 107(b) and 116(1A) JSA Regs
4 Regs 7(9) and 45(1A), (1B), (1C), (4) and (5) HB Regs

2. Whose capital counts
5 **IS/HB/CTB** s136(1) SSCBA 1992; s13(2) JSA 1995
6 para C2.09 GM; para 34020 AOG

7 *R v SBC ex parte Singer* [1973] 1 WLR 713
8 R(SB) 35/83
9 CIS/654/1991
10 Reg 91(1) HB Regs
11 R(SB) 12/86
12 R(SB) 53/83; R(SB) 1/85
13 R(SB) 49/83
14 R(SB) 23/85
15 **IS** Sch 10 para 13 IS Regs;
   JSA Sch 8 para 18 JSA Regs;
   HB Sch 5 para 14 HB Regs;
   CTB Sch 5 para 14 CTB Regs
16 *Peters v CAO* reported as an appendix to R(SB) 3/89
17 R(IS) 1/90
18 R(SB) 23/85
19 *Barclays Bank v Quistclose Investments Ltd* [1970] AC 567; R(SB) 49/83; CFC/21/1989

20 **IS** reg 23(1) and Sch 10 paras 12, 44 and 45 IS Regs;
JSA reg 88(1) and Sch 8 paras 18, 42 and 43 JSA Regs;
HB reg 19(1) and Sch 5 paras 13, 46 and 47 HB Regs;
CTB reg 11(1) and Sch 5 paras 13, 46 and 47 CTB Regs

21 *Thomas v CAO* (appendix to R(SB) 17/87

22 **IS** regs 40 and 46 IS Regs;
JSA regs 103 and 108 JSA Regs;
HB regs 33 and 38 HB Regs;
CTB regs 24 and 29 CTB Regs;
All CIS/559/1991

23 **IS** reg 48 IS Regs;
JSA reg 110 JSA Regs;
HB reg 40 HB Regs;
CTB reg 31 CTB Regs

24 **IS** Sch 9 para 32 IS Regs;
JSA Sch 7 para 34 JSA Regs;
HB Sch 4 para 29 HB Regs;
CTB Sch 4 para 30 CTB Regs

25 **IS** reg 2(1) and Sch 10 para 1 IS Regs;
JSA reg 1(3) and Sch 8 para 1 JSA Regs;
HB Sch 5 para 1 HB Regs;
CTB Sch 5 para 1 CTB Regs;
All R(SB) 3/84; CIS/427/1991

26 **IS** Sch 10 paras 2, 3, 8, 9, 25-28 and 37 IS;
JSA Sch 8 paras 2, 3, 5-9, 13 and 14 JSA;
HB Sch 5 paras 2, 3, 9, 10, 24-27 and 37 HB;
CTB Sch 5 paras 2, 3, 9, 10, 24-27 and 37 CTB

27 CIS 562/1992

28 CIS/7319/1995

29 R(SB) 32/83

30 CIS/7319/1995, para 22

31 R(IS) 6/95

32 CIS/685/1992; CIS/8475/1995; CIS/15984/1996

33 R(SB) 14/85

34 para 34578 AOG

35 CIS/6908/1995

36 **IS** Sch 10 para 4 IS Regs;
JSA Sch 8 para 4 JSA Regs;
HB Sch 5 paras 4 and 24 HB Regs;
CTB Sch 5 paras 4 and 24 CTB Regs

37 **IS** reg 2(1) IS Regs;
JSA reg 1(3) JSA Regs;
HB reg 2(1) HB Regs;
CTB reg 2(1) CTB Regs

38 **IS/JSA** para 34429 AOG; **HB/CTB** para C2.12.ii.a and b GM

39 **IS** reg 2(1) IS Regs;
JSA reg 2(1) JSA Regs;
HB reg 2(1) HB Regs;
CTB: not defined, but the same would be expected to apply

40 CSB/209/1986; CSB/1149/1986; R(SB) 22/87

41 **IS** Sch 10 para 5 IS Regs;
JSA Sch 8 para 10 JSA Regs;
HB Sch 5 para 6 HB Regs;
CTB Sch 5 para 6 CTB Regs

42 CIS/635/1994

43 **IS** Sch 10 paras 11-14, 16, 23 and 24 IS Regs;
JSA Sch 8 paras 16-19, 21, 28 and 30 JSA Regs;
HB Sch 5 paras 12-15, 17, 30 and 31 HB Regs;
CTB Sch 5 paras 12-15, 17, 30 and 31 CTB Regs

44 **IS** Sch 10 paras 7 and 41 IS Regs;

44 **JSA** Sch 8 paras 12 and 39 JSA Regs;
HB Sch 5 paras 8 and 38 HB Regs;
CTB Sch 5 paras 8 and 37 CTB Regs

45 **IS** Sch 10 paras 36, 38 and 40 IS Regs;

JSA Sch 8 paras 35, 36 and 38 JSA Regs;
HB Sch 5 paras 36, 39 and 41 HB Regs;
CTB Sch 5 paras 35, 38 and 40 CTB Regs

46 **IS** Sch 10 para 18 IS Regs;
JSA Sch 8 para 23 JSA Regs;
HB Sch 5 para 19 HB Regs;
CTB Sch 5 para 19 CTB Regs

47 **IS** Sch 10 para 10 IS Regs;
JSA Sch 8 para 15 JSA Regs;
HB Sch 5 para 11 HB Regs;
CTB Sch 5 para 11 CTB Regs

48 CIS/494/1990

49 **IS** Sch 10 para 8(a) IS Regs;
JSA Sch 8 para 13(a) JSA Regs;
HB Sch 5 para 9(a) HB Regs;
CTB Sch 5 para 9(a) CTB Regs

50 **IS** Sch 10 para 6 IS Regs;
   JSA Sch 8 para 11 JSA Regs;
   HB Sch 5 para 7 HB Regs;
   CTB Sch 5 para 7 CTB Regs;
   All: R(SB) 4/85
51 CFC/15/1990
52 **IS** Sch 10 para 19 IS Regs;
   JSA Sch 8 para 24 JSA Regs;
   HB Sch 5 para 20 HB Regs;
   CTB Sch 5 para 20 CTB Regs
53 **IS** Sch 10 para 23A IS Regs;
   JSA Sch 8 paras 28 and 29 JSA Regs;
   HB Sch 3 para 39A HB Regs;
   CTB Sch 5 para 30A CTB Regs
54 **IS** Sch 10 paras 11 and 15 IS Regs;
   JSA Sch 8 paras 16 and 20 JSA Regs;
   HB Sch 5 paras 12 and 16 HB Regs;
   CTB Sch 5 paras 12 and 16 CTB Regs
55 **IS** Sch 10 para 17 IS Regs;
   JSA Sch 8 para 22 JSA Regs;
   HB Sch 5 para 18 HB Regs;
   CTB Sch 5 para 18 CTB Regs
56 **IS** Sch 10 para 29 IS Regs;
   JSA Sch 8 para 31 JSA Regs;
   HB Sch 5 para 32 HB Regs;
   CTB Sch 5 para 32 CTB Regs
57 **IS** Sch 10 para 22 IS Regs;
   JSA Sch 8 para 27 JSA Regs;
   HB Sch 5 para 23 HB Regs;
   CTB Sch 5 para 23 CTB Regs
58 **IS** Sch 10 para 34 IS Regs;
   JSA Sch 8 para 34 JSA Regs;
   HB Sch 4 para 38 HB Regs;
   CTB Sch 4 para 40 CTB Regs
59 **IS** Sch 10 para 21 IS Regs;
   JSA Sch 8 para 26 JSA Regs;
   HB Sch 5 para 22 HB Regs;
   CTB Sch 5 para 22 CTB Regs
60 **IS** Sch 10 para 46 IS Regs;
   JSA Sch 8 para 44 JSA Regs;
   HB Sch 5 para 48 HB Regs;
   CTB Sch 5 para 48 CTB Regs
61 **IS** Sch 10 para 20 IS Regs;
   JSA Sch 8 para 25 JSA Regs;
   HB Sch 5 para 21 HB Regs;
   CTB Sch 5 para 21 CTB Regs
62 **IS** Reg 49(a) IS Regs;
   JSA reg 111(a) JSA Regs;
   HB reg 41(a) HB Regs;
   CTB reg 32(a) CTB Regs
63 R(SB) 57/83; R(SB) 6/84
64 R(SB) 18/83
65 R(SB) 6/84

66 **IS** Reg 49(a)(i) IS Regs;
   JSA reg 111(a)(i) JSA Regs;
   HB reg 41(a)(i) HB Regs;
   CTB reg 32(a)(i) CTB Regs
67 **IS** Reg 49(a)(ii) IS Regs;
   JSA reg 111(a)(ii) JSA Regs;
   HB reg 41(a)(ii) HB Regs;
   CTB reg 32(a)(ii) CTB Regs
68 R(SB) 27/84
69 R(SB) 2/83; R(SB) 31/83
70 **IS** Reg 49(b) IS Regs;
   JSA reg 111(b) JSA Regs;
   HB reg 41(b) HB Regs;
   CTB reg 32(b) CTB Regs
71 **IS** Reg 49(a) IS Regs;
   JSA reg 111(a) JSA Regs;
   HB reg 41(a) HB Regs;
   CTB reg 32(a) CTB Regs
72 **IS/JSA** para 34681 AOG;
72 **HB/CTB** para C2.34 GM
73 **IS** reg 50 IS Regs;
   JSA reg 112 JSA Regs;
   HB reg 42 HB Regs;
   CTB reg 33 CTB Regs
74 **IS** Sch 10 para 21 IS Regs;
   JSA Sch 8 para 26 JSA Regs;
   HB Sch 5 para 22 HB Regs;
   CTB Sch 5 para 22 CTB Regs
75 **IS** Reg 52 IS Regs;
   JSA reg 115 JSA Regs;
   HB reg 44 HB Regs;
   CTB reg 36 CTB Regs
76 CIS/15936/1996; CIS/263/1997;
   CIS/3283/1997 (joint decision); *CAO
   v Palfrey and Others* (CA), *The Times*,
   17 February 1995 (upholding CIS/
   391/1992 and CIS/417/1992
   apparently to be reported as R(IS) 5/
   98)
77 Memo AOG JSA/IS 35, October 1998
78 CIS/7097/1995; CIS/15936/1996;
   CIS/263/1997; CIS/3283/1997 (joint
   decision – common appendix para
   17)
79 **HB/CTB** para 2.42 GM
80 R(IS) 2/93
81 **IS** reg 51(6) IS Regs;
   JSA reg 113(6) JSA Regs;
   HB reg 43(6) HB Regs;
   CTB reg 34(6) CTB Regs
82 **IS** reg 51(1) IS Regs;
   JSA reg 113(1) JSA Regs;
   HB reg 43(1) HB Regs;
   CTB reg 34(1) CTB Regs

83 CIS/124/1990; CSB/1198/1989;
   R(SB) 9/91; CIS/124/1990
84 CIS/40/1989
85 CIS/621/1991
86 CIS/264/1989
87 CIS/7330/1995, para 12(3)
88 R(SB) 38/85
89 R(SB) 12/91
90 CIS/2627/1995
91 CIS/236/1991
92 **IS** reg 51(7) IS Regs;
   JSA reg 113(7) JSA Regs
93 CIS/240/1992
94 CIS/12403/1996
95 **IS** reg 51(6) IS Regs;
   JSA reg 113(6) JSA Regs;
   HB reg 43(6) HB Regs;
   CTB reg 34(6) CTB Regs
96 CIS/30/1993, but other
   commissioners have taken a different
   view (see, eg, CIS/25/1990 and CIS/
   81/1991)
97 **IS** reg 51(1) IS Regs;
   JSA reg 113(1) JSA Regs;
   HB reg 43(1) HB Regs;
   CTB reg 34(1) CTB Regs;
   All R(IS) 14/93
98 R(IS) 14/93
99 para C2.69 GM
100 para C2.97 GM
101 para C2.92 GM
102 **IS** reg 51A IS Regs;
   JSA reg 114 JSA Regs;
   HB reg 43A HB Regs;
   CTB reg 35 CTB Regs
103 **IS** reg 51(2) IS Regs;
   JSA reg 113(2) JSA Regs;
   HB reg 43(2) HB Regs;
   CTB reg 34(2) CTB Regs;
   All CIS/368/1994
104 **IS** reg 51(3)(a)(ii) and (8) IS Regs;
   JSA reg 113(3)(a)(ii) JSA Regs;
   HB reg 43(3)(a) and (7) HB Regs;
   CTB reg 34(3)(a) and (7) CTB Regs
105 **IS** reg 51(3)(a)(i) IS Regs;
   JSA reg 113(a)(i) JSA Regs
106 **IS** reg 51(3)(b) IS Regs;
   JSA reg 113(3)(b) JSA Regs;
   HB reg 43(3)(b) HB Regs;
   CTB reg 34(3)(b) CTB Regs

Chapter 8

Liable relatives – social security

This chapter explains the rules about liability to pay maintenance to people who claim income support (see p93) or income-based jobseeker's allowance (see p125), and how maintenance affects entitlement to income support, income-based jobseeker's allowance, housing benefit (see p102) and council tax benefit (see p111). It covers:
1. Who is liable to maintain you (p211)
2. Pursuing maintenance (p212)
3. The amount of maintenance (p213)
4. How maintenance you receive affects your benefit (p213)
5. How maintenance you pay affects your benefit (p217)

This chapter does **not** deal with the liability to maintain children, for which special rules apply – see CPAG's *Child Support Handbook* and *Welfare Benefits Handbook*.

As a matter of public policy, you are expected to exhaust any remedies for maintenance from a person who is liable to maintain you before relying on the support of the state. This chapter deals with the liability to pay maintenance to someone who is claiming income support (IS) or income-based jobseeker's allowance (JSA). For details of the liability to maintain someone who is receiving assistance from social services for the costs of a care home, see Chapter 17.

If you have separated from your spouse, you may be able to get maintenance. Payments of maintenance could be on a voluntary basis or under a court order. Detailed advice about maintenance orders is beyond the scope of this *Handbook*. You should consult a solicitor if you need advice. If you are on a low income you may be able to get free advice under the Green Form (or, in Scotland, Pink Form) Scheme and apply for legal aid towards the cost of court proceedings.

1. **Who is 'liable to maintain' you**

The Secretary of State can take proceedings against anyone who has a liability to maintain you (or your children) while you are claiming IS or income-based JSA.

There are no similar rules imposing any liability to maintain a person who is claiming housing benefit (HB) or council tax benefit (CTB) or any other social security benefit.

While you are on IS or income-based JSA, **you** must be maintained by your **spouse**, if you are married or separated.[1] This applies even if you and your spouse are separated against your will, and even if your separation is only temporary – eg, because one of you needs residential or nursing care.

For IS/income-based JSA purposes, there is no liability to maintain an ex-spouse if you are now divorced (although any maintenance you receive from an ex-spouse counts in the same way as maintenance by a spouse – see p213). As a result, there may be some unintentional financial incentive for spouses to divorce who may otherwise have no wish to do so – eg, when they are only separated because one of them needs to live in a care home.

If you have to live apart from your spouse because you need care or treatment (eg, in a hospital or a care home) you may be assessed and paid as separate individuals for benefit purposes. However, your spouse is still liable to maintain you and may be asked to make a financial contribution to the Benefits Agency towards the cost of any IS or income-based JSA paid to you (see below) *or* to social services (but not to both[2]) towards the cost of any care home charges paid by them (see Chapter 17). In practice, in order to avoid causing undue distress to couples (particularly pensioners) when one spouse has to live in a care home, both the Benefits Agency and social services tend to take a relaxed view of their responsibilities for pursuing liable relatives for maintenance in such circumstances.

If you are a 'person from abroad' subject to a 'sponsorship undertaking' (see Chapter 9) you must be maintained by your **sponsor**. For IS (but not income-based JSA[3]) this could include your ex-spouse after you are divorced.

Otherwise, no one who is not your spouse has any liability to maintain you.

Your right to claim benefit is not affected by the fact that the Benefits Agency can get money back from someone who is liable to maintain you. You should, therefore, not be refused IS or income-based JSA while maintenance is being pursued. However, maintenance that is recovered may affect your benefit (see p213).

---

2. **Pursuing maintenance**

If you are not receiving any, or enough, maintenance you may be able to apply for a court order and you should seek advice from a solicitor. If, however, you are unable or unwilling to pursue maintenance for yourself the Benefits Agency may take steps to pursue maintenance on your behalf.

Prosecution

A person who is liable to maintain you can be prosecuted if IS or income-based JSA is paid as a result of her/his persistently failing to maintain you. The maximum penalty is three months' imprisonment or a fine of £2,500 or both.[4] Prosecutions, however, are rare. If you are charged with such an offence, you should consult a solicitor as soon as possible. Legal aid may be available to help meet the costs of proceedings.

Maintenance orders

Instead of, or as well as, prosecuting you (see above), the Secretary of State may take court proceedings to enforce a liability for maintenance against any person who is liable to maintain you.[5] This enables the Benefits Agency to pursue maintenance on your behalf while you are on IS or income-based JSA.

The magistrates' (or, in Scotland, sheriff's) court can make an order telling the person who is liable what s/he has to pay. The fact that there was an agreement that you would not ask for any, or any more, maintenance is not a bar to an order being made (even if the former matrimonial home has been transferred to you on condition that you do not make a further claim for maintenance).[6] All the circumstances must be taken into account[7] and the court is entitled to refuse to make an order for maintenance if you have been guilty of adultery, cruelty or desertion.[8]

Collection of maintenance

While you are on IS or income-based JSA, if maintenance is payable through a magistrates' or sheriff's court (including orders made in the county or sheriff's court or High Court but registered in the magistrates' or sheriff's court) it can be paid direct to the Benefits Agency.[9] In return, the Benefits Agency pays you the amount of IS or income-based JSA which you would receive if no maintenance was being paid. The Benefits Agency does not usually agree to this sort of arrangement unless payments have actually been missed, but it may do so if you have good reason for wanting it done and you explain why.

3. **The amount of maintenance**

There is some flexibility about how much maintenance your spouse is required to pay for you. S/he can negotiate with the Benefits Agency to pay an amount s/he can afford given her/his outgoings. As a starting point for negotiations, the Benefits Agency compares your spouse's net income with the total of:[10]

- the IS personal allowances and premiums s/he would qualify for if entitled to IS;
- household expenses including rent, mortgage and council tax (excluding arrears);
- 15 per cent of her/his net wage (to cover expenses for work); *and*
- the balance of any other expenses exceeding the 15 per cent margin that are considered essential.

If your spouse has a new partner, two calculations are performed – one as if s/he was single and the other using joint incomes. The lower figure is used as the basis for negotiation.

If the Benefits Agency feels that your spouse is not paying enough it has the right to take her/him to court (see p212). The Benefits Agency has considerable discretion in deciding what steps to take and how much maintenance it should agree to, and there is wide variation in practice in different areas.

4. **How maintenance you receive affects your benefit**

Most maintenance payments paid by liable relatives are taken into account in working out the amount of benefit to which you are entitled. These are usually treated as income and count in full to reduce your entitlement to benefit.

There are no special rules on the treatment of maintenance payments for HB/CTB (except that if you are a lone parent or a couple with a child, £15 of any maintenance payment made by your former partner, or your partner's former partner, or the parent of any child in your family, is disregarded in working out the amount of your benefit[11]). If you are receiving payments regularly, they are taken into account as income (see p178). If you are paid irregularly or in lump sums, they are taking into account as capital (see Chapter 7).

How a payment of maintenance affects your IS/income-based JSA depends on whether it counts as a periodical or lump sum liable relative payment, or whether it does not count as a liable relative payment at all.

Liable relative payments

Unless it is a payment that does not count, payments from your spouse (including one from whom you are separated or divorced) or from your sponsor if you are a person from abroad subject to a sponsorship undertaking, count as liable relative payments.[12]

The following types of payment from your spouse or ex-spouse (or sponsor) do **not** count as liable relative payments[13] but are treated instead under the normal income and capital rules and may sometimes be disregarded – see Chapters 6 and 7:

- any payment arising from a disposition of property (see below) in consequence of your separation, divorce or the nullity of your marriage;
- any gifts not exceeding £250 in any period of 52 weeks (so long as they are not so regular as to count as periodical payments);
- payments made after the liable relative has died;
- any payment in kind;
- any payment made to someone else for the benefit of you (or a member of your family) – eg, a mortgage capital repayment paid to the building society – which it is unreasonable to take into account;
- any payment which has already been taken into account; *or*
- any payment which you have used before a decision is made on how to treat it – eg, if you have cleared debts or paid your solicitor's bill.

A 'disposition of property' is when it is divided up or your former partner buys out your interest. 'Property' includes a house and land as well as assets such as the contents of your former home or a bank account.[14]

Periodical liable relative payments

Periodical 'liable relative payments' are:[15]

- any payment made, or due to be made, regularly, whether voluntarily or under a court order or other formal agreement;
- any other small payment no higher than your weekly IS or income-based JSA;
- any payment made instead of one or more regular payments due under an agreement (whether formal or voluntary), either as payment in advance or arrears. This does not include any arrears due before the beginning of your entitlement to IS or income-based JSA.

Periodical payments which are received on time are each spread over a period equal to the interval between them – eg, monthly payments are spread over a month. Payments are converted to a weekly amount – eg, monthly payments are multiplied by 12 and divided by 52 to produce a weekly income figure.

Arrears of periodical liable relative payments

If arrears of maintenance are paid for a period before the date of your claim for IS/income-based JSA, they do not count as periodical payments.[16] The Benefits Agency deals with such payments as lump sums treated as income (see p217). This means that they are spread over a future period. You should try to argue that this is wrong and that such payments should be treated as capital. The benefit rules do not exclude arrears from the definition of periodical payments just to have them brought back into the calculation in this way. Any other interpretation is unfair and gives the Secretary of State an unwarranted windfall at your expense.[17]

If a payment is made for a period during your claim, and it includes a lump sum for arrears (or in advance), the payment is spread over a period calculated by dividing it by the weekly amount of maintenance you should have received.[18]

> **Example**
> Tia should receive maintenance of £80 a month. It is not paid for three months and she then receives £200.
> £80 a month is treated as producing a weekly
>
> income of: $\dfrac{£80 \times 12}{52} = £18.46$
>
> The £200 is taken into account for: $\dfrac{£200}{£18.46} = 10.83$ weeks
>
> Tia is assumed to have an income of £18.46 for the next 10 weeks and 6 days. The maintenance payments due are still two weeks and one day in arrears (£40)

If a payment is specifically identified as being arrears of maintenance for a particular period, the Benefits Agency can:

- take it into account for a forward period from the week you report you have received it; *or*
- attribute it to the past period which it was intended to cover, unless it is more practicable to choose a later week.[19] In this case the Secretary of State can recover the full amount of extra benefit paid to you while maintenance was not being received.[20] (This can still be done when you receive a payment after your claim ends which is for arrears of maintenance that should have been paid while your were claiming.)

It is important to work out how you would be better-off financially. You should then argue for the payment to be spread over whichever period is more advantageous to you. This depends on the amount of IS or income-based JSA you would otherwise receive, the amount of the payment and whether any other periodical payments are being made.

Example 1

Connie should have been receiving maintenance at the rate of £25 a week. Her husband misses eight weeks and she has to claim IS at the rate of £15 to top up her pension. On a change of circumstances, her entitlement to IS increases to £30 a week. Her husband then pays her eight weeks' arrears of maintenance (£200).

The Benefits Agency might try to take the maintenance into account for eight weeks at the rate of £25 a week from the date it is paid to Connie. If it does this, she loses £200 (£25 x 8 weeks).

Connie argues that the maintenance should be attributed to the eight-week period it was intended to cover. The Benefits Agency can then recover the IS she was paid for that period. She says she will pay the Benefits Agency what she owes out of the arrears of maintenance. This is a very good case for arguing that it is not 'more practicable' to spread the payment forwards rather than over the past period. She loses £120 (£15 X 8 weeks).

Example 2

Gwen is in exactly the same position as Connie. However, when her husband paid her arrears of maintenance of £200, he also started making regular maintenance payments. She is better off having the payment of arrears spread forwards from the date of payment. The new maintenance payments of £25 a week reduce her IS to £5 a week. If the Benefits Agency takes the arrears into account for eight weeks from the date it is paid to Gwen, she only loses £40 (£5 x 8 weeks).

Lump sum payments

If you are already receiving periodical liable relative payments equal to your IS/income-based JSA, then a lump sum payment of maintenance counts as capital.[21]

If you stop getting periodical liable relative payments or get less than an amount equal to your IS/income-based JSA, any of the lump sum you still have is treated as producing an income equal to your weekly IS/income-based JSA plus £2.[22]

If you are getting periodical liable relative payments and IS/income-based JSA, any lump sum you also receive is treated as producing an income equal to your weekly IS/income-based JSA plus £2 which would be paid if you did not get the periodical payment.[23]

You are then disqualified from getting IS/income-based JSA for a period beginning on the first day of the benefit week in which the payment is received

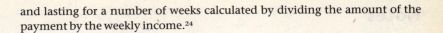

and lasting for a number of weeks calculated by dividing the amount of the payment by the weekly income.[24]

Example
Fiona receives a lump sum of £2,000 from her husband. Her IS is £48. Under the rules, the lump sum is treated as producing a weekly income of £50. She does not receive IS for 40 weeks (£2,000 divided by £50 = 40).

If the periodical payments are varied or stop, or if your circumstances change so that your entitlement to IS/income-based JSA would be higher, you should ask for the calculation to be done again.[25]

5. **How maintenance you pay affects your benefit**

If you are contributing to someone's maintenance you might qualify for an increase of a non-means-tested benefit even if you are not living with her/him. This may then affect your entitlement to IS/income-based JSA/HB/CTB. Paying maintenance may enable you to qualify for:
- child benefit or guardian's allowance; *or*
- a child or adult dependency increase with incapacity benefit, severe disablement allowance, invalid care allowance or retirement pension; or
- a child dependency increase with widowed mother's allowance; *or*
- an adult dependency increase with your maternity allowance.

For details of these benefits see Chapter 3.

There are special rules that allow the Benefits Agency to recover money from you if you are meant to be contributing to the maintenance of someone who is claiming IS/income-based JSA but fail to do so. If you do not pay what you are meant to pay, that person's IS/income-based JSA may be increased to make up the difference, and the extra IS/income-based JSA paid may be recovered from any of the benefits listed above which you receive.[26]

Notes

1. **Who is 'liable to maintain' you**
   1 ss78(6)-(9) and 105 SSAA 1992
   2 CRAG 11.003
   3 ss78(6)-(9) and s105(1)(b) and (4)

2. **Pursuing maintenance**
   4 s105(1) SSAA 1992
   5 s106 SSAA 1992; s23 JSA 1995
   6 *NAB v Parkes* [1955] 2 QBD 506;
      Hulley v Thompson [1981] 1 WLR 159
   7 s106(2) SSAA 1992; s23 JSA 1995 and
      Reg 169 JSA Regs
   8 *NAB v Parkes* [1995] 2 QBD 506
   9 **IS** s106(4)(a) SSAA 1992;
      JSA s23 JSA 1995 and Reg 169 JSA
      Regs

3. **The amount of maintenance**
   10 Residual Liable Relative and
      Proceedings Guide, paras 1630-42

4. **How maintenance you receive
   affects your benefit**
   11 **HB** Sch 4 paras 13(3) and 47 HB Regs;
      CTB Sch 4 paras 13(3) and 46 CTB
      Regs
   12 **IS** reg 54 IS Regs;
      JSA reg 117 JSA Regs
   13 **IS** regs 54, 55 and 60(1) IS Regs;
      JSA regs 117, 118 and 124(1) JSA
      Regs
   14 CSB/1160/1986; R(SB) 1/89
   15 **IS** reg 54 IS Regs;
      JSA reg 117 JSA Regs
   16 **IS** reg 54 IS Regs;
      JSA reg 117 JSA Regs
   17 *Regina v West London SBAT ex parte
      Taylor* [1975] 1 WLR 1048 (DC);
      McCorquodale v CAO (CA) (appendix
      to R(SB) 1/88)
   18 **IS** reg 58(4) IS Regs;
      JSA reg 122(4) JSA Regs
   19 **IS** reg 59(1) IS Regs;
      JSA reg 123(1) JSA Regs
   20 s74(1) SSAA 1992; reg 7(1) SS(PAOR)
      Regs
   21 **IS** reg 60 IS Regs;
      JSA reg 124 JSA Regs

   22 **IS** reg 57(1) IS Regs;
      JSA reg 121(1) JSA Regs
   23 **IS** reg 57(2) IS Regs;
      JSA reg 121(2) JSA Regs
   24 **IS** regs 57(4) and 59(2) IS Regs;
      JSA regs 121(4) and 123(2) JSA Regs
   25 **IS** reg 57(3) IS Regs;
      JSA reg 121(3) JSA Regs

5. **How maintenance you pay affects
   your benefit**
   26 s74(3) SSAA 1992; reg 9 SS(PAOR)
      Regs

Chapter 9

....

Special rules for special groups – social security

This chapter considers some of the special rules which restrict the entitlement of special groups of people to claim certain benefits. It covers:
1. People from abroad (p219)
2. People without fixed accommodation (p222)

Even if you are not entitled to claim any benefits because of the special rules which apply to special groups, you may still be entitled to assistance from social services (see Chapter 18).

Special rules apply to 16/17-year-olds, students, people involved in trade disputes, and prisoners, and to entitlement to benefit for periods when you go abroad. For details of these see CPAG's *Welfare Benefits Handbook*.

---

1. People from abroad

This section provides an outline only of complex rules which apply to people coming from abroad. For details of these rules, see CPAG's *Migration and Social Security Handbook* and *Welfare Benefits Handbook*.

If you have come from abroad there are a number of factors to take into account:
- your immigration status – ie, the extent of your right to enter or remain in the United Kingdom (UK);
- European Community (EC) law which provides additional rights to certain citizens of European Economic Area states, reciprocal agreements providing additional rights to people from certain other countries, and the special rules for people from Northern Ireland, the Isle of Man and the Channel Islands;
- how long you have been, and will be, residing in this country.

Immigration status

Your right to most social security benefits now depends on whether there are any restrictions on your right to be in the country.

If you have **indefinite leave** to enter or remain in the UK you can claim all social security benefits. However, if another person has signed an undertaking to maintain and accommodate you (a 'sponsorship undertaking'), you will not normally be entitled to income support (IS), income-based jobseeker's allowance (JSA), housing benefit (HB) or council tax benefit (CTB), or certain other benefits, for at least five years.

If you have **limited leave** to enter or remain in the UK it will normally be on the condition that you do not have recourse to 'public funds'. 'Public funds' means any weekly means-tested benefit, attendance allowance, disability living allowance, severe disablement allowance, invalid care allowance, child benefit or housing provided by local authorities. It does **not** include assistance provided by social services, whether by way of accommodation in a care home or otherwise. Spouses or dependent relatives of people with indefinite leave are often granted limited leave.

If you have **exceptional leave** to enter or remain you will normally be entitled to claim most social security benefits, but your leave (and right to claim) will normally be periodically reviewed and may therefore only last for a limited period.

Refugees are entitled to claim most benefits. If you are waiting for the outcome of an application for refugee status you are treated as an 'asylum-seeker'. 'Asylum-seekers' are usually only entitled to claim IS/income-based JSA/HB/CTB if it has been continuously in payment since 4 February 1996, or if they applied for asylum as soon as they entered the country, or if they apply for asylum after there has been an 'upheaval declaration' from the Home Office that they cannot be expected to have to return to their home country.

Asylum seekers (and possibly other people from abroad) who are not entitled to social security benefits and have no other means of support may nevertheless be entitled to assistance from social services (see Chapter 18). However, the government is introducing new measures which will exclude all asylum seekers from entitlement to social security and social services assistance from April 2000 (see Chapter 18).

The rights of EEA citizens

EC law provides additional rights to certain European Economic Area (EEA) citizens. EC law aims to:
- prohibit discrimination on nationality grounds in social security matters;
- promote 'the principle of aggregation' – ie, allowing you to rely on periods of employment, residence and contributions paid in one EEA country towards entitlement to benefit in others;
- promote 'the principle of exportation' – ie, allowing you to take certain benefits with you to another EEA country;
- promote 'the single state principle' – ie, requiring you to claim benefit only from the state in which you last worked;

- promote the freedom of movement to enter and take up employment or receive a service in any member state subject to the same tax, housing and social advantages offered to the nationals of that state;
- promote the right to reside in a member state of your choice.

Most of the restrictions on claiming benefits which apply to certain people from abroad (see above), do not apply to EEA citizens who may also be exempt from most of the residence conditions attached to most benefits (see below).

Reciprocal agreements

There are several countries with which Great Britain has reciprocal agreements, which mean you can receive some British benefits while in the other country and *vice versa*. For details see CPAG's *Migration and Social Security Handbook*.

Technically, the rules about benefits described in this *Handbook* apply only to Great Britain, which consists of England, Wales and Scotland. It does not include Northern Ireland, the Isle of Man or the Channel Islands, which have their own social security laws. Great Britain is not the same as the UK, which does include Northern Ireland.

However, because of the close links between Great Britain, Northern Ireland and the Isle of Man, you do not lose any non-means-tested benefit by moving between them and National Insurance (NI) contributions paid in one country count as though they were paid in each of the others. For most practical purposes the systems in Great Britain, Northern Ireland and the Isle of Man may be treated as identical.

The Channel Islands, Jersey and Guernsey have their own social security schemes but there is a reciprocal agreement under which you can receive some British benefits. You also remain entitled to Great Britain benefits (other than jobseeker's allowance) while in the Channel Islands.

Residence conditions

For most social security benefits you must usually be both 'present' and either 'ordinarily resident' or 'habitually resident' in Great Britain in order to qualify, although some periods of temporary absence may be ignored.

To be 'ordinarily resident' there must be a degree of continuity about your residence so that it can be described as settled. Residence in another EEA country may count as residence in Great Britain. This test applies to attendance allowance, disability living allowance, severe disablement allowance and invalid care allowance. Note that the test of 'ordinarily resident' for benefit purposes applies quite differently to the 'ordinary residence' test which social services are required to apply (see Chapter 12).

The 'habitual residence' test applies to IS/income-based JSA/HB/CTB. It requires that you have a 'settled intention' to remain and that you must be actually resident for an 'appreciable period of time'. This is commonly interpreted as being at least three to six months but this should depend on the facts of each case and you should argue that a shorter period should suffice, if necessary. People who were previously habitually resident in the UK but who are now returning to the UK after a period abroad should be treated as habitually resident from the first day of their return. Certain EEA citizens, refugees and people with exceptional leave to enter or remain in the UK (see above) are exempt from this test.

For further details see CPAG's *Welfare Benefits Handbook*.

2. **People without fixed accommodation**

It is not usually necessary for you to have a home to qualify for most benefits. However, special rules apply to IS/income-based JSA for people who are 'without accommodation' so that you are only entitled to the normal personal allowances for yourself and any partner, but not to any premiums for yourself or partner (or any allowances or premiums for dependent children).[1]

'Accommodation' is described in guidance as 'an effective shelter from the elements which is capable of being heated; and in which occupants can sit, lie, cook and eat; and which is reasonably suited for continuous occupation. The site of the accommodation may alter from day to day, but it is still accommodation if the structure is habitable'. This would cover tents, caravans and other substantial shelters, but cardboard boxes, bus shelters, sleeping bags[2] and cars[3] would not count.

If you are only temporarily absent from the accommodation you occupy as your home and are living a lifestyle as though you have no accommodation (eg, you are sleeping rough) you should still be treated as having accommodation.[4]

If the Benefits Agency decides you have an unsettled way of life it may refer you to a voluntary project centre. This should, however, only be done with your consent and if a place is available, and IS/income-based JSA should not be refused or delayed if you are unwilling to take the advice being offered or are not interested in being resettled.[5]

If you are known in an area, you should receive your benefit by giro, payment or order book in the normal way (see p225), but if you are 'likely to move on or mis-spend your money' you may be required to collect your benefit on a daily or part-week basis.[6]

If you are claiming JSA you must be available for and actively seeking work. However, your reduced prospects of finding work, unless you are placing unreasonable restrictions on it, should be taken into account, and although it must be possible for you to be contacted at short notice if you are to satisfy the requirement that you are willing and able to take up any job immediately, this can be achieved by daily visits to the JobCentre or a drop-in centre or support group where a message can be left for you.

Notes

2. **People without fixed accommodation**
    1 **IS** Sch 7 para 6 IS Regs;
       JSA Sch 5 para 3 JSA Regs
    2 paras 29503-504 AOG
    3 CIS/16772/1996
    4 para 29506 AOG
    5 para 15 HC Handbook
    6 para 42 HC Handbook

10

Chapter 10

Administration – social security benefits

This chapter explains how claims for social security benefits are administered, how to claim a social security benefit, how your claim is dealt with, and how to challenge a decision made on your claim. It covers:

1. Administration of benefits (p224)
2. Payment of benefits (p225)
3. Who should claim (p226)
4. How to make a claim (p227)
5. When to claim (p229)
6. How your claim is dealt with and decided (p233)
7. Appeals (p235)
8. Decisions and reviews on housing and council tax benefit claims (p239)
9. Complaints (p240)

1. Administration of benefits

Most social security benefits are administered by the Benefits Agency. Most claims are dealt with by your local Benefits Agency office (unless you live in certain parts of London when your claim may be processed by a special unit elsewhere in the country, although you may still deliver your claim to your local office). However, special units have been set up to process claims for:

- attendance allowance (AA – see p85) and disability living allowance (DLA – see p81), which are administered initially by regional disability centres and then by the Disability Benefits Unit in Blackpool;
- invalid care allowance (ICA – see p88), which is administered by a central unit in Preston;
- jobseeker's allowance (JSA – see pp93 and 125), which is administered by the Employment Service (part of the Department for Education and Employment) on behalf of the DSS at local JobCentres;
- family credit (FC) and disability working allowance (DWA), which are administered from Preston, and working families tax credit (WFTC) and

disabled person's tax credit (DPTC) (see pp125 and 115), which are now administered by the Inland Revenue from central units in Preston and Belfast;

- child benefit, which is administered in Washington, Tyne and Wear.

Although claims for AA/DLA/ICA (and child benefit) are processed elsewhere, they may be paid by your local Benefits Agency office if you are being paid another benefit which is administered locally.

Telephone numbers and addresses of local Benefits Agency offices can be found in telephone directories under 'Benefits Agency'. See Appendix 3 for the numbers and addresses of central units.

Housing benefit (HB) and council tax benefit (CTB) (see pp102 and 111) are administered by local authorities (usually by the housing or finance departments).

2. Payment of benefits

Once awarded, payments of any benefit you are entitled to may be made by giro, order book or by automated credit transfer direct to your bank account.[1] In exceptional circumstances (eg, if you live at an unsafe address) it may be possible for you to be paid cash.[2] Most benefits are paid in respect of your entitlement for a whole week, but AA, DLA and income support (IS) or JSA can be paid at a daily rate if you spend part of a week in hospital or in a care home. Most benefits are usually paid so that they can be cashed every week, but some benefits are usually paid fortnightly (eg, JSA), and some are paid four-weekly (eg, AA/DLA unless they are paid together with a weekly benefit such as IS). Some benefits are paid in advance, some in arrears, and some partly in advance and arrears.[3] Payments of benefit by automated credit transfer are usually paid four-weekly in arrears. Payments may sometimes be made to someone else on your behalf – eg, your appointee, or (for HB) your landlord, or (for DLA mobility component) the Motability scheme (see p142). You may authorise an 'agent' to cash any payment on your behalf.

Once you have been awarded benefit you must cash the payment within a year of it being due (although giros and order books are only valid for one month and three months respectively, and you will have to ask for a replacement if necessary), although this period can be extended if you can show good reasons for the delay.[4]

For further details about payment of benefits, see CPAG's *Welfare Benefits Handbook*.

---

3. **Who should claim**

You generally claim benefit for yourself. However, for IS, income-based JSA, HB or CTB, if you have a partner either one of you can make the claim for both of you. Sometimes it may be better for the claim to be made by one partner instead of the other, so you should check the rules in Chapter 3 to see which is best for you.

If you are 'unable to act' for yourself (eg, because of ill health or disability) someone else, called an 'appointee', can be authorised to act on your behalf.[5] Anyone aged 18 or over may be an appointee – eg, a partner, friend, relative or carer, or in some cases the director of your local social services department. Appointees are not necessary if a court has already appointed someone else to look after your affairs. DSS guidance advises that owners or managers of care homes should only be made appointees as a last resort if nobody else can be appointed and that a social services appointment may be possible instead.[6] This is reinforced in guidance to social services which stresses that 'it is most undesirable that a manager or proprietor should take on this role' and expects that proprietors should be required to notify social services if no one else is available so that they may make a recommendation[7] or take on the role themselves.

An appointee takes on all your rights and responsibilities as a claimant – eg, s/he must report any relevant changes in your circumstances and may have to repay any benefit which may have been overpaid to you. Normally this will only apply from the date your appointment has been agreed, but if someone acts on your behalf before officially becoming your appointee, her/his actions can be retrospectively validated by the appointment.[8]

In the past, it was common practice for a separate appointment to be required for each benefit administered by the Benefits Agency, but common rules now apply to all appointments and it is arguable that only one appointment should have to be made which should cover all benefits. However, local practice still varies and you will need to clarify with the Benefits Agency exactly what the scope of your appointment is considered to be. Sometimes you may prefer not to be appointed to act for all benefits – eg, if a claimant has mental health problems or a drug or alcohol dependency and you want to take care of some of her/his benefits to meet essential living expenses but leave her/him with one benefit to use for personal spending. You may need to try to negotiate suitable arrangements with the Benefits Agency. A separate appointment is strictly necessary for HB/CTB, although in practice the local authority will simply confirm an appointment if the Benefits Agency has appointed you to act for any of the benefits it administers.

Applications to become an appointee must be made in writing. You are expected to give a month's written notice if you no longer wish to act as appointee, although the appointment may in any case be terminated at any time by the Benefits Agency or local authority. This may happen if, for example, an appointee is no longer necessary, or it is considered that you are not acting in the claimant's best interests and someone else (eg, the director of social services) should be appointed instead.

If you are an appointee for a claimant who dies, you must re-apply to be an appointee in order to settle any outstanding benefit matters.[9] An executor under a will can also pursue an outstanding claim or appeal on behalf of a deceased claimant even if any decision on a claim in question was made before the formal grant of probate.[10]

The responsibilities of an appointee are not the same as those which apply to an agent who is merely a person you may authorise to cash or collect any payment of benefit made to you.

4. **How to make a claim**

In order to qualify for a benefit you must make a claim[11] in writing, usually on an appropriate form (except for certain retirement pensions which do not have to be claimed if you are already receiving another retirement pension or widows' benefit – see Chapter 3). Claim forms are available from your local Benefits Agency office or central unit or, for HB/CTB, your local authority. Claims for JSA must usually be made in person at a JobCentre. Except for IS and JSA, any letter or other written communication may be accepted as a valid claim,[12] but in practice it is best to use the proper form if at all possible. The Benefits Agency should respond by sending you the proper form (or returning an incomplete form) and giving you a month in which to complete it (or longer if it is considered reasonable) in order to validate your claim from your initial correspondence or form.[13]

If you request a claim form by telephone, the claim may be registered from the date of the request and provided you then complete and return the form within one month, or six weeks for AA/DLA, or longer if it is considered reasonable, the claim will be treated as if it had been made on the date you first requested the form.

In some limited circumstances your claim may be backdated (see p229). However, the rules can be very strict, and unless you have a good reason for deferring a claim you should claim as soon as you think you might be entitled to a benefit, even if it might take you some time to collect all the information which may be required in support of your claim, as you will be able to send this in later.

If you claim the wrong benefit, but are in fact entitled to another benefit instead, your original claim can sometimes be treated as a claim for the right benefit.[14] This applies to the following benefits:

Benefit claimed	May be treated as a claim for
Income support	Invalid care allowance
Attendance allowance	Disability living allowance
Disability living allowance	Attendance allowance
Severe disablement allowance	Incapacity benefit
Retirement pension	Widows' benefits
Widows' benefits	Retirement pension
Incapacity benefit	Severe disablement allowance

In addition, claims for AA or DLA can be interchanged with claims for constant attendance allowance paid with disablement benefit and *vice versa* (and similar rules allow for maternity allowance claims to be interchanged with claims for incapacity benefit and severe disablement allowance and *vice versa*, and for the interchange of claims for FC and DWA and tax credits, and for the treatment of claims for child benefit and guardians allowance).

Similarly, if you claim a non-means-tested benefit for yourself or an increase for a child or adult dependant, your claim may be treated as a claim by someone else for an increase in her/his benefit for you or for the dependant.[15]

Providing information to support your claim

For all benefits, you are expected to provide information and evidence to support your claim.[16] The type of information and evidence you need is explained the claim form. It includes proof of your identity and your national insurance number (or, if you do not know it or do not have one, you will have to co-operate with the Benefits Agency in attempting to trace it or apply for one).

Special conditions apply to claims for IS and JSA. These impose an 'onus of proof rule' or 'evidence requirement'[17] which mean it is your responsibility to complete your claim form fully and correctly *and* to produce any information and evidence necessary to verify your claim. If your claim is considered to be defective or incomplete, you will be contacted by the Benefits Agency and expected to complete or prove your claim within one month of your initial attempt to claim, otherwise you may lose your entitlement to benefit, which may only be paid from the date you eventually prove your claim. You will be exempt from this evidence requirement only if:[18]

- you could not complete the form or get the information or evidence required because of a physical, mental, learning or communication difficulty *and* it is not reasonably practicable for someone to help you complete the form or get the proof on your behalf; *or*
- the information or evidence required does not exist; *or*
- you could not get the information or evidence required without serious risk of physical or mental harm *and* it is not reasonably practicable to get it in another way; *or*

- you could only get the information or evidence required from a third party *and* it is not reasonably practicable to get it from her/him; *or*
- it is considered that sufficient proof has been provided to show that you are not entitled to IS or JSA – eg, because your capital is too high so that it would be inappropriate to require further proof about your income.

If you think one of these exemptions applies to you, let the Benefits Agency know as soon as possible. If it accepts that you are exempt, it may help you fill in the form or give you longer to complete it or collect evidence or information on your behalf or tell you that you will not have to provide the information after all.

5. **When to claim**

You are not usually entitled to any benefit for any day before your date of claim (although you may sometimes be able to claim in advance if you know you are not entitled now but will be soon – eg, because you will shortly be coming out of hospital). The date of your claim is normally the first day in the benefit week after your claim is received. There are strict time limits for claiming benefits.[19]

Claims for AA and DLA can never be backdated.[20]

For other benefits, however, if you miss the time limit for claiming, your claim can sometimes be backdated for up to three months. Some benefits can be backdated automatically, but some can only be backdated in very limited circumstances. In either case, if you want your claim to be backdated you must ask for this to happen or it will not even be considered.[21]

Benefits which can be backdated automatically

The following benefits can be backdated automatically (ie, regardless of the reasons you may not have claimed earlier, but provided you met the conditions of entitlement throughout the period in question)[22] for up to three months:

- incapacity benefit;
- severe disablement allowance;
- industrial injuries benefits;
- retirement pension;
- widows' benefits;
- invalid care allowance;
- increases of non-means-tested benefits for adult or child dependants, and child benefit and guardian's allowance.

There are exceptions to these rules, however, so that if you miss the time limit for claiming disablement benefit for occupational deafness or asthma or a widow's payment you may lose your right to benefit altogether.

Backdating claims for income support and jobseeker's allowance

Claims for IS and JSA can be backdated for up to one month if there are 'good administrative reasons' – ie, if it is 'consistent with the proper administration of benefit' and one of the following applies:[23]

- your claim is late because the office where you are supposed to claim was closed (eg, due to a strike) and there were no other arrangements for claims to be made;
- you could not get to the benefit office or JobCentre due to difficulties with the type of transport your normally use and there was no reasonable alternative;
- there were adverse postal conditions – eg, bad weather or a postal strike;
- you stopped getting another benefit but were not informed before your entitlement ceased so you could not claim IS or JSA in time;
- you claimed IS or JSA in your own right within one month of separating from your partner;
- a close relative (ie, your partner, parent, son, daughter, brother or sister) of yours died in the month before your claim.

Alternatively, your claim can be backdated for up to three months if you can show that it was not reasonable to expect you to claim before you did and your delay was for one of the following specified reasons:[24]

- you have learning, language or literacy difficulties *or* are deaf or blind *or* were sick or disabled (but not if you are claiming JSA) *or* were caring for someone who is sick or disabled *or* were dealing with a domestic emergency which affected you *and*, in either case, it was not 'reasonably practicable' for you to get help to make your claim form anyone else;
- you were given information by an officer of the DSS (or the Department of Education and Employment) and as a result thought you were not entitled to benefit;
- you were given advice in writing by a Citizens Advice Bureau or other advice worker, a solicitor or other professional adviser (eg, an accountant), a doctor or a local authority and as a result thought you were not entitled to benefit;
- you or your partner were given written information about your income or capital by your employer or a bank or building society and as a result you thought you were not entitled to benefit;
- you could not get to the benefit office or JobCentre because of bad weather.

Even if one of these reasons applies, you might still be paid less than three months' arrears if you claim because of a new interpretation of the law.[25]

If a person is acting as your appointee, then it is your appointee not you who must show that it was not reasonable to expect her/him to claim sooner than s/he did for one of the reasons listed above.[26] If someone is acting on your behalf on an informal basis, then it is still up to you to show that the reasons applied to you, or else you must show that it was reasonable for you to delegate responsibility for your claim and that you took care to ensure that the person helping you did it properly.[27]

Similar rules also apply to backdating claims for FC, DWA and the new tax credits.

Backdating claims for housing benefit and council tax benefit

Unlike other benefits, claims for HB and CTB can be backdated for up to 52 weeks (from the date of your request for backdating, which may be later than the date of your original claim), but only if you can show you have continuous good cause for a late claim. What constitutes 'good cause' is not spelled out in the regulations but it has been held to mean 'some fact which having regard to all the circumstances (including the claimant's state of health and the information which he received and that which he might have obtained), would probably have caused a reasonable person of his age and experience to act (or fail to act) as the claimant did'.[28]

Common examples are where a claimant has been misled by someone s/he could have been expected to rely on (eg, officers of the Benefits Agency or local authority or an independent adviser)[29] or where it may have been reasonable to believe there was no entitlement to benefit and therefore no reason to claim or ask about it.[30] Health problems, disabilities, language difficulties, limited knowledge and experience of claiming benefits, and factors beyond your control (eg, difficulties with the post), may be relevant factors, although they may not necessarily amount to good cause in themselves.[31] It may, for example, be arguable that you have good cause for a late claim for CTB if you are jointly liable for council tax but your name is not on the bill.

In practice, many local authorities have taken a more relaxed view to the backdating of claims than has the Benefits Agency for whom the same rules used to apply. Other local authorities have taken a more rigid view because the subsidies they receive from the DSS are reduced for backdated claims, although that is not a legitimate reason they should take into account in considering whether to allow a backdated claim.

Whether you have good cause for a late claim or not, the date of claim for HB/CTB may also be treated as earlier than the date the claim is actually made if:[32]

- you have claimed IS or JSA and your HB/CTB claim was sent to the Benefits Agency within four weeks of your IS/JSA claim, in which case your HB/CTB claim is treated as made on the same day as your IS/JSA claim;
- you receive IS/JSA and you then become liable to pay rent, in which case you will be allowed four weeks to make your claim for HB/CTB;
- for CTB, if there is a delay in your local authority fixing its council tax rate, so long as you claim within four weeks of being notified of the rate, your claim may be backdated to 1 April (or the date you first become entitled if later).[33]

Claims for HB/CTB may be renewed from the expiry date of a previous award if the renewal claim is made within four weeks of that date.[34]

Backdating of benefits following awards of another qualifying benefit

Special rules apply on backdating claims if your entitlement to a benefit depends on the outcome of a claim for another benefit. They may apply if you wish to claim ICA but it cannot be awarded until the person you are looking after is awarded AA, or if your entitlement to IS depends on you being awarded the severe disability premium which is only payable if you are awarded AA.

If you claim ICA or incapacity benefit or severe disablement allowance (or DWA or DPTC), and your entitlement depends on the outcome of your or another person's claim for a qualifying benefit, you should *not* delay making a claim until that other benefit is finally awarded (even if you are not sure what the outcome of that claim will be), otherwise you may lose benefit. Your claim may initially be refused while that other claim is waiting to be decided but when it is awarded, provided you make a further claim within three months of the decision to award that benefit, your claim will be backdated to the date of your original claim no matter how long ago that may have been.[35] If you delay making a claim until the outcome is known, you may only be entitled to a maximum of three months' arrears of backdated benefit.

It was intended that similar provisions would also apply to claims for IS and JSA. However, the rules appear to have been defectively drafted and it may not be possible to secure any extra backdating in this way if you would not be entitled to any IS or JSA at all for as long as the other qualifying benefit is not yet payable.[36] Nevertheless, you should still not delay making your claim for IS/JSA, but you should make it clear on your claim form that you are awaiting the outcome of a claim for another benefit. Guidance issued to the Benefits Agency asks it, in such circumstances, to hold on to your claim form (unless you would be entitled to at least some IS/JSA, in which case this will be paid to you in the meantime and any extra will be paid in arrears when the other benefit is awarded) and to avoid making a decision on it until the outcome of the other claim is known, so that it can then award you the amount owing to you from the date of your claim.

If, however, the Benefits Agency fails to do this you should still ask for your claim to be backdated as soon as the other qualifying benefit is awarded. Even though the rules may not strictly allow for this to happen, the Benefits Agency may consider making an *ex gratia* payment for the amount that would have been paid had the rules not been defectively drafted.

Delays in dealing with qualifying benefits should count as good cause for a late claim for HB/CTB. Note that HB/CTB claims may not be backdated more than 52 weeks and it may take longer than that to secure awards of qualifying benefits, particularly if appeals are necessary.

If you lose benefit because of the way your claim(s) are dealt with, you should seek expert advice (see Appendix 4).

6. **How your claim is dealt with and decided**

New rules on how claims are dealt with were being gradually introduced by the Social Security Act 1998 at the time this *Handbook* was being written. For all weekly benefits (except HB and CTB or social fund grants and loans – see Chapter 3) the new rules will have taken effect by 29 November 1999. This section considers only the effect of these new rules. For details of the rules which applied previously and any transitional arrangements see CPAG's *Welfare Benefits Handbook* and *Welfare Rights Bulletin*.

Decisions

Except for HB and CTB (see p239), all decisions on all benefits are made in the name of the Secretary of State. You must be given written notice of any decision and told of your right of appeal. If the notice of your decision does not give reasons, you can request a statement of reasons within one month, which must be provided within 14 days.[37]

If you disagree with any decision, you can ask the Secretary of State to revise or supersede it, or you can appeal against it to an independent tribunal. It is not necessary to ask for a decision to be revised or superseded if you want to appeal instead straightaway. However, if you want to ask for a revision or supersession or appeal, you must normally do so within one month of being notified of the decision in question.

Revisions

Asking for a revision may be simpler than an appeal and you could be given a favourable decision more quickly. Also, if your application for a revision is turned down, you can appeal against the new decision.

You do not have to ask for a revision in writing, although it is always best to do so. If you are uncertain about whether your request for a revision is being acted upon, you should consider appealing anyway, making sure you do so within the time limits. If you ask for a revision and also appeal, your appeal could lapse if the decision is revised and is more advantageous to you than the earlier decision, even if you do not get everything you want.

You can ask for a revision (or the Secretary of State may carry one out her/himself):[38]

- on 'any grounds' within a 'dispute period' of one month. This time limit may be extended (up to an absolute maximum of 13 months) but only if it is considered reasonable to do so and your application has merit and there are special circumstances which mean that it was not practicable for you to ask within a month.[39] If you are asked for further evidence or information you must provide this within one month (or longer if reasonable) otherwise your application will be decided only on the information and evidence already provided and your benefit may be suspended or terminated in the meantime;[40] or

- at 'any time' if:
  - there has been an official error[41] (eg, if the Benefits Agency fails to take into account relevant evidence, so long as you have not contributed to the error); *or*
  - you have misrepresented or failed to disclose facts and as a result, the decision is more favourable to you than it would otherwise have been;[42] *or*
  - you have been refused benefit but are now entitled to it because you have been awarded another benefit;[43] *or*
  - you were awarded benefit, but are now entitled to it at a higher rate because you have now been awarded another benefit.[44]

Decisions may only be revised on the basis of your circumstances at the time the decision was made.[45] If your circumstances have changed, you should ask instead for a decision to be superseded.

Any issues not raised by your application for a revision will not have to be taken into account.[46] You should therefore ensure that you provide as much detail as possible in your application to ensure that anything that may be relevant is taken into account.

Any revised decision takes effect from the date on which the original decision with which you disagree took effect – eg, your date of claim. You can be paid arrears of benefit going back to that date. However, if the Secretary of State considers that the date from which the original decision took effect was wrong, the revised decision can take effect from the correct date.[47]

Supersessions

If you think that a decision is wrong but it is more than one month since it was made, you may ask for a supersession (or the Secretary of State may supersede a decision her/himself). A request for a revision or a notification of a change of circumstances can be treated as a request for a supersession.[48] Decisions may be superseded if:[49]

- there has been, or it is anticipated that there will be, a relevant change of circumstances;
- the decision in question was legally wrong or (even if it was made by a tribunal or a commissioner) it was made in ignorance of relevant facts or there was a mistake about the facts of your claim; *or*
- you have been awarded benefit, but from a later date you become entitled at a higher rate because you are awarded another benefit.

As with revisions, any issues not raised by your application for a supersession will not have to be taken into account,[50] and you will be expected to provide any evidence or information requested of you.

Supersessions generally take effect from the date of the decision being replaced or the date your circumstances changed and arrears may be paid accordingly, except that arrears following changes of circumstances will only be paid to you if you have notified the Benefits Agency of the change within one month (or longer if reasonable up to a maximum of 13 months).[51] There are also special rules allowing for decisions affecting allowances for housing costs for IS/JSA to take effect from earlier dates.[52]

There are special rules which may limit the amount of arrears payable to you on a revision or a supersession following a test case. See CPAG's *Welfare Benefits Handbook* for further details.

7. **Appeals**

This section deals with the effects of the new rules made under the Social Security Act 1998. For details of the rules which applied previously and for transitional arrangements see CPAG's *Welfare Benefits Handbook* and *Welfare Rights Bulletin*.

You have the right of appeal to an independent tribunal against most decisions made in the name of the Secretary of State.[53] You can appeal against an original decision or a decision made after an application for a revision or a supersession. You may also appeal against certain decisions about your NI contributions.

You must be given written notice of any decision against which you can appeal, including information on your right of appeal and your right to request a statement of reasons within one month (and which must be provided to you within 14 days).[54]

Time limits

You must appeal within one month of notification of any decision. If you have requested a statement of reasons, you will have a further 14 days from the end of that month within which to appeal. If the Secretary of State revises, refuses to revise, or supersedes a decision, the one-month time limit will run from the date you are sent the new decision.[55]

If you miss the time limit for appealing, a late appeal can only be allowed (up to a maximum of a further 12 months after your one month time limit) if it is considered to have reasonable prospects of success and it is 'in the interests of justice' for it to be allowed late. This will only apply if it was not practicable for you to appeal within one month because:[56]

- you, your spouse or a dependant has died or suffered serious illness;
- you are not resident in the UK;
- normal postal services were disrupted; *or*
- there are other special circumstances which are 'wholly exceptional'.

The longer the delay, the more compelling the circumstances need to be.[57] In deciding whether it is in the 'interests of justice' to allow a late appeal, no account can be taken of the fact that:

- a court or commissioner has interpreted the law in a different way than previously understood and applied;
- you (or your adviser) misunderstood or were unaware of the relevant law, including the time limits for appealing.[58]

Although you will be given a summary of any decision many on any application for a late appeal,[59] there is no right of appeal against a decision refusing to allow it,[60] although you can ask for such a decision to be reconsidered or you may be able to apply to the High Court for a judicial review if the decision is clearly unreasonable.

How to appeal

Any appeal must be in writing. Although it does not have to be on any particular form as long as it contains sufficient detail and reasons, in practice it is best to use the appropriate forms which should be readily available from any Benefits Agency office or advice agency.

The appeal must be signed by you, or by a properly authorised representative,[61] and must include enough information to enable the decision in question to be identified and your grounds for your appeal. If the appellant dies, some other person may apply to be their appointee to proceed with the appeal on their behalf. A grant of probate or letter of administration will not necessarily suffice.[62]

You (or your representative) may withdraw your appeal at any time before it is decided by giving notice in writing.[63]

Any appeal may be struck out, provided that you have been told this may happen, if the tribunal considers that:[64]

- it is 'misconceived' – ie, it is 'frivolous or vexatious' or 'obviously unsustainable and has no prospect of success';[65] *or*
- the tribunal does not have jurisdiction to deal with the appeal because there is no right of appeal against the decision in question;
- you have failed to comply with a direction given to you by the chair or clerk of the tribunal – eg, a request to provide information to support your appeal (although this could include merely failing to respond to a letter asking whether you would prefer a paper or oral hearing).

Appeals struck out may, however, still be reinstated if you apply within one month and if you provide further information and there are reasonable grounds for reinstatement or it is accepted that you may not have received warning that your appeal could be struck out.[66]

Tribunal hearings

Tribunals consist of up to three members drawn from a panel of people with a range of different experience.[67]

Three-member tribunals (a lawyer, a doctor and a person with experience of disability) will hear appeals about disability living allowance and attendance allowance.[68]

Two-member tribunals (a lawyer and a doctor) will hear appeals about whether:[69]

- you are incapable of work; *or*
- you have an industrial disease, or the extent of your disablement; *or*
- you are disabled for the purpose of your claim for industrial injuries benefits, or severe disablement allowance (or DWA or disabled person's tax credit).

Two-member tribunals (a lawyer and a financial expert such as an accountant) will hear complex appeals about relevant financial issues – eg, the accounts of trust funds and profit and loss accounts.

One-member tribunals (a lawyer) will hear all other appeals.

Tribunals may also invite another panel member to assist them as an 'expert'. The expert can attend, give evidence or provide a report, but may not take part in making the decision.

The tribunal service aims to deal with as many appeals as possible in the absence of appellants, and will convene 'paper hearings' in order to do so.

However, you have a right to an 'oral hearing', which will be arranged, but only if you specifically request it. Oral hearings will provide an opportunity for you to state your case in person. You may be accompanied or represented at any hearing. Hearings which have been arranged may be postponed or adjourned at the tribunal's discretion.[70]

Tribunals are not obliged to consider issues that are 'not raised by' your appeal,[71] nor can they look 'down to the date of the hearing' (ie, they can only look at the circumstances which existed at the time of the decision in question and not any subsequent changes such as a deterioration in your health), nor can they carry out physical examinations (unless the appeal relates to the assessment of disablement for severe disablement allowance or industrial injuries benefits).[72]

Tribunal decisions

You should always be given a decision notice by the tribunal confirming its decision. If you have arranged an oral hearing, this should be given to you immediately after your appeal has been decided. You can ask for a full statement of the tribunal's decision and the reasons for it, but you must ask within one month of the decision being notified to you. This time limit may be extended, but only in the same very limited circumstances in which late appeals may be allowed (see p236), and there is an absolute limit of three months.[73]

You may apply for any tribunal decision to be set aside. Decisions may be set aside if the tribunal considers that it is just to do so and there has been some procedural defect – eg, a hearing proceeded in your absence even though you wanted to attend, but you were not given notice of the hearing.[74]

Appeals against tribunal decisions

If you disagree with any tribunal decision you may apply to the chair of the tribunal for leave to appeal to a social security commissioner. However, you must apply within one month from the date the tribunal's decision is sent to you (although the time limit can be extended for up to a further 12 months if there are special reasons for doing so)[75] and appeals to commissioners may only be allowed if the tribunal has made an error of law.

If the tribunal chair agrees that an error of law has been made, s/he *may* set aside the decision.[76] If the Benefits Agency agrees with you that the tribunal has made an error of law, the chair *must* set aside the decision.[77] In either case, arrangements will then be made for your appeal to be heard by another tribunal as soon as possible.

If the chair does not set aside the decision s/he may still grant you leave to appeal. If s/he does not do so, you may then apply for leave directly to the commissioner within a further month (although this time limit may also be extended if there are special reasons for doing so). Decisions of commissioners may also be challenged in the courts.

For details of what constitutes an 'error of law' or special reasons for late appeals to the commissioner, and advice and guidance on preparing and pursuing an appeal, see CPAG's *Welfare Benefits Handbook*.

8. Decisions and reviews on claims for housing benefit and council tax benefit

The local authority must notify any 'person affected' of any decision about a claim for HB/CTB. All decisions must contain specific information which should include details of your right to ask for the decision to be reviewed.[78] A 'person affected' is:[79]

- the claimant;
- an appointee;
- the benefit authority;
- if the decision concerns whether or not to make a payment direct to a landlord or agent, that person;
- if the decision concerns the recovery of an overpayment, any person from whom it is decided to recover the benefit.

Any 'person affected' can make a signed request for reasons for any decision, apply for a review or apply for a decision to be set aside.[80]

You may apply for a review of any decision on any grounds.[81] Applications for a review should be made in writing within six weeks of notification of any decision,[82] although this time limit may be extended if there are special reasons.[83] Local authorities do not in practice tend to apply time limits strictly, but if your request is refused their decision is final.[84] If you are awaiting a written explanation of reasons for any decision, the period between your request for reasons being received and the explanation being posted to you is ignored in applying the time limits.[85]

Decisions on review should take effect from the date of the original decision or from the date of any relevant change of circumstances if that is later,[86] except that under no circumstances may arrears of benefit be paid for more than 52 weeks before the date of an original claim or review request.

If you are still dissatisfied with the outcome of a review, you have a right to request a further review by a review board. Review boards are made up of local councillors and although they are not independent, they are required to act as if they are.[87]

Applications for further reviews must be made within 28 days of a review decision being notified to you, although this time limit may be extended by the chair of the review board if there are special reasons for doing so.[88] Review boards should convene oral hearings within six weeks or as soon as possible after that.[89] You should be invited to attend, and may be accompanied or represented. Decisions of review boards and reasons for them should be sent to you within seven days of a hearing, or as soon as possible afterwards.[90] Decisions take effect from the same date as reviews would do so. Decisions of review boards may be corrected, set aside or even reviewed in certain circumstances,[91] but otherwise they are final and you will have to apply to the courts for a judicial review if you are still dissatisfied with the outcome.

For advice and guidance on applying to review boards and the courts see CPAG's *Welfare Benefits Handbook*.

9. **Complaints**

The review and appeal procedures set out above enables you to challenge the outcome of decisions made about your claim for any benefit. You should consider making use of the formal complaints procedures instead if you wish to challenge the *manner* in which your claim is dealt with rather than the actual decision itself – eg, if you are not happy with:
- delays in processing your claim;
- poor service – eg, failing to answer the telephone or respond to enquiries or losing your papers;
- poor or negligent advice;
- the attitude or behaviour of staff.

All Benefits Agency offices (whether local or based in a central unit) have a customer services manager to whom you should complain if you cannot resolve any problem with the supervisor of the section dealing with your claim. If you are still dissatisfied, you may ask for your complaint to be referred to an independent complaints review panel. These are made up of local people familiar with the difficulties encountered by benefit claimants, and may include representatives from social services or welfare rights agencies. If you are still dissatisfied, you should contact your Member of Parliament (or, in Scotland, Member of Scottish Parliament, or, in Wales, your Member of the National Assembly) and ask her/him to intervene on your behalf or else refer your complaint to the Parliamentary Commissioner for Administration (the Ombudsman). The Ombudsman investigates all complaints of maladministration by central government agencies which may have caused an injustice. Unless you live in Wales, you cannot refer a complaint to the Ombudsman yourself – all referrals must be made through your Member of Parliament.

If your complaint is about the administration of a claim for HB or CTB, you should instead make use of the local authority's formal complaints procedure.

If you are still dissatisfied, you should complain to a local councillor and/or to a councillor who chairs the council committee responsible for administering HB/CTB. Further complaints of maladministration may be made direct to the Local Government Ombudsman.

Either Ombudsman may recommend that you should be awarded compensation, particularly if you have suffered any hardship or loss as a consequence of the grounds for your complaint, and such recommendations are not uncommon in typical cases where there has been some unreasonable delay in dealing with your claim or review. Most local authorities and Benefits Agency offices would prefer not to deal with the Ombudsman, and will often go to great lengths to resolve your complaint themselves rather than have to deal with an investigation.

Notes

2. Payment of benefits
1 Reg 20 SS(C&P) Regs
2 para 5039 IS Guide (payments volume)
3 Regs 22-26A SS(C&P) Regs
4 Reg 38(1) and (2A) SS(C&P) Regs

3. Who should claim
5 Reg 33 SS(C&P) Regs;
 HB Reg 71 HB Regs;
 CTB Reg 61 CTB Regs
6 'Agents, Appointees, Attorneys and Receivers' guide, paras 57-58, April 1998
7 'Home Life: a code of practice for residential care' paras 2.6.4-2.6.5
8 R(SB) 5/90
9 CIS/642/1992
10 CIS/379/1992

4. How to make a claim
11 Reg 3 SS(C&P) Regs
12 Reg 4 SS(C&P) Regs
13 Reg 4(7) SS(C&P) Regs
14 Reg 9(1) and Sch 1 SS(C&P) Regs
15 Reg 9(4) and (5) SS(C&P) Regs
16 Reg 8(2) SS(C&P) Regs; reg 23 JSA Regs

17 Reg 4(1A) SS(C&P) Regs
18 Reg 4(1B) SS(C&P) Regs

5. When to claim
19 Reg 9(4) and (5) SS(C&P) Regs
20 ss65(4) and (6) and 76 SSCBA 1992
21 R(SB) 9/84
22 Reg 19(2) and (3) and Sch 4 SS(C&P) Regs
23 Reg 19(6) and (7) SS(C&P) Regs
24 Reg 19(4) and (5) SS(C&P) Regs
25 s68 SSAA 1992
26 R(SB) 17/83; R(IS) 5/91; CIS/812/1992
27 R(P) 2/85
28 CS/371/1949; para A2.23 and Part A2 Annex A GM
29 R(SB) 6/83; CS/50/1950; R(U) 9/74; CI/146/1991; CI/142/1993
30 R(SB) 6/83; CI/37/1995
31 R(S) 25/52; R(P) 2/85; R(S) 10/59; R(SB) 17/83; CSB/813/1987; R(G) 1/75
32 **HB** reg 72(5) HB Regs;
 CTB reg 62(5) CTB Regs
33 Reg 62(11) CTB Regs
34 **HB** regs 72 and 96A HB Regs;
 CTB regs 62 and 81A CTB Regs

35 Reg 6(16)-(23) SS(C&P) Regs
36 CSIS/80/1995; AM(AOG) 66, 17
February 1998

6. **How your claim is dealt with and decided**
37 Reg 28(1) and (2) SS&CS(D&A) Regs
38 Reg 3(1) SS&CS(D&A) Regs
39 Reg 4 SS&CS(D&A) Regs
40 Reg 3(2) SS&CS(D&A) Regs
41 Regs 1(3) and 3(5)(a) SS&CS(D&A) Regs
42 Reg 3(5)(b) SS&CS(D&A) Regs
43 Reg 3(7) SS&CS(D&A) Regs
44 Reg 3(7) SS&CS(D&A) Regs
45 Reg 3(9) SS&CS(D&A) Regs
46 s9(2) SSA 1998
47 Reg 5 SS&CS(D&A) Regs
48 Reg 6(5) SS&CS(D&A) Regs
49 Reg 6(2) SS&CS(D&A) Regs
50 s10(2) SSA 1998
51 s10(5) SSA 1998; Reg 7 SS&CS(D&A) Regs
52 Reg 7(13)-(23) SS&CS(D&A) Regs

7. **Appeals**
53 s12 and Sch 2 and 3 SSA 1998
54 Reg 28 SS&CS(D&A) Regs
55 Reg 31(1) SS&CS(D&A) Regs
56 Reg 32(1) and (4)-(6) SS&CS(D&A) Regs
57 Reg 32(7) SS&CS(D&A) Regs
58 Reg 32(8) SS&CS(D&A) Regs
59 Reg 32(10) and (11) SS&CS(D&A) Regs
60 Reg 32(9) SS&CS(D&A) Regs
61 Reg 33(1)(a) SS&CSA(D&A) Regs
62 Reg 34 SS&CS(D&A) Regs
63 Reg 40 SS&CS(D&A) Regs
64 Sch 5 para 2 SSA 1998; reg 46 SS&CS(D&A) Regs
65 Reg 1(3) SS&CS(D&A) Regs
66 Reg 47 SS&CS(D&A) Regs
67 ss 6(2) and 7(2) SSA 1998
68 Reg 36(6) SS&CS(D&A) Regs
69 Reg 36(2) SS&CS(D&A) Regs
70 Reg 51 SS&CS(D&A) Regs
71 s12(8)(a) SSA 1998
72 Reg 52 SS&CS(D&A) Regs
73 Regs 53(4) and 54(1) SS&CS(D&A) Regs
74 Reg 57 SS&CS(D&A) Regs
75 Reg 58(5) SS&CS(D&A) Regs
76 s13(2) SSA 1998
77 s13(3) SSA 1998

8. **Decisions and reviews on claims for housing benefit and council tax benefit**
78 **HB** reg 77 and Sch 6 HB Regs; **CTB** reg 67 and Sch 6 CTB Regs
79 **HB** reg 2(1) HB Regs; **CTB** reg 2(1) CTB Regs
80 **HB** regs 77(4), 79(2) and 86(10) HB Regs; **CTB** regs 67(2), 69(2) and 75(1) CTB Regs
81 **HB** reg 79(2) HB Regs; **CTB** reg 69(2) CTB Regs
82 **HB** reg 79(2) HB Regs; **CTB** reg 69(2) CTB Regs
83 **HB** reg 78(3) and (4) HB Regs; **CTB** reg 68(3) and (4) CTB Regs
84 **HB** reg 78 HB Regs; **CTB** reg 68 CTB Regs
85 **HB** reg 79 HB Regs; **CTB** reg 69 CTB Regs
86 **HB** reg 79 HB Regs; **CTB** reg 69 CTB Regs
87 **HB** regs 81 & 82 HB Regs; **CTB** regs 70 & 71 CTB Regs
88 **HB** reg 81 HB Regs; **CTB** reg 70 CTB Regs
89 **HB** reg 82(1) HB Regs; **CTB** reg 71(1) CTB Regs
90 **HB** reg 83(5) HB Regs; **CTB** reg 72(5) CTB Regs
91 **HB** regs 85-87 HB Regs; **CTB** regs 74-76 CTB Regs

Chapter 11

Common problems – social security

This chapter explains some of the problems which commonly occur when claiming social security benefits and how to deal with them. It covers:

1. Not claiming and underclaiming (p243)
2. Underpayments (p244)
3. Overpayments (p245)
4. Poverty and unemployment traps (p245)
5. Overclaiming (p247)
6. Competing claims (p248)
7. The 'domino' effect (p250)
8. Timing of claims (p251)
9. Poor or negligent advice (p252)
10. Delays (p252)
11. Fraud (p254)

1. Not claiming and underclaiming

It is well known that many people do not claim all the social security benefits to which they are entitled and much research has been undertaken to examine why. It is widely recognised that there are a variety of causes, ranging from the complexity of the social security scheme (particularly relating to means-tested benefits), a lack of available reliable information and sources of advice, dissatisfaction with previous experiences of claiming benefits, and a reluctance amongst certain eligible claimants (particularly older people) to subject themselves to what is perceived as the stigmatising and intrusive effect of means-testing.

Even if people do claim all the benefits to which they are entitled, it is not uncommon for them to 'underclaim' – ie, to claim a rate of benefit that is lower than that which should be payable to them. For example, they may claim attendance allowance (AA) but not declare all of their personal care needs so that only the lower rate instead of the higher rate is awarded to them; or they may claim a retirement pension, but not claim an increase of that benefit payable in respect of a dependant. Similarly, they may not ensure that a notification of an award of one benefit (eg, AA) is passed on to the agency responsible for dealing with a claim for another (eg, housing benefit) which could result in a higher award of that benefit (see Chapter 3). The interdependence of awards of different benefits is also a common cause of underpayments (see below).

There are very restrictive rules on the backdating of claims for all benefits (see Chapter 6) so you may lose money if you do not claim at the earliest opportunity. If possible, you should seek advice (see Appendix 4) as soon as you can. If in doubt, you should go ahead and claim any benefit you might possibly be entitled to (but first see overclaiming, p247).

2. Underpayments

Even if people claim all the benefits to which they are entitled, it is also well known that claims are not always processed or decided upon in the way that they should be. This is often the result of poor or indifferent administration, inadequate claim forms, and the complexities of the rules on which entitlement to certain benefits depend. For example, local Benefits Agency offices responsible for assessing entitlement to claims for income support (IS) are often not informed, or overlook notifications provided, by the Disability Benefits Unit of awards of AA or disability living allowance (DLA) which may effect entitlement to IS (eg, because the severe disability premium may have become payable). Local authority offices responsible for administering claims for housing benefit and/or council tax benefit (HB/CTB) also often fail to appreciate or act on the effect of an award of AA/DLA or awards of overlapping benefits (see p69). Claim forms are often confusing or ambiguous and claimants may be unclear what information is required from them, or decision-makers misunderstand the information provided to them, often to the claimant's disadvantage. Also, entitlement to some benefits is dependent on judgmental questions (eg, the extent of a claimant's 'incapacity for work' or 'personal care' needs) which often results in unreliable and inconsistent decision-making.

If you disagree with a decision made on any claim for benefit, you should always challenge it as soon as possible (see Chapter 10). If you identify an error in the way your benefit has been calculated or assessed, you should ask for the error to be corrected, and for payment of any missing amounts, as soon as possible. If the procedures for revising your award of benefit do not apply or do not properly compensate you for the effects of the mistake, you should ask for compensation. You may be paid an *ex gratia* payment equal to the amount you have lost, as well as additional amounts for any hardship you may have suffered, extra expenses you may have incurred, and interest on any arrears of benefit owing to you. If you feel you are not being offered adequate compensation, you should complain (see Chapter 10).

You should always use this *Handbook*, other sources of information and seek as much independent advice as possible (see Appendices 4 and 5) before and after claiming social security benefits so that you are sure you have claimed and been awarded all the benefits to which you are entitled.

3. **Overpayments**

It is also not uncommon for claimants to be paid more benefit than they are entitled to. Sometimes this is through no fault of their own – eg, due to poor administration or an error or oversight in a calculation or in the interpretation of complex rules. Sometimes it is through an accidental or innocent mistake on their part – eg, failing to report a change of circumstances by an oversight or through failing to appreciate the significance of it. Sometimes it may even be a more culpable failure to disclose some relevant information.

If you have been overpaid any benefit you will usually be *asked* to repay it even if it is the result of an official error. Sometimes you will *have* to repay overpaid benefit, sometimes you will not, and this will often (but not always) depend on the extent to which you may be considered to be responsible for the overpayment having occurred. Overpaid benefit may be recovered by deductions from benefits to which you are entitled. The rules on the recovery of overpayments can be very complicated. See CPAG's *Welfare Benefits Handbook* for further details, or seek advice as soon as possible (see Appendix 4).

4. **Poverty and unemployment traps**

One of the unintentional problems caused by the current scheme of social security benefits is that means-testing creates 'poverty traps' and 'unemployment traps'. Poverty traps occur when your dependency on means-tested benefits is such that you are unable to improve your financial circumstances by your own endeavours (eg, by increasing your income from earnings or other means) because your means-tested benefits may reduce by the same amount, or only slightly less, or sometimes by more, than any increase in income you are able to secure for yourself. Unemployment traps occur when the amount of income available to you from claiming means-tested benefits is more than would be available to you if you took up work.

Example:

Ranbir is 35 years old and lives in supported accommodation for single people with learning disabilities. £65 of the weekly rent is eligible for housing benefit (HB). The council tax is £17.50 a week.

He has been treated as incapable of work since he left school and has since then been receiving severe disablement allowance (SDA) and income support (IS) which includes a disability premium totalling £73.30 a week. As he gets IS, he is also awarded maximum HB and council tax benefit (CTB) so that he has no eligible housing costs and so can use all of his £73.30 to meet all of his other needs.

He is then paid £15 a week for work undertaken as part of a sheltered work scheme for people with disabilities. He is still treated as incapable of work and his £15 earnings are disregarded in his claims for SDA/IS/HB/CTB. He therefore now has £88.30 to meet his other needs.

He then decides instead to take on work for an employer for which he is paid net earnings of £160 for 25 hours a week. He loses entitlement to SDA (as he can no longer be treated as incapable of work) but applies for disabled person's tax credit (DPTC) instead. Because of the level of his earnings he only qualifies for a small award of DPTC worth £4.80 a week. Because of his total income (£164.80) he is no longer entitled to IS and his HB/CTB (which nevertheless includes a disability premium because he gets DPTC so that he still qualifies for an earnings disregard of £15) is reduced, so that he now has to pay £49.73 towards his rent and £15.30 towards his council tax (totalling £65.03). This leaves him with £99.77 to meet his other needs.

He then takes an opportunity to increase his earnings to £170 a week. However, his earnings are now too high to qualify for any DPTC. As a result he no longer qualifies for a disability premium with HB/CTB and is therefore also only entitled to a lower earnings disregard of £5 a week. Consequently, he is no longer entitled to HB/CTB at all and must pay all of his rent and council tax (totalling £82.50) out of his earnings (£170), which leaves him with £87.50 to meet his other needs.

Although he may be better off in work than if he was not working at all (not counting the value of any eligibility for social fund grants and other sources of financial assistance which are only payable to those on IS), when he earns £170 a week he is £0.80 worse off than when he was only earning £15 a week, and £12.27 worse off than when he was earning £160.

Similar effects can apply even if you are not dependent on means-tested benefits, as your entitlement to non-means-tested benefits may be adversely affected by taking up work or increasing earnings.

Example:

Andy has received a redundancy payment of over £16,000 so is not entitled to any means-tested benefits. He lives with his wife and two dependent children for whom child benefit is payable. His wife is severely disabled and receives the middle rate care component of disability living allowance. Andy cares for his wife so he is entitled to invalid care allowance (ICA). This is worth £39.95 a week. He is also entitled to claim a dependency increase for his wife (worth £23.90 a week) and children (worth £21.25 a week) because his wife has no earnings. The total value of his claim for ICA is £85.10 a week. Andy takes up a part-time job which will not affect his entitlement to ICA if it pays no more than £50 a week. But if he increases his earnings to £50.01, he will lose all £85.10 of his entitlement to ICA.

In some circumstances, it may not be possible to avoid poverty traps and unemployment traps, particularly because of the rules on notional income (see p182). However, you should always at least consider the consequences of taking up work or increasing your income or earnings before doing so by referring to all the different rules set out in this *Handbook* and other sources of information or by seeking advice (see Appendices 4 and 5).

5. **Overclaiming**

It is usually best to claim all the benefits to which you may be entitled in order to maximise your income. However, one of the effects of current means-testing is the risk of overclaiming, which means that if you claim everything to which you may be entitled you might be worse off than if you did not. In other words, not claiming or underclaiming benefits (see p243) could leave you better off, and overclaiming could leave you worse off.

The main problem is when you make a claim for a non-means-tested benefit (either for yourself or in respect of a dependant) which, when awarded, means that because of your increased income you are no longer entitled to income support (IS). Although your weekly income may actually be slightly higher than when you were getting IS, you may still find you are actually worse off because you will no longer be eligible for social fund grants (see p117) and other sources of financial assistance (see Chapter 4) which may only be paid to those in receipt of IS.

Example:
Brian is 45 years old and lives alone in rented accommodation. He cares for his mother who has claimed attendance allowance (AA). As her claim for AA has not yet been decided he is not entitled to invalid care allowance (ICA) but he is able to claim IS and receives £51.40 a week and maximum HB/CTB. His own health deteriorates and he is advised that he is entitled to incapacity benefit (IB). He claims IB and is awarded £57.40 a week. Because his income now exceeds his IS applicable amount he is no longer entitled to IS and his HB/CTB is reduced by a total of £5.10. Although he may have

£0.90 a week more than when he was on IS to meet his other needs, he will not be eligible for a social fund grant or other sources of financial assistance and so may have greater difficulties in managing than when he was on IS (at least until the AA/ICA claims are decided).

Similar problems occur when opportunities arise to take up work or increase earnings (see poverty traps and unemployment traps, p245). There is also a risk that claiming some benefits may sometimes adversely affect the income of another person, and *vice versa* (see competing claims below).

In some circumstances, it may not be possible to avoid the effects of overclaiming, particularly because of the rules on notional income' (see p182). However, you should always at least consider the consequences of claiming other benefits before doing so by referring to all the different rules set out in this *Handbook* and other sources of information or by seeking advice (see Appendices 4 and 5).

6. **Competing claims**

Generally, your entitlement to any benefit depends on and affects only your own circumstances and those of any partner or dependent children who live with you. Sometimes, however, your entitlement to benefit may depend on or be affected by the circumstances of another person who is not part of your family. This is because some benefits compete with others in that if you claim one benefit this may remove or reduce the entitlement of another person to another or the same benefit, and *vice versa*. This may occur as a consequence of:

• claims by carers; *or*
• claims by non-dependants; *or*
• claims by liable relatives.

Claims by carers

If you are a carer of another person who is entitled to the severe disability premium (SDP), that person will lose that SDP if you are paid ICA (see p88). It is possible that the extra gains to you of an award of ICA (or carer's premium) may be worth rather less than the value of the SDP to the person you are looking after.

If you claim ICA you may prevent another carer from being awarded ICA for looking after the same person (see p87). It is possible that the extra gains to you of an award of ICA or carer's premium may be worth rather less to you than the value of an award of ICA or carer's premium to another carer.

Claims by non-dependants

If you are a non-dependant living in the home of another person who receives help with their housing costs and/or council tax by claiming IS/HB/CTB, any increase in your income may increase their non-dependant deduction and therefore reduce their benefits (see pp99, 109 and 114). It is possible that the value of any increase in your income may be worth rather less than the value of their lost benefits.

Example:
Peter lives with his mother, who receives HB/CTB. Peter has earnings and other income (from which he pays no tax or NI contributions) worth £150 a week. A non-dependant deduction is applied to reduce his mother's HB by £22.65 and her CTB by £4.40 (totalling £27.05). Peter learns that he is entitled to disabled person's tax credit because he has a disability and works 20 hours a week. He is awarded DPTC worth £10.30 a week. Because his gross weekly income has now increased to £160.30, his mother's HB non-dependant deduction increases to £37.10, although the deduction for CTB remains at £4.40. This totals £41.50. By applying for DPTC Peter has increased his income by £10.30 a week. However, his mother's HB/CTB has reduced by £14.45 a week.

Claims by liable relatives

Any maintenance you receive from a liable relative (see Chapter 8) may reduce any means-tested benefit to which you may be entitled. The amount of maintenance your liable relative may have to pay will usually depend on her/his income. If her/his income increases (eg, because s/he has been awarded a social security benefit to supplement her/his other income) the amount of maintenance liability may also increase. If you are dependent on IS, you may sometimes lose your entitlement altogether as a result of any payment or increase in maintenance. Although your weekly income may actually be slightly higher than when you were getting IS, you may still find you are actually worse off because you will no longer be eligible for social fund community care grants and other sources of financial assistance (see Chapter 4) which may only be paid to those in receipt of IS.

There is a particular risk of this happening if your spouse is in a care home and claiming IS and/or help from social services with the costs of the accommodation. The rules on income (see p175 and Chapter 13) provide an incentive for your spouse to pay you half of certain private pension payments s/he may receive. However, if the amount paid to you would mean that you are no longer entitled to IS for yourself, you may find that you are worse off than if you did not receive the payment.

In some circumstances, it may not be possible to avoid the effects of competing claims, particularly because one person may still wish to claim a competing benefit even though the value to that person may be less than to another and they may not share the same common interest, and because of the rules on notional income (see p182). However, you should always at least consider the consequences of claiming other benefits before doing so by referring to all the different rules set out in this *Handbook* and other sources of information or by seeking advice (see Appendices 4 and 5).

7. The 'domino' effect

Whether or not you are entitled to a benefit, and the rate at which it should be paid, is sometimes dependent on you or another person (ie, your partner, or dependent child, or carer, or person you are caring for, or someone else who lives in your home) being entitled to another qualifying benefit (for further details, see Chapter 3). An award of one qualifying benefit may significantly increase your total income by increasing your entitlement to other benefits (for examples, see p130). However, if that 'qualifying benefit' is withdrawn, your entitlement to your other benefits may be reconsidered and even withdrawn. This is known as the 'domino' effect because if entitlement to one benefit collapses, entitlement to other benefits may also do so.

For example, it may have been accepted that you are disabled enough to qualify for the higher rate care component of disability living allowance (DLA – see p81). As a result, you may have been treated as 'incapable of work' and '80 per cent disabled' so that you qualify for severe disablement allowance (SDA – see p79). Because of this, you will not have been required to sign on as available for work and are able to claim IS (see p93). Your award of DLA (and SDA) entitles you to the disability premium and may entitle you to the severe disability premium when calculating how much IS should be paid to you (see p97). And because you receive IS, you are automatically entitled to the highest rates of HB or CTB (see pp104 and 113) and assistance with certain health and other benefits (see p143) and you may be able to apply for community care grants from the social fund (see p117). Your award of DLA may also entitle you to assistance from the independent living fund (ILF) (see p143) and may even affect any charges you may be expected to contribute for community care services (see p49). It will also determine whether a carer may claim ICA (see p88) for looking after you and affect your carer's entitlement to other benefits or the rate at which they should be paid (eg, IS/HB/CTB) may also be dependent on continuing entitlement to ICA which in turn depends on your continuing entitlement to DLA.

If, however, it is then decided that you no longer meet the conditions of entitlement to DLA, your award of DLA will be stopped. You may then no longer qualify for SDA and your IS may be reduced or stopped, so that you may have to reclaim HB/CTB. Any assistance you receive from the ILF and any ICA your carer may be claiming may also be stopped. In such circumstances, you will need to challenge the decision to stop your DLA as soon as possible (see Chapter 10) so that all your (and your carer's) benefits and services can be reinstated. In the meantime, you (and your carer) will have to consider what other benefits you may still be able to claim – eg, you may be able to persuade the Benefits Agency that you are still incapable of work so that you can continue to claim IS, or else you may have to sign on to claim jobseeker's allowance (JSA) instead, or claim a reduced rate of IS while you are appealing, and/or re-claim HB/CTB and any health and other benefits which may have depended on your award of IS. You will also need to notify the ILF that you are appealing against the refusal of your award of DLA so that ILF payments may still continue, and you may need to ask for any community care services and charges to be reassessed so that proper arrangements for your care can still be made.

You may need to seek expert independent advice in such circumstances (see Appendix 4).

8. **Timing of claims**

For most benefits, it is nearly always important to claim any benefit to which you are entitled as soon as possible otherwise you may lose money because of the restrictions on the backdating of benefits (see p229). This also applies to claims for benefits to which you may not yet be entitled, but to which you will become entitled following an award of another qualifying benefit which has not yet been decided (see p232).

Sometimes, however, it may be advantageous to defer a claim for benefit.

For example, you may be entitled to the severe disability premium while claiming IS, HB or CTB but only while a carer is not being paid ICA for looking after you. However your entitlement to the severe disability premium is not affected by backdated awards of ICA. It may therefore be advantageous to you, yet still not disadvantageous to your carer, if your carer delays any claim for ICA to which s/he may be entitled to (see p88).

Similarly, awards of tax credits (see pp115 and 125) are paid for fixed periods and it may be advantageous to delay your claim until a change in your circumstances or an uprating of benefit occurs so that these can be taken into account when calculating your entitlement.

Some complicated situations can arise requiring careful consideration if you want to maximise your entitlement to benefits. If in doubt you should consider all the rules on any benefits you may be entitled to, as set out in

Chapters 3 and 10 of this *Handbook* and in CPAG's *Welfare Benefits Handbook*. Alternatively seek expert advice (see Appendix 4).

9. **Poor or negligent advice**

In order to ensure that you are paid all the benefits to which you may be entitled, you may be dependent on the advice you are given. If you discover the advice you are given is poor or negligent and as a result you have lost money, you may be entitled to compensation. This can apply whether the advice you were given was from the Benefits Agency or local authority dealing with claims for benefits or an independent advice agency. For example, the Benefits Agency has been ordered to compensate a claimant when it gave misleading information about time limits which led the claimant to miss a deadline for challenging a decision which would have caused a loss of benefit.[1] Social workers assisting with other matters have also been held liable for incomplete or misleading benefits advice.[2] Although social services have a duty to offer appropriate advice and information to people with disabilities,[3] it has been held that they 'cannot be expected to offer expert advice on [a social security benefit] which is not part of the council's responsibility, but can be expected to point the way to getting sound advice' and that they 'certainly should not offer advice unless justifiably content as to the extent of [their] knowledge'.[4]

If you have lost benefits due to poor or negligent advice, you may have a remedy by using the complaints procedures of the agency responsible, or referring to the ombudsman (see p240), or applying to the courts. You may therefore need the further assistance of a different advice agency or solicitor (see Appendix 4).

10. **Delays**

The administration of the social security scheme has long been the source of widespread criticism. Delays in processing claims or changes in circumstances or issuing payments, or in the handling of appeals, are still common. These can be caused by genuine oversight, poor or indifferent administration, inadequate resources or deliberate policy decisions. They invariably cause claimants considerable frustration and hardship. Nevertheless, a number of remedies exist in cases of delay, and often the mere threat of taking action against those responsible for the delay will result in a prompt response.

Local authority HB/CTB units have a duty to make a decision on properly made claims, tell you in writing what the decision is, and pay you any HB or

CTB you are entitled to, within 14 days or, if that is not 'reasonably practicable', as soon as possible after that.[5] If you are a private tenant and it has not been possible to assess your HB within the required period (eg, if the delay has been caused by a rent officer or other third party), there is a further duty to issue you with an interim payment or payment on account while your claim is being investigated[6] (and if this later proves to be less than your full entitlement you will be paid the extra, or if it proves to be more it may be recovered as an overpayment[7]). In practice, many local authorities take considerably longer than 14 days to deal with claims and do not always comply with the duty to make payments on account. If this applies to your claim, you should consider making a complaint to the ombudsman (see p240). Alternatively, seek the advice of a solicitor with a view to applying for a judicial review in the High Court to seek an order to compel the authority to make a decision and/or payment. Strictly speaking, these duties apply to how a local authority deals with a claim for benefit, rather than to a review of an existing award, but in practice the local authority can be held accountable by the Local Government Ombudsman and the courts on a review if the delay is unreasonable.

For benefits administered by the Benefits Agency, there is no longer a similar statutory duty to decide on any claim within any set period or to make an interim payment,[8] although the Benefits Agency intends to set target times for dealing with claims. According to the Benefits Agency's own official guidance,[9] it should consider any request for compensation for long delays if:

- the Benefits Agency was significantly at fault for the delay; *and*
- the amount of benefit involved was more than £100; *and*
- any compensation would be £10 or more; *and*
- the delay was more than the relevant 'delay indicator'.

'Delay indicators' are different for each benefit and provide for a very significant period of delay before the Benefits Agency will readily accept any responsibility to pay compensation. For example, for IS it is two months; for AA and DLA it is seven months (or two months if the claim is made under the special rules for the terminally ill); and for ICA it is nine months. Nevertheless, it is likely that the Parliamentary Ombudsman and the courts would take a less tolerant view of delays, and if you are likely to suffer hardship even if benefit has been delayed by only a few days (eg, because you have no other income and are dependent on an award of IS) you should consider using the complaints procedure or taking legal advice straightaway.

If your claim for benefit has been decided, but there is a delay in issuing payment, you may have an additional remedy by suing for payment in the county court (or in Scotland, the sheriff's court) and should seek advice (see Appendix 4).

You may be entitled to a crisis loan from the social fund (see p123) while you are waiting for a claim for benefit to be decided or paid.

If you are suffering hardship due to a delay in the way any appeal is being dealt with by a review board (for HB/CTB), the tribunal service or the social security commissioners, you should consider complaining to the Ombudsman or by applying for a judicial review in the courts. In cases of exceptional delay there may be a remedy by applying to the European courts on the grounds that 'in the determination of his civil rights and obligations... everyone is entitled to a fair and public hearing *within a reasonable time* by an independent and impartial tribunal established by law'.[10]

11. **Fraud**

You may commit an offence if you deliberately mislead the Benefits Agency or local authority, or if you deliberately fail to notify a change in your circumstances which you know could affect the amount of benefit payable to you.

If you commit a fraud you may be at risk of being prosecuted and you could be cautioned, fined or even imprisoned. Sometimes you will be asked to agree to pay a penalty payment as an alternative to being prosecuted (although this option will probably only be offered to you if the prospects of a successful prosecution are considered to be weak). In either case, you may also have to repay any benefits overpaid to you as a consequence of any fraud.

You should always seek expert advice, preferably from a solicitor, if you have any reason to believe that you are suspected of fraud or are being investigated for fraud by the Benefits Agency or local authority. For further information see CPAG's *Welfare Benefits Handbook*.

Notes

9. **Poor or negligent advice**

1 Parliamentary Ombudsman investigation No.C.421/98
2 Local Government Ombudsman reports on investigation No 93/A/ 3738 into a complaint against East Sussex County Council, 20 March 1995 and investigation No 98/C/ 1842 into a complaint against Stockport MBC, 30 March 1999
3 s29 NAA 1948 and s1 CSDPA 1970; DHSS Circular 13/74
4 Local Government Ombudsman report on investigation No 91/C/ 1246 into a complaint against Wakefield Metropolitan District Council, 9 December 1993

10. **Delays**

5 **HB** regs 76(3), 77(1)(a) and 88(3) HB Regs
CTB regs 66(3), 67(1)(a) and 77(3)(b) and (c) CTB Regs
6 Reg 91(1) HB Regs; R v Haringey LBC ex parte Azad Ayub [1992] 25 HLR 566, QBD; para A6.36 GM
7 Reg 91(2) and (3) HB Regs
8 The duties have been removed on the implementation of the SSA 1998
9 Financial Redress for Maladministration
10 Article 6, European Convention on Human Rights. For further information, contact European Commission of Human Rights, Council of Europe, BP 431 RG 67006 Strasbourg Cedex, France.

Part 4

....

General provisions for social services and health authorities and care homes

This Part explains the rules which will apply to you if you need residential or nursing home care and whether you will be able to get help with funding of such care.

Chapter 12 covers the duties of social services and health authorities to arrange care in a home, the different types of home, and in choosing a home. The following chapters then explain the rules that social services use to work out how much you will need to pay for the care they have arranged.

It covers the rules for the way income (see Chapter 13) and capital and property (see Chapter 14) are treated. It explains how much money you should be left with each week to cover buying personal items (see Chapter 15).

It explains what happens if you choose to go into a home that is more expensive than social services thinks necessary for someone with your level of needs (see Chapter 16) and the rules for deciding whether your husband or wife remaining at home will need to make a contribution towards the costs of your care (see Chapter 17). It also covers the rules for asylum-seekers.

This Part also covers how your charge is collected, and the rules that can be used if it is thought that you have deliberately deprived yourself of income or capital in order to pay less (see Chapter 18), how the financial assessment is carried out, how they are reviewed and your rights to complain about the charge.

Part 4

General provisions for social services and health authorities and care homes

Chapter 12

Arranging for accommodation in care homes

This chapter explains what you need to consider or do if you think you might need residential or nursing care. It covers:

1. Who can have accommodation arranged by social services or the NHS? (p259)
2. Deciding if you need to be provided with care in a residential or nursing home (p263)
3. The different types of accommodation (p268)
4. Who has to pay and what should be covered in the fees (p271)
5. Accommodation arranged by social services (p277)

1. Who can have accommodation arranged by social services or the NHS?

The legal provisions – social services (in England and Wales)

When social services provide or arrange residential or nursing home accommodation for either a temporary or permanent stay it is nearly always under the National Assistance Act 1948. Social services departments have a *duty* under this act to provide or arrange residential or nursing care:

- if you are 18 or over (those under 18 come under the Children Act 1989); *and*
- if you need care and attention due to:
  – age;
  – illness;
  – disability;
  – or any other circumstance (which specifically includes mental disorder, and drug and alcohol dependency). Recently, asylum seekers unable to claim benefits have been able to use this provision; *and*

12

Chapter 12: Arranging for accommodation in care homes
1. Who can have accommodation arranged by social services or the NHS?

- if it is not otherwise available to you; *and*
- if you normally live in that local authority area; *or*
- if you do not but your need is urgent.[1]

Even if you were to come under the above list, and if you were already in a residential or nursing home at 1 April 1993, you will not be able to have your accommodation arranged by social services unless there are specific circumstances. These are explained in Chapter 22.

Social services departments have a *power* to provide or arrange residential or nursing home care if you:

- are an expectant or nursing mother (it does not matter if you are under 18); *or*
- ordinarily live in another authority's area, provided that authority agrees.[2]

They also have the power to provide hostel accommodation for disabled people who work in workshops provided by the department.[3]

Legal provisions in Scotland

The Social Work (Scotland) Act 1968 provides the legal basis for social work departments to provide or arrange residential and nursing home accommodation. The National Assistance Act 1948 provides the legal basis for charging. Social work departments have a *duty* to provide or arrange this kind of accommodation if you are:

- 18 or over;
- a person in need[4] of community care services due to needing care and attention because of infirmity or age;
- suffering from illness or mental disorder or are substantially handicapped by disability; *or*
- are in need of care and attention because of drug or alcohol dependency or release from prison or other forms of detention.

If you are already living in a residential or nursing home by 1 April 1993, then the social work department is strictly limited in its powers to help you (see Chapter 22).

The Community Care Residential Accommodation Act 1998

Since August 1998 the law has been amended to make sure that social services departments do not count capital under £16,000 (the current capital limit – see p293) when deciding whether it needs to provide you with accommodation.[5] This change in the law came about because one authority decided that if a person had more than £1,500 s/he could afford her/his residential or nursing home fees and, therefore, it did not need to make the

Chapter 12: Arranging for accommodation in care homes
1. Who can have accommodation arranged by social services or the NHS?

12

arrangements.[6] All social services departments now have to follow the rules and help with fees if a person has less than £16,000, as long as they have assessed the person as needing that sort of care (see p263).

Ordinary residence

This is not defined and so does not follow the rules for habitual residence used by the DSS (see p221). In order to avoid disputes between different local authorities about which should be responsible, there is guidance.[7] If you have freely chosen to move into an area with the intention of settling there, you are 'ordinarily resident' in that area. However, if your residential or nursing care is provided by social services, you will be deemed to continue to be ordinarily resident in that authority even if you live in another area. But if you move to another authority and make your own arrangements with a care home, you will be ordinarily resident in the area where the care home is. You will need to apply to the social services department where the home is, if you later need any help with the funding. In England there is a determination by the Secretary of State where a woman moved from one authority, having been assessed by another as needing residential care, to a home in another authority. The social worker in the first authority took her to the home, but as the woman had over £16,000 capital, social services did not make the arrangements. She later needed financial help and applied to the new authority which considered that the first authority should be responsible. The determination was that as she had moved of her own volition and there had been no need for the first authority to make the arrangements, then she could not be deemed to be ordinarily resident in an area where she no longer lived.[8]

If you are told by the social services department that you are the responsibility of another authority, you should not be left without help during the time it takes to sort out which authority should be responsible for you. Seek advice if this happens. If you have no settled residence, have come from another local authority or from abroad, the social services department where you are now should provisionally accept responsibility and provide you with services you need.[9]

Aftercare provision – social services and health (England and Wales)

If you have been detained in hospital under any of the following sections of the Mental Health Act 1983:
- Section 3
- Section 37
- Section 47
- Section 48

12

Chapter 12: Arranging for accommodation in care homes
1. Who can have accommodation arranged by social services or the NHS?

and have left hospital, there is a joint duty on health and social services departments to provide aftercare services until such time as it is jointly decided that such services are no longer needed.[10] Aftercare services under Section 117 are not defined but can include residential services.[11] If you need residential or nursing care because of your mental condition, then unless that condition improves, it is likely you will continue to need Section 117 aftercare residential services. Just because you have settled in the home does not necessarily mean that you no longer need residential after-care services; the relevant question of whether you continue to need after care services should be addressed.[12]

The High Court recently (28 July 1999) addressed the question of how long aftercare services continue, especially if you still need residential care. It found that there may be cases where, in due course, there will be no need for aftercare services for the person's mental condition, but services are still needed for other needs such as physical disability. Each case will have to be examined on the facts. Where the resident has dementia, the Court found it difficult to see how the mental condition could improve to the point where aftercare services would no longer be needed.

The main point at issue in that case was whether s117 of the Mental Health Act acts as a gateway for using s21 of the National Assistance Act to actually provide the accommodation or whether it is a stand-alone provision. The Court found that it is a stand-alone duty, that residential accommodation is provided under s17 and so cannot be provided in these cases under s21. This being the case, there can be no charge for the accommodation.[13] It is estimated that about half the authorities in England and Wales have charged for residential care provided under s117. Seek advice if you have been detained in hospital under any of the sections listed on p261 and you are now being, or have been, charged for residential or nursing care.

Aftercare provision (Scotland)

In Scotland, if you are or have been suffering from a 'mental disorder' it is the duty of the social work department to provide aftercare.[14] Local authorities can charge for these services.

Legal provision – NHS

If you need continuing in-patient care, either in hospital or in a nursing home then your health authority should arrange it.[15] You will still be considered to be a hospital in-patient and so will have limited choice about which home or hospital you can go to. Guidance has been issued in England, Wales and Scotland which sets out four national eligibility criteria:

- you have a complex medical, nursing or other clinical need, or need frequent not easily predictable interventions under the supervision of a consultant or specialist nurse or other NHS team member; *or*

Chapter 12: Arranging for accommodation in care homes
2. Deciding if you need to be provided with care in a residential or nursing home

12

- you need routine specialist health care equipment or treatments which need specialist staff; *or*
- you have a rapidly degenerating or unstable condition; *or*
- you have a prognosis which suggests you are likely to die in the very near future.[16]

But within national guidance each health authority draws up its own eligibility criteria to decide who it will provide health care for and whether it will be in a hospital or nursing home.

The guidance also makes it clear that the NHS should be prepared to fund rehabilitative and palliative care. Later English guidance pointed out concerns about health authorities setting tight time limits on how long they will fund rehabilitative or palliative care.[17]

The Court of Appeal recently ruled that although the guidance is lawful, North and East Devon Health Authority's eligibility criteria was not lawful because it placed rigorous limits on what it considered to be NHS services. This meant that social services were left providing health care beyond the scope of an authority whose primary responsibility is to provide social services.[18]

The national guidance, produced by the Department of Health, which was criticised by the Court of Appeal as not being clear, is to be reviewed. The outcome of this review is expected early in 2000. In the meantime authorities (at present in England only) have been advised to ensure that their eligibility criteria are in line with the judgment and existing guidance, and if the guidance is revised they should consider how they will reassess individuals against the revised criteria.[19]

If you are in a nursing home, or have been told you need nursing home care, you should ask what your health authority has done in relation to this judgment. If the NHS takes responsibility for arranging your care you will not have to pay (see p272)

Ordinary residence

If you are taken ill and are in hospital, away from home or in a specialist unit in a different health authority area, the health authority in which you live will be responsible for your care.[20]

2. Deciding if you need to be provided with care in a residential or nursing home

Social services

If you are going to need help with funding your stay in a residential or nursing home, you will need to be assessed by social services (see p40). Since 1993 social services departments act as gatekeepers to funding for residential and nursing home care (although in some cases the NHS will arrange your nursing home care (see p272)). Each social services department has its own eligibility criteria for deciding who needs residential or nursing care.

If social services decide you need nursing home care they need the consent of the health authority (health board in Scotland) before they can arrange your accommodation. In an emergency, social services can place you in a nursing home without the consent of the health authority but it must be obtained as soon as possible.[21] In Scotland, guidance states that a joint assessment of health and social care needs should be carried out within at least five working days of admission.[22]

If your situation is very urgent social services can place you in a residential or nursing home care without an assessment[23] and do one as soon as possible afterwards.

If you want help from social services with funding residential care or nursing care but are told you do not need it, or that you only need residential care when you think you need nursing care, you can complain and ask for a reassessment (see p54). It is important to get a copy of your needs assessment to show why you need the particular care you think you do. Any medical evidence you can get to support you will be helpful.

If you can afford to pay for residential and nursing home care

Even if you know you can afford to pay the fees of the care home, it is useful to get assessment of your needs. The assessment should not just look at the type of home that would be suitable but should look at all the other options, such as help at home, sheltered accommodation, aids and equipment that could help you. You may decide after the assessment that there are ways for you to manage at home.

Social services have been told that they cannot refuse to assess the needs of anyone on the grounds that the person has financial resources of over £16,000 and that they should give the person advice about the type of care they require and what services are available.[24] It is very useful to get an assessment if you are likely to need help with funding in the relatively near future, as you need to be sure that social services have agreed that you need the type of care you are going into.

If you have capital over £16,000 you could choose to make your own arrangements. However, social services departments have been told in guidance that they must satisfy themselves that you are *able* to make your own arrangements with a care home, or have others who are *willing and able* to do so for you.[25] If you are not able and there is no one else who is willing and able, then social services must arrange your care in a residential or nursing home. They will then charge you the full cost until your capital is reduced to £16,000.

Chapter 12: Arranging for accommodation in care homes
2. Deciding if you need to be provided with care in a residential or nursing home

12

Some social services departments are very reluctant to provide residential or nursing care accommodation if you have a property which can be sold and which is worth more than £16,000. Although you are considered to have more than £16,000, you might not be able to get hold of the money until the property has been sold. This can cause considerable difficulties in meeting the fees while the property is on the market. The guidance described above may help if you can show you are unable to make your own arrangements and there is no one who is willing and able to do so. If the social services department has a policy of never making the arrangements until your available capital is down to a certain level this may be open to challenge as it is a blanket policy which takes no notice of individual circumstances. Seek advice if you are told you cannot have help with funding whilst your property is for sale. But see p359, as you might want to consider whether you would be better off financially by making your own arrangements.

If social services agree that you need residential or nursing care, it is useful for you to know the type of care it thinks you need and also how much it would usually pay for that type of care. If you make your own arrangements with a residential care or nursing home, you will need to make you own contract with them. It may help to know how much social services pay and what this covers. Sometimes proprietors charge more if you make your own arrangements than if you have a contract arranged by social services. Some homes are prepared to negotiate on their fees. If you decide to go into a home that is more expensive than social services would normally pay, especially if you are going to need to have help with funding in the future, it is useful to know what the shortfall will be so that you can work out if you would be likely to find a third party to make up the difference, or whether it would be likely you might have to move (see p278 and Chapter 16).

The NHS

If you want the NHS to fund your place in a nursing home, you will need to show that you come within the local eligibility criteria for NHS funding in a nursing home for 'continuing in-patient' care, rehabilitation, or palliative care. The guidance suggests that such options should always be considered[26] but currently only about 8 per cent of places in nursing homes are arranged by the NHS. Although there is national guidance (see p262), health authorities have different interpretations of it. In one area you might be considered to be the responsibility of the NHS, but in another area you may not. If you think the NHS should be responsible for your care in a nursing home, a useful start is to have a copy of the local eligibility criteria. You should be able to get one from your local health authority or hospital. Your community health council (health council in Scotland) should be able to help if you have problems getting the criteria.

12

Chapter 12: Arranging for accommodation in care homes
2. Deciding if you need to be provided with care in a residential or nursing home

Since the recent Court of Appeal judgment (see p262) all authorities in England should be looking at their eligibility criteria and as a result of the judgment may need to change them.

If you are about to be discharged from hospital

It is very often a stay in hospital which precedes the need to go into residential or nursing care. Unless the NHS agrees to arrange your place in a nursing home, the cost of care in a residential or nursing home will fall on you – either completely if you can afford it, or with some help from social services. It is, therefore, very important that you are aware of your rights and understand the process what should happen, before you are discharged.

Hospitals in England and Wales work to the *Hospital Discharge Workbook* which emphasises the multi-disciplinary nature of decisions about discharge and the need for a keyworker, and that planning for discharge should come at an early stage and not at the point you are ready to leave hospital. Guidance[27] in England, Wales and Scotland also stresses the following points.

- You and your family should be kept informed of the discharge process.
- You should receive information in writing to enable you to take key decisions about continuing care.
- You should be given written details of the likely costs of any of the options being considered, including the availability of social security benefits.
- You should get a written statement of which aspects of your care will be arranged and funded by the NHS.

Although you do not have the right to stay in hospital indefinitely if it has been decided that you no longer need hospital care, you do have the right to refuse to be discharged into a nursing home or residential care home. A small number of people under mental health legislation do not have this right. Other options should be explored but if you reject these, the guidance says that it may be necessary to implement your discharge home with a package of health and social care. You will probably be charged for your social care (see p49).

The right to review (England and Wales)

If you are in hospital and disagree with the decision to discharge you, you have the right to ask for a review if you think the health authority's eligibility criteria have not been correctly applied.[28] The review is in two stages. The initial stage is an internal review of the decision. If you are not satisfied with that decision, you must be given information about the formal review procedure and information about advocacy services, and put in touch with them if you wish. Your request to a designated officer should be dealt with urgently and you should get a response in writing within two weeks. Normally

Chapter 12: Arranging for accommodation in care homes
2. Deciding if you need to be provided with care in a residential or nursing home

12

the health authority will seek advice from an independent panel which should check that the proper procedures have been followed, and ensure that the eligibility criteria have been properly and consistently applied. The review process cannot be used to complain about the content of the eligibility criteria. During the time of the review you should not be discharged from hospital. This type of review is separate from the NHS complaints procedure (see p54), which can be used to complain about the eligibility criteria.

The right to appeal (Scotland)

If you are in hospital in Scotland you have the right to appeal against a clinical decision to discharge you from continuing NHS care.[29] Information on this procedure and on any advocacy service must be available from the hospital staff on request. The appeal is in two stages. Once the consultant has decided that you can be discharged, you or your carer/advocate have ten days to request a review of the decision by the Director of Public Health. This should be completed within two weeks. If it is decided that you should be discharged, you have the right to request a second opinion from an independent consultant from another health board area. You cannot be discharged during the appeal process. This appeal process is to ensure that the criteria set out in the guidance has been correctly applied. The appeal process cannot be used to complain about the content of the criteria. The appeal procedure is separate from the NHS complaints procedure and there is nothing to stop you using both procedures at the same time.

Part funding by the NHS

If it is agreed that you need continuing in-patient care in a nursing home funded by the NHS, this is provided under the National Health Service Act 1977 (or, in Scotland, the 1978 NHS (Scotland) Act).[30] It is quite clear that in such cases the NHS bears all of the cost. However an increasing number of health authorities offer other arrangements, often via social services departments whereby the health authority will meet some of the costs of a nursing home. It is frequently referred to as 50/50 funding.[31] This type of funding can and does cause confusion regarding a person's status. Some social services departments that have received such a payment from a health authority will calculate their charges to you only on the 50 per cent they have to pay, but others may charge based on the full cost. If the DSS becomes aware of any NHS funding, it may still consider that you are a hospital in-patient (see p125).

If the health authority is prepared to pay some of your nursing home fees, then it is worth checking whether you should in fact have all of your fees met, as it may be that you are borderline for fitting into the eligibility criteria for continuing in-patient care. This is especially so since the recent Court of

12

Chapter 12: Arranging for accommodation in care homes
2. Deciding if you need to be provided with care in a residential or nursing home

Appeal judgment (see p262). It may however be that the health authority is just trying to make a sensible arrangement with social services to free up much-needed hospital beds.

If your benefits are affected by such an arrangement it is important to appeal. As yet, there have not been any commissioners decisions on this type of funding arrangement. In an earlier case where a health authority had entered into a contractual arrangement with a nursing home to provide beds for ex-patients, it was found that the individuals were still to be regarded as in hospital for benefits purposes.[32] Guidance was issued to health authorities following this case reminding them that where the NHS made a contract with a nursing home it had to be for the full cost, not just the part of the fees not met by benefits.[33]

3. **The different types of accommodation**

Recently, English cases have established that social services can arrange your accommodation in ordinary housing,[34] but in the vast majority of cases care is provided in:

- local authority residential homes;
- independent residential care homes;
- nursing homes;
- independent or local authority hostels not providing board.

Health authorities can arrange your accommodation in nursing homes or hospices. It is very important that you go into a home which most suits your needs.

It is important to be aware that different benefits are payable depending on whether you are in a local authority home or independent sector home. It is particularly important if you will be funding the cost yourself in full, as you cannot get attendance allowance (AA) in a local authority home (see p358). You should also compare the costs of local authority homes with those of independent sector homes, as local authority homes can be more expensive.

Local authority residential homes

These are homes which are owned and managed by local authority social services departments. The homes are often for older people, or people with learning disabilities or with a mental illness. Some social services departments do not provide board for homes for younger people as they want to encourage independence (see p270).

At present local authority homes do not have to be registered, but they are regularly inspected by the local authority inspection unit.

Some social services departments are either closing their homes or transferring them to the independent sector. As long as there are sufficient independent homes in the area, local authorities do not have to provide them directly.[35]

Independent residential care homes

Independent residential care homes can be provided by:
- private organisations or individuals; *or*
- voluntary organisations such as charities or not-for-profit organisations.

They vary in size, from less than four people, to over 30 residents.

In England and Wales all independent residential homes which provide board and personal care have to be registered, including small homes of less than four people.[36] Regulations specify the facilities and services which should be provided in all homes.[37] Personal care is defined as care which includes assistance with bodily functions where such assistance is required.[38] Guidance[39] suggests that personal care is the sort of care which might be provided by a caring relative responding to physical or emotional needs. Board is not defined. Both board and personal care have to be provided to fulfil the requirements of registration.

In Scotland it is the level and type of care provided which determines whether establishments providing accommodation are required to be registered under the Social Work (Scotland) Act 1968. This includes any establishments where the whole or substantial part of their function is to provide personal care or support.[40] Personal care is defined as including 'the provision of appropriate help with physical and social needs' and support is defined as 'counselling or other help provided as part of a planned programme of care'.

Inspection units based in social services departments are responsible for inspecting independent residential homes. The reports of these inspections are available to the public.

Nursing homes

Nursing homes can be run by health authorities, NHS trusts or privately by individuals or organisations. Some nursing homes are run by not-for-profit organisations.

The health authority is responsible for registering nursing homes, which are described as homes:
- for the nursing of people suffering from sickness, injury or infirmity;
- for pregnant women or women immediately after childbirth; *or*
- where various specified treatments such as dialysis or endoscopy can be carried out.[41]

Nursing homes which are intended for nursing mentally disordered patients have to be registered as mental nursing homes.[42]

The person in charge of a nursing home must be a registered medical practitioner or a qualified nurse, and in addition the registering authority must be satisfied that there will at all times be sufficient, suitable qualified staff in attendance.[43]

Inspections should be carried out on a regular basis and reports must be available to the public.

Dual registered homes

It is becoming increasingly common for homes to have dual registration as both residential and nursing homes. Being in such a home could avoid a move later if you become more disabled. However, although it is simple to move from one part of the home to another, it will cost you more if you fund yourself. It is therefore worth asking for an assessment of your needs to see if you really need to move to the nursing section. If social services made the arrangements for you and are still funding your care, they will need to agree that you now need nursing care and seek permission from the health authority.

At present such homes have to be registered with both the health authority and local authority inspection units.

Independent or local authority homes not providing board

Most residential care is in homes which provide board and personal care. However, some people have their accommodation provided in ordinary housing or in homes (hostels) which are not required to be registered. Social services run homes where the cost of board is not included and you can buy your meals as you want them – sometimes known as pay-as-you-eat schemes. There are also independent providers who specialise in offering supported services to different client groups, with a view to encouraging independence. The way the accommodation is set up will affect benefits (see p271) and also the way you are charged (see p390). In these situations you will count as a 'less dependent resident'[44] and social services do not have to use the national regulations to work out your charge. Each local authority will decide what is reasonable to charge you, given your commitments for buying food or fuel, and your incentive to work if you do not lose so much of your money in charges.[45]

Choosing your home

Moving into a residential or nursing home is a very important step to take, emotionally and financially. Although there are many different types of homes, the registration standards mean that the basic requirements of care should be available in all homes. Some charities provide factsheets or booklets giving information about what you should look for when choosing a home. Everyone is different and what suits you might not suit someone else.

You should ask to see the home's brochure and, if possible, the contracts they use. This should give you an idea of the way the home is run and what it will and will not allow. Some homes allow you to take pets or your own furniture for your room, or they have a kitchen area where you can make yourself a light meal. Make sure the home will take notice of your likes and dislikes. It is also very important to establish exactly what is covered by the fees quoted and whether there are any extra costs that you might have to meet (see p271).

Try to go to several homes before you make a decisions. What may sound ideal in a brochure might not be so. A visit will help you get a feel for whether you would be comfortable there and get on with the staff and other residents. If you cannot go yourself, make sure someone goes who knows your tastes. Many homes will send staff to visit prospective residents if they cannot go themselves.

Try to resist being hurried into making a decision and going into the first home you see. This may be difficult if you are in hospital and you know your bed is needed, but remember it's your life and it's vital that you are comfortable in the home you live in.

If you are unhappy with the home you are in

Even if you choose a home where you think you could be happy, you may find that you have some concerns. The home might change hands and the new management have different ideas. Or there may be some aspect which you did not consider when you moved in. It is usually best to sort out problems informally as far as possible. If you cannot, then use the home's complaints procedure. All independent residential care homes must have a complaints procedure. Although it is not required for nursing homes, many do. If this does not resolve the problem then:

- if you are in a local authority home or social services have arranged your care, then you can use their complaints procedure if you have a complaint against the home they have provided or arranged (see p57);
- if you are in a home where you have arranged the accommodation yourself, you can contact the inspection unit which covers the home and raise your concerns with them.

---

4. Who has to pay and what should be covered in the fees

Who pays for residential or nursing care depends on whether it has been arranged by the resident or arranged by social services or the NHS. The present system means that residential and nursing care is provided either free of charge, or the resident pays all or part of the fees.

Getting your residential and nursing home care free of charge

There are three groups of people who can get their residential or nursing home care free of charge:
- people in a nursing home arranged by the NHS;
- war pensioners who need skilled nursing care because of disability (depending on the cost of the home);
- in England and Wales, people in a residential or nursing care home which is part of section 117 aftercare services (see p261).

Nursing home care arranged by the NHS

If your nursing home care has been arranged by the NHS then it will be free of charge at the point of delivery.[46] This means, however, that you will be treated as a hospital in-patient and your benefits will be affected accordingly, including any DLA mobility component (see p348). As with any hospital setting you will not have a choice of nursing home but you should ask that your wishes be taken into account as far as possible.

There are times when the DSS might regard you as a hospital in-patient when the NHS is not funding you. If you are treated for benefit purposes as if you are in hospital but your nursing home care is not free, seek advice.

The fact that nursing care is free if arranged by the NHS means it is important to be aware of local criteria for providing such care (see p262).

War pensioners who need skilled nursing care

The War Pensions Agency can (but in practice very rarely does) pay up to a maximum of £411 (£467 in London) if you need 24 hour nursing care because of your disability.[47] It will only pay this if social services have not been involved in assessing your needs for nursing care. The level of fees that can be met can be higher if no other nursing home is suitable. Fees are paid without a means test. Your basic war pension will continue to be paid but other benefits are reduced or withdrawn – eg, constant attendance allowance stops after four weeks, and some other war pension benefits after eight weeks.

There are other provisions allowing you to claim nursing breaks up to four weeks a year. In some circumstances you can claim nursing home fees to give your carer a break.

If you get a war pension, particularly if it is paid at a high rate, it is worth discussing the possibility of help with nursing home fees with your local War Pensioners' Welfare Officer at an early stage. It may be one of the few circumstances where it could be advantageous not to have social services assess your needs for nursing care.

This is at the discretion of the Secretary of State and so there are no appeal rights.

Residential section 117 Mental Health Act aftercare services (England and Wales)

A recent case in the High Court made it quite clear that if residential care is part of aftercare services, there is no power which allows local authorities to charge you (see p261).[48] However, some social services departments are making charges in those circumstances.

It is important to seek advice if you are receiving section 117 services but are being charged for your residential accommodation. Even if social services did not make the arrangements for you because you have over £16,000, you should still seek advice as, technically, you are being means-tested and if you had less than £16,000, social services would have had to make the arrangements for you and not charged.

Aftercare services in Scotland

Accommodation provided as part of 'aftercare' under section 7 of the Mental Health (Scotland) Act 1984 comes under the same charging procedures described in Chapter 23.

Getting help with your fees

Social services

Since 1993, the most common way to get help with your fees is from social services departments. If you are assessed as needing residential or nursing care social services will make the arrangements and work out how much you need to pay according to the rules which are described in the following chapters. Social services are liable for the full fees (or in the case of their own homes, the cost of running them). The cost to social services is known as the standard charge. If you have over £16,000 you will have to pay the standard charge. If you cannot afford the standard charge then you will be assessed to decide how much you should pay.[49]

If social services make the arrangements for you they are liable for the full costs of your care (see p279 if you are in a home more expensive than social services would normally pay). Social services make a contract with the home which should specify what will be provided. It has been suggested in a recent report by the Office of Fair Trading that residents should have a copy of that contract.[50] It is always useful for you to know what services have been contracted for you, in order that there is no misunderstanding about what should be provided.

NHS services to residential and nursing homes

If you are getting help with fees from social services and are in residential care, you should still receive NHS services free of charge. Local authorities have been specifically told not to contract with independent residential homes for any service which is an NHS responsibility, such as district nursing, incontinence supplies, chiropody and specialist equipment.[51] Whether you will get these services depends on whether your health authority provides them to the community. Many residents find they have to pay out of their personal expenses allowance (see Chapter 15) for adequate supplies of incontinence pads or chiropody services as these are not supplied by the health authority.

Residents in nursing homes are supposed to have their general nursing needs met by the home. However, the health authority should still supply specialist services to you in a nursing home – eg, physiotherapy and incontinence advice. In England and Wales incontinence services, however, are not supplied by the NHS to residents in nursing homes. Guidance states that these should be included in the basic price of the home rather than provided by the NHS.[52] In Scotland GP's can prescribe continence products for people living in nursing homes.

If you receive help with fees from social services you should qualify for full help for those NHS services which incur a charge via health benefits (see p137).

Paying for extras

You may wish to pay for extra services supplied by the home which are not part of the basic care package contracted for by social services. In England the Department of Health's view is that as long as you have the legal capacity to do so, and you are not facing any pressure from either the home or social services, then there is no reason why you cannot enter into a contract with the home owner to provide extra services outside the package to meet your assessed needs.[53] Before you enter into such a contract you should be clear that you know what will be provided. Some local authority contracts specifically exclude owners of care homes entering into any contract in relation to you outside of the local authority's own contract. This is to avoid the possibility of owners of care homes entering into private contracts with residents or relatives to boost the amount of money they receive for looking after you.

Sometimes social services departments arrange non-residential services even if you live in a residential or nursing home – eg, for daytime activities. If they have been negotiated as part of the residential or nursing home care package, they should be included in the standard charge. If it is a separate package, then social services can decide whether or not to charge you under its discretionary charging powers (see p49). However, guidance points out that as residents only have personal expenses allowance and any disregarded income available, the charge, if any, should be minimal.[54]

Other help with the fees

As well as help from social services there are other sources of help with funding. These are:

- preserved rights to income support (see Chapter 22);
- using the benefits that are available if social services does not make the contract with the home (England and Wales) (see p359);
- friends, relatives and charities.

There is nothing to stop you getting help from friends, relatives or charities. In some cases, if you have not been assessed as needing residential care you may need to turn to them. Relatives may feel they should help with your fees if there is a waiting list for social services funding, but you should be careful of allowing social services to avoid their duties if they have assessed you as needing residential or nursing care (see p278).

Charities are normally precluded from paying for services that are the responsibility of the local authority. They may consider topping up your fees if you are in accommodation more expensive than social services consider necessary for your needs, or they may help if you have been assessed as not needing residential or nursing care. Charities often help people with preserved rights who have a shortfall from IS in meeting their fees (see Chapter 22).

Paying the full fees yourself

If you are not entitled to help from social services or the NHS, you will have to pay the full fees. In some circumstances social services may still make the arrangements for you even though you pay the full cost (see p273). In this case you will have the security of a social services contract. Otherwise you will need to make your own arrangements with the home you have chosen.

As well as making sure you feel that you will be happy in the home, it is very important to be clear about, and have written information on, all the financial implications. These include:

- exactly what is included in the fees (eg, laundry, hairdressing, newspapers, incontinence supplies, and chiropody are sometimes included in the fees but sometimes not);
- the cost of services not included in the fees;
- whether a deposit is required, what it is for and when is it returnable;
- how often the fees are reviewed and what notice is given;
- the minimum period of notice you have to give to leave the home;
- whether you can have a trial period;
- what effect a period in hospital or away on holiday would have on your fees.

Although it is not always easy to ask, it is also important to be sure what payment the home would continue to expect if you die, and how soon your room would need to be cleared. It is important that relatives are aware of this to avoid the distress of finding that fees still need to be paid for a short while.

The Office of Fair Trading has recommended that all residents should have a copy of their contract and that a standard contract should be made available before you move in so that you have time to seek advice about the terms and conditions.[55] It is essential to have a written contract to avoid later misunderstandings.

You should still be able to get any NHS services which are supplied in the community if you are in a residential care home, and specialist NHS help if you are in a nursing home. However, in England and Wales you will have to pay for your incontinence supplies in a nursing home. These should be included in the fee.

The level of the fees

Recent research has backed up anecdotal evidence that people making their own arrangements may be charged more for exactly the same facilities as those residents who are funded by social services.[56] Homes will sometimes negotiate their fees, so it can be useful to know what social services would normally pay for someone with your needs. You can then use this to compare the fees of the homes you visit.

It is also important to establish (especially if you are likely to need help from social services in the future) whether the home will drop its fees to social services level if they take over the arrangements. Some homes are prepared to do this, but others will keep to the fees they set and so you would need to find someone to make up the difference (see p278).

Getting help if you have been funding yourself

Even if you make your own arrangements with a residential or nursing home you may later need to approach social services to get help with funding once your capital approaches £16,000. You will normally need to approach the local authority where you now live. The social services department will assess you to see if you need the type of care you are getting. This can sometimes take several weeks so it is worth approaching them several months before your capital reaches £16,000 so they have time to assess your needs and undertake a financial assessment by the time your capital gets down to £16,000. Social services have been told that when residents whose capital is approaching £16,000 apply to them, they should undertake the assessment as soon as reasonably practicable, and if necessary take over the arrangements to ensure that the resident is not forced to use up capital below £16,000.[57] You should also apply for IS when your capital reaches £16,000.

Occasionally social services will decide you do not need residential or nursing care and will not make the arrangements and not help to fund you. If they do not think you need nursing care you may need to move from a nursing home to a residential home. This does not happen very often. If it does, you can ask for a review of the assessment to make sure social services have taken all your needs into account. You should also seek advice.

Couples

If you are one of a couple with a joint account of over £32,000, and you are funding yourself in residential or nursing home care, it may be worth considering splitting your account. This is because you will not get help from social services until your joint capital is down to £32,000 (when you are counted as each having £16,000). For example if you have a joint account of £42,000 you will need to spend £10,000 on fees before you can get help. If you split your account so you each have £21,000, you will only need to spend £5,000 before you can get help.

Getting help from the NHS

If your condition worsens while you are in a residential or nursing home you may meet the eligibility criteria for NHS-funded care. If you are in a residential care home and become a patient in hospital you should then be assessed under the normal hospital discharge rules (see p266). If you are in a nursing home you may continue to be nursed through your worsening condition without going to hospital. You should ask your GP for an assessment to see whether you now come under the local eligibility criteria for NHS-funded nursing home care. If you do, then the NHS should take over the funding of your care, although it may not agree to do so at the home you are in.

Note: Following the Court of Appeal case *R v N and E Devon ex parte Coughlan* (see p262) some health authorities may change their eligibility criteria. You might find that although your condition has not worsened you are now eligible for NHS-funded nursing care. It is worth checking if the eligibility criteria has been changed as a result of the judgment and to ask for a reassessment of whether you fall within NHS-funded care.

5. **Accommodation arranged by social services**

If social services have agreed that you need residential or nursing care arranged by them, the following points should be considered:
- how quickly should accommodation be arranged;
- your right to choose accommodation;
- will it involve moving to a home in another area;

- seeing if you like the home (trial periods);
- how you pay your assessed contribution.

How quickly should accommodation be arranged?

Once social services has decided that you need residential care arranged for you, then it should be done as soon as you have found a suitable place and you are able to move in. There may be delays if there are no vacancies in the home of your choice and you might need to move into another home while you are waiting. Wherever possible you should try to avoid several moves. Much will depend on your circumstances and whether you can arrange suitable care at home while you are waiting for a vacancy or whether you can stay in hospital during this time.

Delays sometimes occur because social services do not have the resources to fund you and they have placed you on a waiting list. But social services cannot use their lack of resources as a reason for not making the arrangements once a decision has been made that you need the care.[58] They also have a duty to provide the accommodation from the date the decision is made.[59] Guidance states that social services should make arrangements without 'undue delay' and if there is going to be a delay they should ensure that suitable arrangements are in place to meet your needs and those of your carer.[60] If you are waiting for funding from social services and have been told that the delay is because of lack of resources you should seek advice.

The right to choose accommodation

You have the right to choose which home you live in as long as:
- it is suitable to your assessed needs;
- a bed is available;
- the person in charge is willing to provide the accommodation subject to the usual terms and conditions laid down by social services;
- it would not cost social services more than it would normally cost for your assessed needs.

You also have the right to go into accommodation that is more expensive than social services would be prepared to pay as long as you have a third party to meet the difference in cost.[61] See Chapter 16 for how third party top-ups work.

If you are already in a home and want to move, you can do so on the same basis as anyone moving into a home for the first time.

Social services have been told they must have a clear, justifiable reason which relates to the criteria of the direction, if they decide not to arrange accommodation in the home of your choice.[62] There have been reports that some authorities, because of lack of financial resources, will only place you in one of their own homes, or one where they have a block contract – ie, where they have contracted for a number of beds. Lack of resources is not part of the criteria in the Choice of Accommodation Directive, so you should argue that you should be given your choice. The Local Government Ombudsman found maladministration where a local authority had not explained the provisions in the Choice of Accommodation Directive.[63]

Having a number of homes to choose from

Social services have also been told that they must not set arbitrary ceilings on the amount they are willing to pay for residential or nursing homes, and must not routinely expect third parties to make up the difference. They must be able to show that there are homes which could provide you with the services you need within the usual cost.[64] If you think that your choice has been limited because only a few homes are within the cost social services will normally pay, then you should seek advice.

Reasons for going to a particular home

You may have reasons for going to a home which is more expensive than social services will normally consider. If your needs can only be adequately met in a home which is more expensive, then social services should meet the full cost of that home, as it is not a question of choice but one of 'paying what the law required' to meet your assessed needs.[65] The Local Government Ombudsman in the same case above (see p278) reminded local authorities that they have the discretion to exceed the normal amount they would pay, and that they should not fetter this discretion.[66] It is important to establish that something which is very important to you should be considered as part of your assessed needs. For instance, it may be important to be in a home which respects your religious beliefs, or where there are staff who speak your language, or where you can remain in close contact with your friends and neighbours. Social services have to take into account your psychological and social needs when making their assessment. In some cases a very strongly held preference could be considered to be a psychological or social need.

What if the home you are in increases its fees by more than social services will pay?

Sometimes homes which have been within the social services level of fees, increase them to above the amount social services will pay for your level of need. In such circumstances you could:
- ask for a re-assessment to see if social services agree that it is an integral part of your needs to remain in that home; *and/or*
- find a third party to meet the difference; *or*
- ask social services to negotiate on your behalf for the home to only charge what social services will pay; *or*

- move to another home with fees which social services will pay.

It is important to establish whether social services will meet the full cost of the fees if the home you are living in increases them above the normal fee level. If the home is meeting your needs and you are settled there you should ask for an assessment about the level of risk involved in your having to move. This, along with your social and psychological needs, should be taken into account in your assessment. If social services agree that it is part of your assessed need to stay in that particular home then it should meet the full cost.

If they disagree then you will need a third party to top up the fee. This could be a relative or a charity (see Chapter 16). You should ask social service to help you find a third party and to explain why one is now needed. Social services will remain responsible for the full fees and will arrange with the third party for their contribution to be paid.

The home should not make its own arrangements with either yourself or a relative outside of the social services contract in order to have the increase in fees met. Social services must be involved as it is responsible for the fees (see p273).

If you do not want to move it is important to seek help so that every avenue can be explored, including seeing if the home will only charge you what social services will pay and complaining to local councillors and MPs/MSPs/National Assembly Members in Wales, if you think that social services should pay the full cost. You can also use the social services complaints procedure (see p57).

Moving into a home in another area

If you may want to move into a home in another area you should be allowed to exercise your choice to do so. However, because of the differences in costs of homes around the country, you could find difficulties if the area you are moving to only has homes which are much more expensive than your social services will normally pay. The direction tells social services departments that there might be circumstances where the need to be in another area is an integral part of the person's assessed needs – eg, being near relatives.[67] Some authorities will only pay to their own area's levels. If this is a blanket policy it could be challenged as it implies they are not prepared to look at an individual's assessed needs.

Cross-border placements

Although the Direction on Choice says you can move anywhere in the UK, in practice this is not the case. There is no provision for social services to pay for residential care in Northern Ireland or for Northern Ireland health and social services boards to pay for accommodation arranged by authorities in England.

Further guidance was issued in 1993[68] to clarify what should be done if someone wants to move from England or Wales to Scotland. If you want to move to Scotland you can ask your social services department to arrange for a Scottish authority to arrange a place for you. The two authorities should ensure that the Scottish authority is reimbursed by the English or Welsh authority.

If you are moving from Scotland your own authority can arrange a place for you in England or Wales if it is a residential home. If you need to go into a nursing home, your authority in Scotland can ask the social services department where you plan to move, to make the arrangements for you. Arrangements should be agreed between authorities to recover the costs.

Both sets of guidance make it clear that full co-operation is expected between authorities if people want to move across the borders.

Seeing if you like the home (trial periods)

Normally you are given a little time to see if you like the home you have moved into and there is a trial period before any permanent decision is made. You need to be clear whether social services regard this trial period as a:
- temporary stay (ie, you might go home); *or*
- temporary stay in that particular home to see if you like it, but as there is no possibility of your going home, you are a permanent resident.

This is important as it will affect the way you are charged (see p390) and it could also affect your benefits (see p349). You also need to be sure that social services and the DSS are treating you in the same way and that you agree with the basis of your trial period.

Guidance states that a stay which is expected to be permanent might turn out to be temporary and equally a stay which is temporary might turn out to be permanent. In the former case it suggests that it would be unreasonable to continue to apply the rules as if you were permanent, especially those about the way your own home is treated. If your stay is temporary but later becomes permanent, then you should only be charged as a permanent resident from the date that decision is made.[69]

A Local Government Ombudsman has said there should be clear criteria for establishing when changes from temporary to permanent status are made and how clients and relatives should be informed of such changes.[70]

How you pay your assessed contribution

Once social services have decided how much you have to pay, they should inform you of the amount. Normally social services will pay the home the full cost and you pay your contribution direct to social services.

You can pay your contribution direct to the home with social services paying the remainder. This can only be done if there is agreement to do this from all three parties – ie, yourself, the home and social services.[71] If you would prefer to pay direct to social services then you cannot be made to pay your contribution direct to the home.

Social services remain liable for the whole amount of the fees, so if you do not pay your share they will need to pay the full amount, but will take steps to recover your contribution from you (see Chapter 18).

Notes

1. **Who can have accommodation arranged by social services or the NHS?**
   1 s21 and 24 NAA 1948 and LAC (93) 10; WOC 35/93
   2 LAC (93)10; WOC 35/93
   3 s29 NAA 1948 and LAC (93)10; WOC 35/93 Appendix 2.
   4 s12 SW(S)A 1968
   5 CC(RA)A 1998 and LAC (98)19; WOC 27/98; SWSG2/99
   6 *R v Sefton Metropolitan Borough Council ex parte Help the Aged* (CCLR) December 1997
   7 LAC (93)7; WOC 41/93; SWSG1/96
   8 Determination by the Secretary of State, 8 March 1996
   9 LAC (93)10; WOC 35/93; SWSG 1/96
   10 s117 MHA 1983
   11 *Clunis v Camden and Islington Health Authority* (CCLR) March 1998
   12 Ombudsman Investigation 97/0177 and 97/0755 Clywd and Conwy
   13 *R v LB Richmond, R v Redcar and Cleveland. R v Manchester, R v LB Harrow* (CCLR) December 1999
   14 s8(1) MH(S)A 1984
   15 s3.1 and s23 NHSA 1977; NHS(S)A 1978
   16 HSG (95)8; LAC (95)5; WHC (95)7; WOC 16/95; NHS MEL (1996)22 but note that this guidance may change early in 2000
   17 EL (96) 8
   18 *R v N and E Devon ex parte Coughlan* (CCLR) September 1999
   19 HSC 1999/180/LAC (99)30
   20 s24(6) NAA 1948

2. **Deciding if you need to be provided with care in a residential or nursing home**
   21 s26 NAA 1948
   22 SWSG 10/98
   23 s47(5) NHS&CCA 1990; s12A(5) SW(S)A 1968
   24 LAC (98)19; WOC 27/98; SWSG 2/99
   25 LAC (98)19; WOC 27/98; SWSG 2/99
   26 HSG (95)8; LAC (95)5; WHC (95)7; WOC 16/95; MEL (1996)22 but note that this guidance could change early in 2000
   27 HSG(95)8; LAC(95)5; WHC(95)7; WOC 16/95; MEL (1996)22 but note that this guidance could change early in 2000
   28 HSG(95)39; LAC (95)17; WHC 95 (7)
   29 MEL (1996) 22
   30 s23 NHSA 1977
   31 The legal basis of such payments is uncertain. Health authorities can make payments various statutory and voluntary bodies under s28A NHSA 1977, which cannot be used for any health function, only in connection with the functions of the organization receiving the payment. From April 2000 there will be some changes to this caused by the HA 1999 and some functions of the NHS will be able to be delegated, and it will be easier for money to be passed from the NHS to

local authorities and vice versa. Under s64 of the HSPHA 1968 grants can be made to voluntary organizations (only) which provide services similar to services provided by the NHS

32 *White and others v Chief Adjudication Officer* 1993 (CCLR) June 1999

33 HSG (95)45; (WOC95)52

3. The different types of accommodation

34 *R v Bristol City Council ex parte Penfold* (CCLR) June 1998 and *R v Wigan MBC ex parte Tammadge* (CCLR) December 1998

35 *R v Wandsworth LBC ex parte Beckwith*

36 s1 RHA 1984; s61 SW(S)A 1968

37 Reg 10 RCH Regs 1984

38 s20 RHA 1984

39 LAC (77)13

40 s61(1) SW(S)A 1968

41 s21 RHA 1984

42 s22 RHA 1984; s1 NHR(S)A 1938

43 s25 RHA 1984

44 Reg 2(1) and 5 AoR Regs 1992

45 CRAG 2.010; SWSG 2.005

4. Who has to pay and what should be covered in the fees

46 s1(2) and s23 NHSA 1977

47 Article 26 Naval, Military and Air Forces etc (Disablement and Death) Service Pensions Order 1983 (as amended 1999)

48 *R v LB Richmond, R v Redcar and Cleveland, R v Manchester, R v Harrow* (CCLR) December 1999

49 s22 NAA 1948; AoR Reg 1992

50 Office of Fair Trading Older People as Consumers in Care Homes, October 1998

51 LAC (92)24 WOC 6/92

52 HSG (95)8; LAC (95)5; WHC (95)7; WOC 16/95, but note this guidance is being reviewed and may change early in 2000

53 Letter from the Department of Health to the Association of County Councils. November 1996.

54 CRAG 1.024A; SWSG 1.017A

55 Older People as Consumers in Care Homes. Office of Fair Trading 1998

56 Disparities between market rates and state funding and residential care. JRF Findings 678, June 1998

57 LAC 98/19; WOC 27/98; SWSG 2/99

5. Accommodation arranged by social services

58 *R v Sefton MBC ex parte Help the Aged and Blanchard (CA)* (CCLR) December 1997

59 *R v Wigan MBC ex parte Tammadge* (CCLR) December 1998

60 LAC (98)19; WOC 27/98; SWSG 2/99

61 LAC (92) 27; WOC 12/93; SWSG 5/93 Choice of Accommodation Directions

62 LAC (92) 27; WOC 12/93; SWSG 5/93 para 7

63 Local Government Ombudsman Report 97/1/3218

64 LAC (92)27; WOC12/93; SWSG 5/93 para 10

65 *R v Avon County Council ex parte M* (CCLR) June 1999

66 Local Government Ombudsman Report 97/A/3218

67 LAC (92) 27; WOC 12/93; SWSG 5/93 para 7.6

68 LAC (93)18; SWSG 6/94

69 CRAG 3.004 and 3.004A SWSG 3.004 and 3.004A

70 Humberside County Council 1992 (91/C/0774)

71 s26(3A) NAA 1948 and 1.023 CRAG; 1.015 SWSG

Chapter 13

Income – financial assessments

This chapter explains the rules on how income is treated by social services when they undertake a financial assessment to determine the amount you will be required to contribute to your accommodation and care costs. For how this information, and the information about capital and property in Chapter 14, is used in the financial assessment process itself see Chapter 23.

Legislation provides for the assessment of income by social services for placements made after 31 March 1993 to establish the amount you will be required to contribute to the cost of your placement in a local authority or an independent care home.[1] For placements made prior to 1 April 1993, see Chapter 22.

Income is treated in a similar way to that for income support (IS) purposes (see Chapter 6). Therefore, this chapter concentrates on the key differences. It covers:

1. General (p284)
2. Treatment of income (p285)
3. Income fully taken into account (p285)
4. Income partially disregarded (p286)
5. Income fully disregarded (p286)
6. Capital treated as income (p287)
7. Tariff income (p287)
8. Trust income (p288)
9. Notional income (p288)
10. Deprivation (p289)
11. Less dependent residents (p290)

1. General

Whatever the amount of your income you will generally be left with no less than a £14.75 personal expenses allowance per week in addition to any income disregarded in the assessment[2] (see Chapter 15). The rest of your income will go towards meeting the standard rate for your accommodation.

In general, all your income will be included as assessable income in the social services financial assessment unless it is partially or fully disregarded.[3] Your income is calculated on a weekly basis and includes capital treated as income (see p287), tariff income (see p287) and notional income[4] (see p288). The most common forms of income for people going into care are:

- state retirement pension and other social security benefits such as income support (IS), housing benefit (HB), council tax benefit (CTB), incapacity benefit (IB), severe disablement allowance (SDA), disability living allowance (DLA), attendance allowance (AA);
- occupational or personal pensions;
- trust income;
- tariff income from capital.

2. Treatment of income

The treatment of income for financial assessment purposes is very similar to the treatment of income for the calculation of IS[5] (see Chapter 6). The following three sections covering income fully taken into account (see p285), income partially disregarded (see p286) and income fully disregarded (see p286) will also examine the **key** differences between the treatment of income for financial assessments and treatment of income for IS.

The treatment of income for temporary (including respite and trial period – see p390 for definitions) residents and permanent residents is the same except that for temporary residents a disregard can be allowed to enable you to continue to meet any financial commitments that you may have in connection with your usual home in the community. These are often called outgoings[6] (see p305). There is also a difference in the way DLA care component and AA are treated for temporary and permanent residents (see pp286 and 286).

3. Income fully taken into account

Most income that is fully taken into account for IS purposes (see Chapter 6) is also fully taken into account for social services financial assessment purposes, with the important additions of:

- Third party payments made to meet higher fees (see Chapter 16). This type of payment is considered to be notional income[7] (see p288);
- IS and income-based jobseeker's allowance (JSA) minus any amount for housing costs[8] (see p99);
- AA/DLA care component (including constant attendance allowance and exceptionally severe disablement allowance payable with industrial injury

disablement benefit or war disablement benefit – see pp89 and 93) aid to permanent residents only[9] (for temporary residents these are fully disregarded – see p286);
- HB where the resident has been admitted permanently into unregistered accommodation or local authority accommodation not providing board so HB is being paid to meet the accommodation charge[10] (see Less dependent resident, p290).

Note: Where any social security benefit is being subjected to a reduction (other than a reduction because of voluntary unemployment) – eg, because of an earlier overpayment – the amount that is taken into account is the gross amount of benefit before reduction.[11]

4. **Income partially disregarded**

Most income that is partially disregarded for IS purposes (see Chapter 6) is also partially disregarded for social services financial assessment purposes:
- As for IS in preserved rights cases only (see Chapter 22), 50 per cent of an occupational pension or personal pensions or payment from a retirement annuity will be disregarded if you pass at least this amount to your spouse with whom you are not residing (if you pass nothing or less than 50 per cent then there is no disregard).[12] However, unlike for IS preserved rights cases, for financial assessment purposes, where you are an unmarried partner rather than a spouse, social services can use their discretionary powers to vary the personal expenses allowance to achieve a similar effect[13] (see p304).

Note: If you are one of a married couple, the guidance given to social services departments states that you should be given advice about the 50 per cent disregard including the fact that you have a choice of whether to pass 50 per cent of your pension to your spouse or not, and whether your spouse would be better off after taking account of the effect of the pension on social security benefits.[14]

5. **Income fully disregarded**

Most income that is fully disregarded for IS purposes (see Chapter 6) is also fully disregarded for social services financial assessment purposes with the important additions of:
- AA/DLA care component (including constant attendance allowance and exceptionally severe disablement allowance payable with industrial injury disablement benefit or war disablement benefit – see pp89 and 93) paid to

temporary residents only[15] (for permanent residents these are fully taken into account – see p285);
- housing costs paid as part of IS/income-based JSA (see p99) for your home in the community;[16]

child benefit (see p92) and child support maintenance payments unless the child is accommodated with you.[17]

Note: As with IS, contributory benefits dependants' additions, DLA mobility component, war widow's special pension and HB/CTB paid for your home in the community, are also disregarded.[18]

6. **Capital treated as income**

Most capital treated as income for IS purposes (see p174) is also treated as income for social services financial assessment purposes with the addition that:
- Capital will be treated as income where social services agree to place you in a higher cost home on the grounds that there is a third party (see Chapter 16) willing to contribute towards the higher cost. A lump sum payment made by the third party will be divided by the number of weeks for which the payment is made and taken fully into account as part of your income.[19] However, any third party payments made to social services to help clear arrears of charges for your residential accommodation will not be treated as income but as capital.[20]

7. **Tariff income**

As for IS (see p174), a tariff income amount of £1 for every £250 or part thereof is added to your weekly assessable income for financial assessment purposes where your capital is from over £10,000 to £16,000,[21] – eg, for £13,200 capital you would be assessed as having a tariff income of £13 a week. For financial assessment purposes this applies to both temporary and permanent residents (see Chapter 6).

Many social services departments only review financial assessments yearly and therefore if your capital of more than £10,000 has reduced within that period, and as a result your tariff income reduces, it is not applied until the yearly review is undertaken. However, the correct tariff income should be applied as soon as the reduction in your capital occurs. You should make sure you inform social services each time your capital reduces by an amount that would reduce your tariff income and seek advice if your financial assessment is not reviewed accordingly. If you are in receipt of IS you will also need to inform the Benefits Agency.

8. **Trust income**

As for IS (see p193), where you are the beneficiary of income only, produced by a non-discretionary or absolute entitlement trust fund, (known as a life interest or, in Scotland, a life rent) this will be taken fully into account for financial assessment purposes.[22] The value of the right to receive income is a capital asset but it is fully disregarded for financial assessment purposes[23] (see p299).

If you are the beneficiary of a discretionary trust fund where payments are made wholly at the discretion of the trustees and there is no absolute entitlement to either capital or income, the trust fund itself will not be treated as a capital asset.[24]

If you have an absolute entitlement to capital and income from a trust fund, see p299.

Income or payments from a discretionary trust are treated as voluntary payments[25] and as such they are treated in the same way as for IS (see p172). If the payments are regular in nature they are treated as income and if the payments are irregular in nature they are treated as capital. Regular payments of up to £20 per week are disregarded as income provided that a disregard has not already been applied to another income.[26] Regular payments which are intended and used for any item which was not taken into account when the standard rate was fixed for the accommodation provided, are also disregarded – eg, a payment to enable you to have your own telephone or television.[27]

Official guidance explains in some detail the different types of trust funds and how they should be treated for financial assessment purposes.[28]

9. **Notional income**

As for IS (see p182) in certain circumstances you are treated as having income which you do not actually have.[29] There are five types of income which are treated as notional income for financial assessment purposes. They are:

- income which is paid to social services by a third party to contribute towards the fees of a home where they are higher than the normal amounts that social services will pay (see Chapter 16).[30] However, payments made by a third person directly to social services in respect of a resident's arrears of charges for residential accommodation should not be treated as the resident's notional income;[31]

- income which is paid to a third party in respect of you or a member of your family for any item which was taken into account when the standard rate was fixed for accommodation provided;[32]
- income which would be available on application[33] (see below);
- income which is due but has not yet been paid;[34]
- income which you have disposed of/deprived yourself of in order to avoid a charge or to reduce the charge payable (see p289).[35]

Income available on application

For income which you have not yet acquired to be taken into account, social services must be satisfied that it would in fact be available to you if you made an application. As for IS, some types of income cannot be taken into account as notional income. These include income payable under a discretionary trust, income payable under a trust derived from a payment made in consequence of a personal injury, working families or disabled persons tax credit, severe disablement allowance, and employment services. In addition, any income which would be fully disregarded (eg, HB) will not be included as notional income.[36]

If an income that would be available if you applied is taken into account as notional income (eg, occupational pension not claimed) social services will assume that the application was made on the date that they first became aware of the possible income.[37]

Some social services departments assume an amount of IS as part of your income in the financial assessment when it is not only not in payment, but also you have not been advised to make a claim. If you are not aware that a source of income (eg, IS) would be available to you upon application, it will be difficult for social services to argue that it can be treated as notional income. However, if this has happened to you, you may need to seek further advice.

10. **Deprivation**

The rules on deprivation of income for financial assessment purposes are similar to the rules for IS (see p183). Any income which you have disposed of or deprived yourself of in order to avoid a charge or to reduce the charge payable, will be considered by social services to be notional income and as such will be treated as actual income and taken into account in the financial assessment in addition to any other assessable income.[38]

You will be considered to have deprived yourself of a resource if, as a result of your own act, you cease to possess that resource[39] and you would have continued to receive it had you not relinquished or transferred it.[40] The onus of proof is on you to prove that you no longer have an income, otherwise social services will treat you as still possessing the actual income.[41]

Social services should only consider the question of deprivation where the income concerned would have been taken into account in the financial assessment. Income such as a charitable payment of less than £20 per week would not lead to deprivation being considered.

Guidance to social services on questions for consideration in deciding whether the deprivation was *in order to avoid or reduce the charge*, makes it clear that the purpose of the deprivation should be examined.[42] If there is more than one reason why you deprived yourself of an income and one of the reasons was to avoid or reduce the charge, it does not matter whether it was the main reason or not as long as it was a significant reason.[43] The guidance also states that the timing of the deprivation should be considered[44] although under the regulations[45] deprivation can be considered for resources disposed of at any time as it is only in some circumstances[46] that the six-month restriction applies (see p326).

If you have sold the right to receive an income resource for the purposes of avoiding or reducing the charge, then your income has been converted into a capital asset and social services can either take account of the former income resource or, where applicable, the difference between the former income resource and the tariff income or the increase in tariff income.[47]

See p300 for more information on the issues of deprivation.

11. **Less dependent residents**

You are a less dependent resident if you are a prospective resident or a resident in:

- independent sector accommodation which is not required to be registered under the Registered Homes Act 1984 or in Scotland the Social Work (Scotland) Act 1968 or Nursing Homes (Scotland) Act 1938 as a residential care or nursing home; *or*
- local authority accommodation that does **not** provide board ('board' is defined as at least some cooked or prepared meals, cooked or prepared by someone other than the resident and eaten in the accommodation and the cost of which is included in the standard rate fixed for the accommodation).[48]

In these circumstances the local authority has complete discretion to ignore the whole of the charging assessment if it is 'reasonable in the circumstances'. This is because it has been recognised that to live as independently as possible, you will need to be left with more than the personal expenses allowance.[49] For further details on the special rules which apply to less dependent residents see pp159 and 391.

Notes

1 Part II NA(AR) Regs 1992

1. General
2 s22(4) NAA 1948
3 Sch 2 (earnings) and Sch 3 (income other than earnings) of the NA(AR) Regs 1992
4 Reg 9 NA(AR) Regs 1992

2. Treatment of income
5 ISG Regs 1987
6 Sch 3 para 27 NA(AR) Regs 1992

3. Income fully taken into account
7 Reg 17(4) NA(AR) Regs 1992
8 Reg I5(1) and Sch 3 para 26 NA(AR) Regs 1992 and para 8.006 CRAG; para 8.006 SWSG 8/96
9 Reg I5(1) NA(AR) Regs 1992 and para 8.006 CRAG; para 8.006 SWSG 8/96
10 Reg I5(1) NA(AR) Regs 1992 and para 8.006 CRAG; para 8.006 SWSG 8/96
11 Reg IS(3) NA(AR) Regs 1992 and para 8.007 CRAG; WOC 29/27; para 4 SWSG 7/97

4. Income partially disregarded
12 Reg 10A NA(AR) Regs 1992
13 para 5.005 CRAG; para 5.005 SWSG 8/96
14 para 4 LAC (97)5, Annex H, CRAG; para 4 SWSG 7/97

5. Income fully disregarded
15 Sch 3 para 6 NA(AR) Regs 1992
16 Sch 3 para 26 NA(AR) Regs 1992
17 Sch 3 para 28A NA(AR) Regs 1992
18 Sch 3 paras 3, 4 and 28 NA(AR) Regs 1992

6. Capital treated as income
19 Reg 16(4) NA(AR) Regs 1992
20 Reg 22(8) NA(AR) Regs 1992

7. Tariff income
21 Reg 28 NA(AR) Regs 1992

8. Trust income
22 para 10.017 CRAG; para 10.017 SWSG 8/96
23 Sch 4 para 11 NA(AR) Regs1992

24 para 10.020 CRAG; para 10.020 SWSG 8/96
25 para 10.021 CRAG; para 10.021 SWSG 8/96
26 Sch 3 para 10(1) NA(AR) Regs 1992
27 Sch 3 para 10(2) NA(AR) Regs 1992
28 s10 CRAG; s10 SWSG 8/96

9. Notional income
29 Reg 17 NA(AR) Regs1992
30 Reg 17(4) NA(AR) Regs 1992
31 Reg 17(5) NA(AR) Regs 1992
32 Reg 17(3) NA(AR) Regs 1992
33 Reg 17(2) NA(AR) Regs 1992
34 Reg 17(2) NA(AR) Regs 1992
35 Reg 17(1) NA(AR) Regs1992
36 para 8.065 CRAG; para 8.065 SWSG 8/96
37 para 8.069 CRAG; para 8.069 SWSG 8/96

10. Deprivation
38 Reg 17(1) NA(AR) Regs 1992
39 para 8.072 CRAG; para 8.072 SWSG 8/96
40 para 8.075 CRAG; para 8.075 SWSG 8/96
41 para 8.076 CRAG; para 8.076 SWSG 8/96
42 paras 8.073 – 8,080 CRAG; para 8.073 to 8.080 SWSG 8/96
43 para 8.077 CRAG; para 8.077 SWSG 8/96
44 para 8.078 CRAG; para 8.072 SWSG 8/96
45 Reg 17(1) NA(AR) Regs 1992
46 s21 HASSASSAA 1983
47 para 8.080 CRAG; para 8.080 SWSG 8/96

11. Less dependent residents
48 Reg 2(1) NA(AR) Regs 1992 and para 2.009 CRAG; para 2.004 SWSG 8/96
49 Regs 5 NA(AR) Regs 1992 and para 2.007 CRAG; para 2.005 SWSG 8/96

Chapter 14

....

Capital and property – financial assessments

This chapter explains the rules on how capital and property are treated by social services when they undertake a financial assessment to determine the amount you will be required to contribute to your accommodation and care costs. For how this information, and the information about income in Chapter 13, is used in the financial assessment process itself, see Chapter 23.

Legislation provides for the assessment of the value of capital and property by social services for placements made after 31 March 1993, to establish the amount that you will be required to contribute to the cost of your placement in a local authority or an independent care home.[1] For placements made prior to 1 April 1993, see Chapter 22.

Capital and property are treated in a similar way to that for income support (IS) purposes (see Chapter 7). Therefore, this chapter concentrates on the key differences. It covers:

1. General (p292)
2. Treatment of capital (p293)
3. If your home is for sale (p295)
4. Capital disregarded indefinitely (p296)
5. Capital disregarded for 26 weeks or longer (p298)
6. Capital disregarded for 52 weeks (p298)
7. Capital treated as income (p298)
8. Trust funds (p299)
9. Notional capital (p299)
10. Deprivation (p300)
11. Diminishing notional capital (p301)

---

1. General

Capital includes property and savings in or outside the UK unless it is disregarded.[2] Capital also includes income treated as capital (see p298) and notional capital[3] (see p299). Some of the most common forms of capital are:

- property (buildings and land)
- savings
- National Savings Certificates
- Premium Bonds
- stocks and shares
- trust funds

2. **Treatment of capital**

The value of your capital remaining after the appropriate disregards (p296) have been applied will be assessed by social services and may affect the amount you will be required to contribute to the cost of your placement.

Social services will not assume any tariff income on the first £10,000 of your capital.[4] Unlike for IS, the £10,000 applies to both temporary (including respite and trial periods – see p390 for definitions) and permanent residents.

If you have between £10,000 and £16,000 social services will assume a tariff income of £1 a week for every £250 or part thereof above £10,000, thus increasing your assessable income[5] (see p287). Again, unlike for IS, this £16,000 upper limit applies to both temporary and permanent residents. If you have capital of more than £16,000 you will be expected to meet the whole cost of your placement (ie, the standard rate) yourself until your capital drops to £16,000 or less.[6] This means that you will be 'self-funding' which affects some social security benefits that may be payable to you (see p351). If you have savings of £16,000 or less, social services should not take this into account when determining whether they should be providing residential accommodation to meet your needs or whether 'care and attention is otherwise available' to you.[7]

The treatment of capital for financial assessment purposes is the same whether you are a temporary (including respite and trial periods, see p390 for definitions) or permanent resident (except for the treatment of your own home as capital – see p293). The rules are very similar to the treatment of capital for the calculation of IS[8] (see Chapter 7). The three sections covering capital disregarded indefinitely (see p296), capital disregarded for 26 weeks or longer (see p298), and capital disregarded for 52 weeks (see p298), will examine the **key** differences between the treatment of capital for financial assessments and the treatment of capital for IS.

The value of your home in the community

If you are a permanent resident or you become a permanent resident and the value of your home in the community is not disregarded (see p296), then it will be taken into account as capital as soon as you enter the care home or once it is agreed that you will not be returning to your home. As for IS, the value of your home in the community will be based on the current selling price, less any debts (eg, a mortgage) charged on it,[9] and less 10 per cent in recognition of the expenses that would be incurred in selling it. Once your home is sold the capital realised, less any debts and the expenses involved in the sale, are taken into account.[10] Any other property that you own (or jointly own) will also be taken into account as capital and will be valued in the same way as a home in the community. If you decide to sell your property, see p295 for what happens while your home is up for sale.

Note: Social services departments do not have the power to enforce a sale of your property and it may not withdraw services if the charge is not met as the duty to make residential provision where there is an assessed need is not conditional upon the payment of the assessed contribution.[11] However, if the charge is not paid you will be accruing a debt to social services which may be pursued (see p321).

Jointly owned land or property

Where you jointly own land or property (including your home in the community), unlike for IS where it is a 'deemed' share based on the number of owners rather than the 'actual' share, social services must assess the value of your actual interest/share in the property.[12] Official guidance deals with joint beneficial ownership of property.[13] It states that the value of the interest is governed by your 'ability to re-assign the beneficial interest to somebody else' and 'there being a market ie, the interest being such as to attract a willing buyer for the interest'.

The guidance further states that the value would be heavily influenced by whether the other joint owner(s) would be able to buy your share. If the joint owner(s) cannot or does not want to do this, in many cases it would be unlikely that an outsider would be willing to buy into the property. Even if someone was willing to buy into the property, the value of this interest could be very low or effectively be nil.

Social services departments are advised to get a professional valuation if they are unsure of your share or if you dispute the valuation. The cost of any valuation should be borne by social services as they do not have any power to charge for costs incurred in connection with the financial assessment process.

In practice, valuing your share in a jointly owned property is very difficult. It is important to seek advice if you think your share has been overvalued. It is often useful to establish with local estate agents if they would be prepared to put your share on the market. It is likely that they would not be prepared to try to sell such a part share of a property as there may not be any willing buyer.

Jointly owned capital (other than property)

If you are one of a couple and you jointly own capital (except any interest in property or land – see p294) with your partner, it will be divided in equal shares for financial assessment purposes, regardless of what your actual share is. Unlike for IS, this is the case for both temporary and permanent residents as social services have no power to assess a couple according to their joint resources.

If you jointly own capital (except any interest in property or land – see p294) with any other person, the same rule will apply regarding dividing it into equal shares, regardless of what your actual share is, in order to determine the assessable income.[14]

This means that if you have, for example, a joint bank account with your sister containing £23,000 and £8,000 belongs to you whilst £15,000 belongs to your sister, social services will assess £11,500 as your share. An adviser, anticipating this decision, may advise that the joint account should be closed and two separate accounts opened for each person so that you would have the £8,000 belonging to you in an account in your sole name. The notional capital rules (see p299) should not be applied in these circumstances as this would not constitute a deprivation of capital because you are still in possession of your actual beneficial entitlement.[15]

Ownership

In some cases there may be a difference between the legal and the beneficial ownership of capital such as a property. If another person has been contributing toward the mortgage and/or running costs of your property (including your own home) they may be able to establish a beneficial interest in your property, even if it is legally owned by you. If a beneficial ownership is established, then the property will be valued as if it is jointly owned.

Property owned but rented to tenants

If you rent your property to tenants and the value of your property is not disregarded, social services will include its capital value in your financial assessment. If the value takes your capital level to above £16,000, then you will be charged the full standard rate for your accommodation and care. Guidance states that it will then be for you to agree to pay the rental income (along with any other income) to social services in order to reduce the accruing debt.[16]

3. **If your home is for sale**

Unlike for IS, social services cannot disregard the value of an unoccupied property (or any occupied property which is not disregarded, see p296) for 26 weeks or longer where reasonable where you are taking steps to sell it.

If you cannot pay your accommodation and care costs (which will usually be the full standard rate charge if your property plus any other capital to be taken into account is valued at above £16,000), until your property is sold and you receive the proceeds of the sale social services can help meet your accommodation and care costs. You will, however, have to pay back the full amount once your property is sold.

In these circumstances social services will usually put a 'charge' on your property in order to recover the amount that they have paid toward the care accommodation and costs when your property is sold. If the 'charge' was placed on your property prior to April 1996 (when the capital limit changed from £8,000 to £16,000), then it will be the £8,000 capital limit that will be applied up to April 1996 (see p324).

Note: There is an alternative way forward in this situation if you are going into independent residential or nursing care. This is often referred to as the 'loophole' provision or the 'self-funding option' (see p351) and it means you may be able to get extra benefits to help meet your accommodation and care costs as long as social services do not contract with the care home for your placement. In this situation, social services would not be helping with the payment of your care costs until your home was sold, therefore there would be no money owed to social services from the proceeds of the sale.

4. **Capital disregarded indefinitely**

Most capital that is disregarded indefinitely for IS purposes (see p195) is also disregarded indefinitely for social services financial assessment purposes, with the important addition that:

- social services have discretionary powers to allow a disregard of the value of your former home where you are a **permanent** resident and it is occupied, wholly or in part, if they think it is reasonable to do so[17] (see p297). This is in addition to the 'defined circumstances', most of which also apply to IS.[18]

The 'defined circumstances' for a disregard of the value of your home to apply where you are a permanent resident are where it is occupied wholly or in part by:

- your spouse/partner or former partner (except where you are estranged or divorced); *or*
- a relative aged 60 or over; *or*
- a relative who is 'incapacitated'; *or*
- a child under 16 for whom you are responsible[19] (for financial assessment purposes only, not for IS purposes).

'Relative' means parent, parent-in-law, brother, sister, son, son-in-law, daughter, daughter-in-law, step-parent, step-son, step-daughter (or the partner of any of these), a grandchild, grandparent, uncle, aunt, niece or nephew.

'Incapacitated' is not defined in the regulations, but guidance states that it is reasonable to conclude that a relative is incapacitated if they are receiving one of the following benefits: incapacity benefit, severe disablement allowance, disability living allowance, attendance allowance or constant attendance allowance, or they would satisfy the incapacity conditions for any of these.[20]

Note: If your partner, children or relatives continue to live in your home, the help they can receive for their housing costs depends on their circumstances. If they are paying the housing costs, even though you are the person liable for them, they can claim housing benefit (HB) or IS housing costs instead of you (see pp102 and 99).

Discretion to disregard

Guidance is provided to social services departments on their discretionary powers to disregard the value of your former home, in which another person continues to live, in circumstances other than those specified in the legislation. The guidance suggests that this could be where your home is the sole residence of someone who has given up their own home in order to care for you, or an elderly friend especially if they have given up their own home.[21] Social services' discretion could also be applied where you were permanently living with a lesbian or gay partner or an adult son or daughter in your home and they are remaining there. Where social services have used their discretion in these types of circumstances, they can review their decision at any time. Guidance suggests that it would be reasonable to begin taking account of the value of a property when the carer dies or moves out.[22]

If you intend to return home

As for IS (see p195), the value of a dwelling (only one dwelling) normally occupied as your home will be disregarded if your stay is **temporary** (including respite and trial period basis – see p390 for definitions) and you intend to return to your home which is still available to you, or you are taking reasonable steps to dispose of your home in order to acquire another property to return to.[23]

The value of any other property that you own (or jointly own) besides your own home will be taken into account as capital.

If your stay is initially thought to be permanent but turns out to be temporary, your home should be treated in the same way as if you had been temporary from the outset.[24] This is an important provision which means that the financial assessment undertaken by social services would have to be retrospectively reviewed and any excess payments made refunded or any charges placed on your property lifted.

5. **Capital disregarded for 26 weeks or longer**

Most capital that is disregarded for 26 weeks or longer for IS purposes (see p195) is also disregarded for 26 weeks or longer for social services financial assessment purposes, with the important exception that:

• social services does not have the power to disregard property that is up for sale (see p295).

6. **Capital disregarded for 52 weeks**

Most capital that is disregarded for 52 weeks or longer for IS purposes (see p195) is also disregarded for 52 weeks or longer for social services financial assessment purposes, with the important addition that:

• IS is included in the list of benefits for which the balance of any arrears paid or any compensation paid due to non-payment is disregarded as capital for a period of 52 weeks.[25] Any payment of this type should be treated as income over the period for which it is payable and any amount left over after the period for which it is treated as income has elapsed should be treated as capital.[26]

Example
You are assessed as being able to pay £75 per week toward the cost of your placement on the basis of your current income pending receipt of IS.
It is explained to you that the charge will be re-assessed or retrospectively reviewed once IS is received and that back payments will be required.
Although not required to do so, you choose to make payments of £90 per week.
After six weeks, arrears of IS at £35 per week (£210) are received.
The charges are re-assessed/retrospectively reviewed, and you are required to pay £110 per week, from the start of your placement.
As you have been paying £15 per week more than required, the arrears payable to the local authority are £120 rather than the full £210 IS arrears.
The remaining £90 becomes capital and is disregarded for 52 weeks.

7. **Capital treated as income**

As for IS purposes (see p195), any income derived from capital (eg, rental income) is normally treated as capital rather than income, from the date on which it is normally due to be paid[27] unless it is income derived from capital disregarded – eg, any capital held in trust which is as a result of a personal injury.[28]

Interest paid on capital will be treated as capital from the date on which it is paid. However, there is an assumed income from any capital over £10,000[29] (see tariff income, p287).

8. Trust funds

The rules about capital placed in a trust fund for social services financial assessment purposes are the same as for IS purposes (see p193). If you are a beneficiary of a non-discretionary or absolute entitlement trust, the value of the capital asset and any income derived from the capital is normally taken into account as capital in the calculation of your contribution.[30]

The important exception to this is where the capital held in trust is derived from a personal injury compensation payment, in which case both the capital and the capital value of any right to receive income are fully disregarded.[31] However, any payments of income made to you from the capital will be taken into account as income for financial assessment purposes.[32]

If you are a beneficiary of a trust where the deed directs that you are to receive income produced by the trust capital only, then you only have an absolute entitlement to the income. These trusts are known as life interests (or, in Scotland, life rents). The right to receive the income from a life interest has a capital value but it is disregarded for financial assessment purposes.[33] For the treatment of the income see p288 chapter 13.

A discretionary trust fund where payments are made wholly at the discretion of the trustees and there is no absolute entitlement to either capital or income will not be treated as a capital asset[34] (see p288 for the treatment of payments made from a discretionary trust fund).

Official guidance explains in some detail the different types of trust funds and how they should be treated for financial assessment purposes.[35]

9. Notional capital

The notional capital rules are similar to the notional income rules (see p288) and the notional capital rules for IS (see p202). In certain circumstances you may be treated as possessing a capital asset even where you do not in fact possess it.[36] The important difference is that the notional income rules are mandatory but the notional capital rules for financial assessment purposes are discretionary. You **will** be treated as possessing income of which you have deprived yourself for the purpose of decreasing the amount that you may be liable to pay for your accommodation; but you **may** be treated as possessing capital of which you have deprived yourself for the purpose of decreasing the amount that you may be liable to pay for your accommodation.

There are three main circumstances in which you **may** be treated as having notional capital:

- where you deliberately deprive yourself of capital in order to reduce the amount of charge you have to pay;
- where you fail to apply for capital which is available to you (capital payable under a trust derived from a payment made in consequence of a personal injury cannot be taken into account as notional capital);
- where someone else makes a payment of capital to a third party on your behalf unless it is for an item which was not taken into account when the standard rate was fixed for the accommodation provided.[37]

10. **Deprivation**

The rules on deprivation for financial assessments are similar to the rules for IS (see p203). Any capital which you have disposed of or deprived yourself of in order to avoid a charge or to reduce the charge payable, may be considered by social services to be notional capital and as such may be treated as actual capital and taken into account in the financial assessment in addition to any other assessable capital.[38] This is an equivalent provision to that for notional income (see p288). However, unlike for deprivation of income, for deprivation of capital social services has discretion – ie, it **may** treat you as possessing actual capital of which you have deprived yourself.

Social services should only consider questions of deprivation of capital when you cease to possess capital which would otherwise have been taken into account.[39] As with deprivation of income, it is up to you to prove that you no longer have the resource, otherwise it will be treated as actual capital.

Guidance to social services sets out the questions for consideration in deciding whether the deprivation was *in order to avoid or reduce the charge*.[40] You, as the resident, should not be treated as depriving yourself of capital in order to reduce your residential accommodation charge if you enable your spouse to purchase a smaller property by making available to her/him part of your share of the proceeds from the sale of the property you shared as your home.

As for notional income, the purpose and timing of the deprivation should be considered. The guidance suggests it would be unreasonable to decide that a resident had disposed of an asset in order to reduce her/his charge for accommodation when the disposal took place a time when s/he was fit and healthy and could not have foreseen the need for a move to residential accommodation.[41] There is, however, a Scottish Court of Session case[42] which has cast some doubt on the use of this argument in many cases.

If you have used capital to acquire personal possessions to avoid or reduce the charge, then the market value of those personal possessions would not be disregarded.[43]

As the rules on deprivation are similar for IS (see p203), some social services departments may look to the decision on any IS claim you have made before considering what action to take, although it has been confirmed by the courts that social services should make independent decisions and may decide that notional capital should be taken into account even where it had not been taken into account for means-tested benefits.[44]

There have been few reported decisions on the scope of the notional capital rules applying to social services financial assessments and reference is often made to social security commissioner decisions on the meaning of the equivalent IS notional capital rules. One issue considered significant by commissioners was whether the person actually knew of the capital limit rule or whether the knowledge could be inferred. This may now be less significant following the decision in the Scottish Court of Session case which held that it was not necessary to find that a person knew of the existence of a capital limit or that s/he had foreseen the making of an application for the relevant benefit in order to apply the notional capital rule. In some cases an elderly person will be incapable of forming any intention and may be assisted by relatives and in such circumstances the true purpose of any transfer may be ascertained or inferred by social services on the basis of information provided to it without any ready admission or specific finding as to the state of knowledge or intention of the elderly person.[45]

See p326 for what happens when deprivation has been decided and notional capital has been taken into account in your financial assessment.

11. **Diminishing notional capital**

Where you have been assessed as having notional capital, social services should reduce the amount of that notional capital each week by the difference between the rate which you are paying for the accommodation and the rate you would have paid if you were not treated as possessing the notional capital.[46]

Notes

1 Part III NA(AR) Regs 1992

1. General
2 s4 (capital to be disregarded) of the NA(AR) Regs 1992
3 Regs 21, 22 and 25 NA(AR) Regs 1992

2. Treatment of capital
4 Reg 21 NA(AR) Regs 1992
5 Reg 28 NA(AR) Regs 1992
6 Reg 20 NA(AR) Regs 1992
7 s21 NAA 1948 and *R v. Sefton MBC ex parte Help the Aged and Others* (1997) I (CCLR) 57 CA; para 11 LAC(98)8, Annex H CRAG; WOC 12/98; s12 SW(S)A 1968 and SWSG 6/98
8 ISG Regs 1987
9 Reg 23(1)(b) NA(AR) Regs 1992 and para 6.011B CRAG; para 6.011b SWSG 8.96
10 Reg 23(1)(a) NA(AR) Regs 1992; para 6.011a and 6.015 CRAG; para 6.010a SWSG 8/96 and para 6.014 SWSG 2/99
11 s22(1) and s25(2) NAA 1948
12 Reg 27(2) NA(AR) Regs 1992
13 paras 7.012 to 7.014a CRAG
14 Reg 27(1) NA(AR) Regs 1992
15 para 6.010 CRAG; para 6.009 SWSG 8/96
16 para 7.017 CRAG

4. Capital disregarded indefinitely
17 Sch 4 para 18 NA(AR) Regs1992
18 Sch 4 para 2 NA(AR) Regs 1992
19 Sch 4 para 2 NA(AR) Regs 1992
20 para 7.005 CRAG; para 7.005 SWSG 8/96
21 para 7.007 CRAG; para 7.007 SWSG 8/96
22 para 7.008 CRAG; para 7.008 SWSG 8/96
23 Sch 4 para 1 NA(AR) Regs 1992
24 para 7.002 CRAG; para 7.002 SWSG 8/96

6. Capital disregarded for 52 weeks
25 Sch 4 para 6 NA(AR) Regs 1992
26 para 6.030 CRAG; para 6.029 SWSG 8/96

7. Capital treated as income
27 Reg 22(4)NA(AR) Regs 1992
28 para 14 sch 3 NA(AR) Regs 1992
29 Regs 9 and 28 NA(AR) Regs 1992

8. Trust funds
30 Reg 22(4) NA(AR) Regs 1992
31 Sch 4 para 10 NA(AR) Regs 1992 and para 10.025 CRAG
32 para 10.026 CRAG; para 10.026 SWSG 8/96
33 Sch 4 para 11 NA(AR) Regs 1992 and para 10.015 CRAG; 10.015 SWSG 8/96
34 para 10.020 CRAG; 10.020 SWSG 8/96
35 s10 CRAG

9. Notional capital
36 Reg 25 NA(AR) Regs 1992
37 Reg 25(3) NA(AR) Regs 1992

10. Deprivation
38 Reg 25(1) NA(AR) Regs 1992
39 para 6.058 CRAG; para 6.057 SWSG 8/96
40 paras 6.057 to 6.066 CRAG; para 6.056 to 6.066 SWSG 8/96
41 para 6.064 CRAG; para 6.063 SWSG 8/96
42 *Yule v. South Lanarkshire Council* 12 May 1999
43 para 6.065 CRAG; para 6.064 SWSG 8/96
44 *Yule v. South Lanarkshire Council* 12 May 1999
45 *Yule v. South Lanarkshire Council* 12 May 1999

11. Diminishing notional capital
46 Reg 26 NA(AR) Regs 1992

Chapter 15

Personal expenses allowance and outgoings

This chapter explains the rules about the personal expenses allowance, which is usually the amount of money you will be left with from your income after you have made your contribution to social services for the cost of your accommodation and care. This chapter also explains the rules about outgoings that you may have in connection with your own home. It covers:

1. Personal expenses allowance (p303)
2. Outgoings (p305)

1. Personal expenses allowance

Legislation requires social services to allow you to retain specified amounts out of your assessable resources for personal expenses.[1] The minimum amount of personal expenses allowance (PEA) is set by regulations made each year.[2] For 1999/2000 the minimum amount is £14.75 per week.

You will get the same amount whether you are a temporary or permanent resident in a local authority or an independent residential care or nursing home. In the past, if you were in a local authority home you would have received a lower PEA, but you were not expected to meet expenditure on personal items (eg, clothing) out of that allowance. Current guidance states that the resident will normally supply their own clothes, but in cases of special need or emergency (eg, if all your clothes are lost in a fire), the local authority may supply replacement clothing.[3]

It is intended that your PEA should be spent as you wish on personal items – eg, toiletries, stationery, gifts. If you are not able to manage your personal expenses allowance because of ill health, social services may (subject to your agreement or that of your attorney or appointee) deposit it in a bank account on your behalf and use it to provide for your smaller needs. Many social services departments have set up a savings account system that is administered by them. Any money that is unspent on your death will form part of your estate.

Social services cannot allow you to use your PEA to help pay for more expensive accommodation even if you wish to do this[4] (see Chapter 16). In addition, care homes should not expect you to use your PEA for services which either are, or ought to be, covered by social services contract with the home. If in doubt, you should contact your social services department.

Increasing the personal expenses allowance

An increase in the PEA is usually called a 'variation'. Social services have discretion to allow more than the minimum amount (currently £14.75) in 'special circumstances'.[5] Guidance gives examples of where a local authority might consider allowing a different amount:

- where you need to keep more of your income to help you lead a more independent life. This may be appropriate if you do not qualify as a 'less dependent' resident (see p290) solely because you live in an independent care home or in local authority accommodation where board is provided;
- where you have a dependent child, the needs of the child (whether or not they are placed with you) should be considered in the PEA;
- where you are temporarily in residential accommodation and you receive income support (IS) which includes an amount for a partner, social services should consider the needs of your partner in the PEA. Social services should not request a charge that would leave your partner without enough money to live on. However, social services could consider the appropriate applicable amount of IS for your partner as being enough to live on.
- where you are one of an unmarried couple, social services is not required to disregard 50 per cent of any works or private pension that you pay to your partner. However, where you are the main recipient of your overall income, they can use their discretion to increase your PEA to enable you to pass some of your income to your partner. Social services are advised to bear in mind the effects that increasing your partner's income could have on benefits such as IS.[6]

Further guidance states that where you are temporarily absent from your care home, social services have the discretion to vary the PEA upwards to enable you to have more money while staying with family or friends.[7]

If you are a permanent resident the PEA is the amount that you will normally be left with out of your income when you have made your contribution to social services for the cost of your accommodation and care. However, if you are in receipt of attendance allowance (AA) or disability living allowance (DLA) care component, which is normally payable for the first four weeks of your stay (see p356) and you are a temporary resident, you will have this income in addition to your PEA. If you are in receipt of, or claim DLA mobility component or any other disregards income (eg, war widow's special pension)[8], this will continue in payment and will be additional income on top of your PEA, whether you are a temporary or permanent resident.

2. **Outgoings**

If you are a temporary resident, social services can disregard a reasonable amount of your income to meet outgoings that you may have in connection with your home in the community. This also includes outgoings on a home you are taking steps to sell in order to acquire another more suitable home to which you will return.[9]

If you are a permanent resident, you are normally not considered to have outgoings as you would no longer have a home in the community. However, it may be that you still have outgoings, for example while your home is up for sale. If this is the case, social services can consider a variation of your PEA (see p304) to allow you to meet these commitments. It is only temporary residents who are eligible for a disregard on their income to meet outgoings in respect of their home in the community.

Guidance sets out a list of examples of outgoings. Where IS and/or housing benefit (HB) are in payment, extra costs not met by benefit might be:
- a fixed heating charge;
- water rates;
- mortgage payments or rent not met by IS/HB;
- service charges not met by IS/HB;
- insurance premiums;[10]

Where neither IS or HB are being paid, your outgoings might include:
- interest charges on hire purchase agreement to buy the dwelling you occupy as your home;
- interest charges on loans for repairs or improvements to the dwelling;
- ground rent or other rental relating to a long tenancy;
- service charges;
- standard charges for fuel;
- payments under co-ownership scheme or tenancy agreement or license of a Crown tenant.[11]

If you share your home in the community with a partner or other adults, outgoings allowed will normally be divided equally and only your share will be included in the extra amount allowed for outgoings in the financial assessment.

Notes

1. Personal expenses allowance

  1 s22(4) NAA 1948
  2 NA(SPR) Regs
  3 Para 5.001 CRAG; para 5.001 SWSG 8/96
  4 para 8.018 CRAG; para 8.018 SWSG 8/96
  5 s22(4)NAA 1948
  6 para 5.005 CRAG; para 5.005 SWSG 8/96
  7 para 8 LAC (97)5; Annex H CRAG, WOC 29/27; para 15 SWSG 7/97
  8 Sch3 NA(AT) para 25 Regs 1992 and para 8.046 CRAG; para 8.046 SWSG 8/96

2. Outgoings

  9 Sch 3 para 27 NA(AR) Regs 1992
 10 para 3.011 CRAG; para 3.011 SWSG 8/96
 11 para 3.012 CRAG; para 3.012 SWSG 8/96

Chapter 16

Third party top-ups

This chapter explains the rules about having a third party top-up your fees when social services has arranged for your care in a residential or nursing home which is more expensive than it would normally pay for someone with your level of needs. It covers:

1. Who can be a third party (p307)
2. Responsibilities of the third party (p308)
3. How third party payments are treated in assessing your charge (p309)

1. Who can be a third party

If you are planning to move into, or are already in, a residential care or nursing home which is more expensive than what social services would normally pay for someone with your level of needs, you will need to have someone else (ie, a third party) to make up the difference. For your rights to choose your accommodation (see p278).

A third party may be any person, relative or friend or organisation (eg, a charity or your employer) willing to make up the difference, other than:

- yourself, because the National Assistance Act 1948 does not permit a resident to use her/his own resources in this way. Guidance was issued in 1994 to state that you cannot use your personal expenses allowance (see Chapter 15).[1] Further guidance was issued in 1998 in England and Wales regarding other resources and correcting the Choice of Accommodation Directive.[2]
- your spouse, unless s/he has the resources to meet her/his liability to contribute towards your care (see Chapter 17) and make an additional third party payment.[3]

In addition, a third party must reasonably be expected to continue to contribute throughout the duration of your care arrangements. Social services have been told to assure themselves there is every chance that the third party will continue to have the resources to make the payments.[4]

Yourself as a third party

Until recently there was some doubt as to whether you could act as your own third party. It has been quite clear for several years that you cannot use your personal expenses allowance (PEA) to pay for more expensive accommodation. However the guidance in England and Wales correcting 'misleading' information (see Footnote 2) was only issued just over a year ago. Many local authorities had entered into arrangements which meant residents used their savings to pay for the accommodation of their choice. If you are being expected to use your savings in this way, you may want to query it with your local authority as it may be contrary to guidance.

It begs the question of what should happen if you want to go into a more expensive residential or nursing home but you do not have anyone to pay the difference. You may feel that if you have capital of up to £16,000 you should be able to use it to pay for the home of your choice. However, the current view of the government is that to allow your savings to be used in this way would require primary legislation. If the law changes in the future there will need to be safeguards to ensure that residents are not put under pressure from either social services or owners off care homes to routinely deplete their remaining savings to pay for more expensive accommodation.

2. Responsibilities of the third party

Social services contract to pay the full fees of the care home and the third party agrees to pay social services the difference between what the department normally pays and the cost of the accommodation. This can be done by:

- the third party paying social services; *or*
- the third party paying the home direct, if your third party, yourself and the homeowner agree.[5]

Social services should tell you and your third party that as the fees and the amounts that social services are prepared to pay do not necessarily increase at the same rate, increases may not be evenly split. If the home's fees rise faster than the level social services will pay, then that increase will fall on the third party. Third party contributions should be regularly reviewed.[6]

Any failure by your third party to pay the level of contribution means you may have to leave the home of your choice. It is suggested that social services should make legally binding contracts with third parties (although charities have restrictions on such contracts) specifying:

- that failure to keep up payments will normally result in the resident having to move;

- an increase in a resident's income will not necessarily mean the third party paying less, as the resident's own income is subject to charging in the normal way;
- that a rise in the accommodation fees will not automatically be shared equally between the authority and the third party; *and*
- if the accommodation fails to honour its contractual conditions, the authority must reserve the right to terminate the contract.[7]

3. How third party payments are treated in assessing your charge

When a third party makes a payment to meet the difference between what social services will pay and the actual cost of your accommodation, that payment is treated as your notional income and taken into account in full.[8] The social services department retains the liability to pay the full costs of the home, but can recoup more money from you because of the third party payment.

Example:

The home you have chosen costs £380 and social services will normally only pay £340. Your son has agreed to pay the extra £40. Your own weekly assessed income is £250 per week, but you are counted as having £290 because the amount your son pays is notionally treated as your income. Social services charge you £275.25 (so leaving you with £14.75 personal expenses allowance), which you and your son pay the home. Social services only has to pay the home the difference of £104.75.

Notes

1. Who can be a third party
1 LAC (94) 1; WOC 4/94 Annex H, CRAG; para 13 SWSG 5/94
2 CRAG 8.018 and LAC (98)8 WOC 12/98, which corrected a 'misleading' sentence in LAC (92)27. No equivalent guidance has been issued in Scotland referring to the equivalent sentence in SWSG 5/93
3 LAC (92) 27; WOC 12/93; para 11.14 SWSG 5/93
4 LAC (92)27; para 11.3 WOC 12/93 SWSG 5/93

2. Responsibilities of the third party
5 LAC (92)27; WOC 12/93; para 11.4 SWSG 5/93
6 LAC (92)27; WOC 12/93; para 11.8 SWSG 5/93
7 LAC (92)27; WOC 12/93; paras 11.9 and 10 SWSG 5/93

3. How third party payments are treated in assessing your charge
8 AoR Regs 1992 Reg 17(4); CRAG 8.062 and SWSG 8.062

Chapter 17

Liable relatives – social services

This chapter explains the rules about the liability to pay maintenance to people whose accommodation and care are funded wholly or partly by social services and how maintenance affects the financial assessment. It covers:
1. Who is a liable relative (p310)
2. Assessment forms (p310)
3. Pursuing liable relative payments (p311)
4. The treatment of liable relative payments (p312)
5. How maintenance you pay affects your financial assessment (p313)

There are similar rules for people who claim income support or income-based jobseeker's allowance (see Chapter 8).

1. Who is a liable relative

Legislation states that spouses are liable to maintain one another (and their children).[1] No one else, including an unmarried partner or, unlike for income support, if you are a 'person from abroad', a sponsor, is liable to maintain you.

Your spouse has a duty to maintain you (ie, make a payment of maintenance which is called a liable relative payment) if your accommodation and care are being provided wholly or partly at public expense by social services. In these circumstances, social services may seek complete or partial reimbursement of the expenditure.[2]

2. Assessment forms

Social services departments have no power to assess couples jointly under the National Assistance Act 1948. This means that even if you have a spouse who is a liable relative, the social services financial assessment form should not ask for information about your spouse's resources.[3]

Social services are advised in guidance that they should first asses your ability to pay based solely on your resources to establish the contribution you are able to pay without assistance from your spouse.[4] Only if you are unable to pay the full charge should social services consider whether it is worth pursuing your spouse for maintenance toward the shortfall.[5]

Some social services departments have a separate form which your spouse may be asked to complete. Social services cannot insist on the completion of such a form or on your spouse disclosing any information about her/his resources. Your spouse should not feel pressured into giving this information. If your spouse has been asked to provide this information and is worried about it, s/he should seek advice.

3. **Pursuing liable relative payments**

Social services departments are advised by guidance that, if you are in receipt of income support (IS) and they pursue maintenance, the Benefits Agency will merely reduce your IS. This would reduce what social services can charge to the original amount so that it may not be worth social services pursuing maintenance where IS is in payment to you.[6] Therefore, the guidance advises that where your spouse is in receipt of IS no action is necessary.[7]

Although it is not clear in the guidance whether this applies to both permanent and temporary residents, not pursuing those spouses in receipt of IS probably refers to permanent residents only as if your spouse was in receipt of IS and you were a temporary resident, s/he would be receiving IS for both of you as a couple and social services may wish to ask for the amount that is payable in respect of you.

Social services cannot force your spouse either to give information about her/his resources or to make a payment. Even if your spouse has already given information about her/his resources social services still cannot insist on your spouse making a liable relative payment. Neither can social services refuse to provide a service or delay arranging a service for you because your spouse refuses to disclose financial information or make a payment (England and Wales only).[8]

Ultimately only the courts can enforce an appropriate payment and legislation provides for social services to refer a case to the magistrates court or sheriff court in Scotland.[9] However, as with all enforcement measures, social services will have to decide whether in terms of the cost and the potential for adverse publicity, the recoupment of expenditure it is worth pursuing to this stage.

If social services approach your spouse and s/he is happy to disclose her/his resources and/or to make a liable relative payment, then the question that arises is the amount. There are no national rules governing the amount of a liable relative payment although some social services departments may operate their own means test.

Any amount that is arrived at by a social services means test is not enforceable by them. You may wish to offer a different amount. The guidance states that social services should consider what would be 'appropriate' and that this will involve discussion and negotiation with your spouse, and will be determined to a large extent by her/his financial circumstances in relation to her/his expenditure and normal standard of living. The guidance states that it would not necessarily be appropriate to expect spouses to reduce their resources to IS levels in order to pay maintenance.[10]

4. **The treatment of liable relative payments**

A liable relative payment is the payment made by your spouse who is liable to maintain you.[11] Certain payments are not treated as liable relative payments even though they are made by a liable relative. These are the same as for IS (see p214).[12]

A liable relative payment can be considered as a periodical or non-periodical payment by social services. Periodical payments and arrears of periodical payments are made for an identifiable period and a weekly income figure is calculated accordingly. The rules for the treatment of non-periodical payments, which are payments that are not made for identifiable periods, are slightly different from the rules which apply for IS. The rules are as follows:

- If you are on IS the Benefits Agency calculates the number of weeks for which IS will be withdrawn. Social services should work out the same number of weeks by dividing the payment by the amount of IS normally in payment (plus any disregards which would be applicable if the payment was a regular payment of earnings). Any remaining amount should be taken into account in the assessment of the final week.[13]
- If you are not on IS the payment is divided by the difference between the standard charge (ie, the full charge) and the contribution you have been assessed to make from your own resources. Any remaining amount should be taken into account as income for the final week.[14]

Example
Mrs Webster is paying a charge (A) of £120.
The standard charge (B) is £250.
She receives a lump sum maintenance payment (C) of £750
The number of weeks over which the payment should be taken into account is calculated as follows:
C (B-A) = 5.77 weeks

Mrs Webster therefore pays the standard charge at £250 for 5 weeks.

In week 6 Mrs Webster will have £100 left from the payment (having used £130 (B-A) a week for the five weeks to meet the extra charge). This should be used to calculate the charge for week 6.[15]

Periodical and non-periodical payments may be made at the same time. If the periodical payment is less than the difference between the standard charge and the amount you would be liable to pay if you did not receive any liable relative payment, the non-periodical payment should be taken into account over a number of weeks calculated by dividing the payment by the difference between the standard charge and the amount you had previously been contributing.[16] Where the weekly liable relative payment is equal to or more than the difference between the standard charge and the contribution you would be assessed as paying if you did not receive a liable relative payment, then the non-periodical payment should be treated as capital.[17]

5. **How maintenance you pay affects your financial assessment**

If you are a resident in a care home and you are contributing to the maintenance of someone there is no specific provision to allow a disregard of the amount that you pay from the assessment of your income unless it is a payment of at least 50 per cent of an occupational pension, personal pension or retirement annuity made to your spouse who is not living with you. In these circumstances 50 per cent of your occupational pension, personal pension or retirement annuity will be disregarded as income in your financial assessment (also see p286).[18]

There is also a provision not to treat any part of an occupational pension, personal pension or retirement annuity that your spouse is legally entitled to receive (eg, by means of a Court Order) as income belonging to you and therefore it would not form part of your income for financial assessment purposes.[19] If, in addition, you pass at least 50 per cent of the part of the occupation pension, personal pension or retirement annuity belonging to you, to your spouse, the 50 per cent disregard will still apply.[20]

If you pay maintenance as a liable relative from income other than an occupational pension, personal pension or retirement annuity then you may need to seek advice about whether the change in your circumstances (ie, becoming a resident in a care home) will affect your liability.

If you remain liable to make maintenance payments, social services may, in special circumstances, be able to use their discretion to increase your personal expenses allowance in order to enable you to continue to meet the commitment.[21]

Notes

1. Who is a liable relative
1 s42 NAA 1948; s97(3) SW(S)A 1968
2 paras 11.001 and 11.002 CRAG; paras 11.001 and 11.002 SWSG 8/96

2. Assessment forms
3 para 11.005 CRAG; para 11.005 SSG 8/96
4 para 11.006i CRAG; para 11.006i SWSG 8/96
5 para 11.006ii CRAG; para 11.006ii SWSG 8/96

3. Pursuing liable relatives payments
6 para 11.003 CRAG; para 11.003 SWSG 8/96
7 para 11.004 CRAG; para 11.004 SWSG 8/96
8 para 11.001 CRAG; para 11.001 SWSG 8/96
9 s43 NAA 1948
10 para 11.006iii CRAG; para 11.006iii SWSG 8/96

4. The treatment of liable relative payments
11 s42 NAA 1948
12 para 11.008 CRAG; para 11.008 SWSG 8/96
13 Reg 18(2) NA(AR) Regs 1992 and para 11.021 CRAG; para 11.021 SWSG 8/96
14 para 11.022 CRAG; para 11.022 SWSG 8/96
15 Reg 32(1) NA(AR) Regs 1992 and para 11.022 CRAG; para 11.022 SWSG 8/96

16 Reg 32(2) NA(AR) Regs 1992 and para 11.023 CRAG; para 11.023 SWSG 8/96
17 Reg 34(1) NA(AR) Regs 1992 and para 11.024 CRAG; para 11.024 SWSG 8/96

5. How maintenance you pay affects your financial assessment
18 Sch 3 NA(AR) para 10A Regs 1992 and para 8.024A CRAG; para 8.024A SWSG 8/96
19 para 8.024C CRAG; para 8.024C SWSG 8/96
20 para 8.024C CRAG; para 8.024C SWSG 8/96
21 s22(4) NAA 1948 and para 5.005 CRAG; para 5.005 SSG 8/96

Chapter 18

Special rules for special groups – social services

This chapter considers the responsibilities of social services to provide accommodation and assistance to special groups of people without other means of support.

It covers:
1. People from abroad (p315)
2. Other special groups (p317)
3. Types of assistance (p318)

Special rules apply to special groups of people so that they are not entitled to claim social security benefits (see Chapter 9). Even if you are not entitled to claim benefits because of these special rules, you may still be entitled to assistance from social services. Indeed, being denied benefit may be the very reason why you need help from social services.

1. People from abroad

As a result of changes in government policy and the law in 1996, many people from abroad are no longer entitled to means-tested benefits (see Chapter 9). These changes were mainly concerned with restricting the right to state support for asylum-seekers and other people from abroad who are subject to immigration control, but many others may also be affected if they fail the habitual residence test (see p221). Many people who are subject to immigration control are also now excluded from local authority housing, even when homeless.

In England and Wales, a person in need of 'care and attention' with no other means of obtaining it may nevertheless apply to social services for accommodation and other assistance.[1] The Court of Appeal has now decided that social services' responsibilities may extend to people whose need for care and attention arises only because they have been excluded from benefits, even if they are not otherwise in need of residential care due to old age, ill health or disablement[2] (those who are in need of residential care for those reasons should be provided with it regardless of whether they are entitled to benefit or not).

The court's decision was concerned with the very exceptional circumstances of asylum-seekers who would otherwise be destitute and in need of 'shelter, warmth and food'. However, it is arguable that the same principles could apply to other special groups (see below).

The court's decision does not mean that every asylum seeker is entitled to assistance. Social services must carry out individual assessments of need to see if assistance is required and how those needs may be met. The courts have decided that social services would no longer have responsibilities towards any person in need who unreasonably refuses to comply with their reasonable requirements in the meeting of that need. This has been held to include an asylum seeker whom they had already accommodated but who had been evicted from two different types of accommodation provided for him due to his threatening behaviour (although social services may still have had a responsibility to assist if there had been any evidence (eg, of mental health problems) to excuse the behaviour).[3]

Social services' responsibilities may apply to asylum-seekers even if they have not applied for asylum in the UK.[4]

In Scotland, destitute asylum-seekers are treated as 'persons in need' who are 'eligible for assistance' under specific legislation.[5] Any help (which may include cash payments) which may be provided is subject to an individual assessment of need.

The existing arrangements for asylum-seekers (whereby those who are not entitled to social security benefits may instead rely on social services for accommodation and support) will be replaced by new measures when the Asylum and Immigration Act 1999 is fully in force from April 2000. The Act aims to implement the government's stated commitment to 'providing a safety net but . . . to do so in a way which minimises the incentive for abuse by those who do not really need the support or who would make an unfounded asylum application in order to obtain the provision'.[6] The Act intends to remove all existing financial and care responsibilities from both the Department of Social Security and social services (including those duties under the National Assistance Act 1948, and the Children Act 1989). The Home Office will instead take on all responsibility for co-ordinating, planning and contracting out a new national scheme of assistance. The Home Office will have powers to direct local authorities to provide accommodation as required (although asylum-seekers will be given no choice as to what part of the country they may be housed in) and will arrange for other needs (such as food) to be met by vouchers or small cash payments. It is not yet clear what level of assistance will be made available or the extent to which additional needs (eg, for health, language or educational facilities, or for family responsibilities) will be met.

2. **Other special groups**

In England and Wales, the very exceptional circumstances of asylum-seekers (see above) have now been given special consideration by the courts in deciding that social services have duties to provide accommodation and assistance to them even though they may not otherwise be in need of care due to old age, ill health or disablement. However, it is still not clear how far the same duties could extend to other special groups.

Although it is not clear, it is at least arguable that social services could have the same responsibilities to other people from abroad who are denied benefit – eg, those who are not (or not yet) habitually resident, or those who are subject to sponsorship undertakings but whose sponsors are not able (or willing) to support them. It has, however, been held that the duties would not generally apply to people who are homeless but not entitled to accommodation from local authority housing departments, except that the duties could apply when accommodation (and other assistance) would meet a need which would otherwise have to be met by other community care services (see Chapter 2).[7] It has also been held that social services do not have any such duties to people who have entered the country illegally or to overstayers, as such people are considered to be not entitled to benefit because of their own wrongdoing (unless they have been prevented from leaving the country due to factors beyond their control).[8]

Because the law is currently unclear in its application to special groups other than asylum-seekers, you will need to seek specialist advice if you are not an asylum seeker and have been denied benefits and have no other means of support.

In Scotland, social work departments have wide powers which allow 'advice, guidance or assistance' (including 'facilities') to be given to anyone with an assessed need, although cash payments may only be made to specified groups of 'persons in need'.[9]

Different duties apply to social services in England, Wales and Scotland whenever the needs of a child are involved. Social services have duties to promote the welfare of 'children in need'[10] and will usually need to make arrangements to ensure that a child is accommodated with her/his family.[11] This may mean that in appropriate circumstances payments can be made to meet the accommodation costs and living expenses not only of the child, but also of the parent(s) and/or other carer(s).

3. **Types of assistance**

If social services have a duty to provide you with residential accommodation, they should not wait until you are actually roofless before helping you and they must also provide you with other assistance to meet your essential needs for 'shelter, warmth and food'.[12] A person for whom accommodation is provided by social services must also be given 'board and other services, amenities and requisites provided in connection with the accommodation.[13]

However (except in respect of children in need), no other assistance must be provided unless there is a duty to provide you with accommodation.[14]

In all cases (except in respect of children in need), social services must deliver the services directly. They have no powers to pay cash to applicants for them to make their own arrangements.[15]

The types of assistance provided by social services vary considerably. Accommodation has been provided from local authority housing stock, or bed and breakfast, or by way of payments direct to the applicant's landlord. Food has been provided by way of food parcels, vouchers or hot meals at a particular site within the area (such as a hospital canteen). Vouchers have been provided for toiletries and some have provided vouchers to obtain winter clothing. In one case, social services were to be challenged when they had provided bed and breakfast only and directed the individual to the nearest soup kitchen, but they agreed at the last minute to provide meals instead.[16]

In Scotland, help may be given in either cash or kind o or for adults or children in need.[17]

Special arrangements exist between the Home Office (or, in Scotland, the Scottish Executive) and social services departments for the reimbursement of expenditure incurred on supporting asylum-seekers. All arrangements for support for asylum-seekers, including the types of assistance available and whether there are children in need, will change from April 2000 (see p315).

Notes

1. People from abroad

1   S21(1)(a) NAA 1948 and LAC (93)10, Appendix 1
2   *R v London Borough of Westminster and others ex parte 'M'* [1996] QBD *Times* 10 October 1996, CA, 17 February 1997
3   *R v Kensington & Chelsea LBC ex parte Muriqi Kujtim* [1999] QBD *Times* 5 August 1999, CA, 9 July 1999
4   *R v Lambeth LBC ex parte Sarhangi* [1998] QBD *Times* 8 December 1998 CA, 17 November 1998
5   s12 SW(S)A 1968; SWSG 3/98
6   'Fairer, Faster and Firmer' – A Modern Approach to Immigration and Asylum', CA 4018, July 1998
7   *R v Bristol CC ex parte Penfold* [1998] QBD, CA 23 January 1998; *R v Wigan MBC ex parte Tammadge* [1998] QBD, CA, 30 July 1998
8   *R v Lambeth LBC ex parte Sarhangi* [1998] QBD *Times* 8 December 1998 CA, 17 November 1998
9   s12 SW(S)A; SWSG 3/98
10   s17 CA 1989; s22 C(S)A 1995
11   s20 CA 1989; s25 C(S)A 1995

3. Types of assistance

12   See footnote 2
13   s21(5) NAA 1948, para 4 Secretary of State's Directions and Approvals; *ex parte Gorenkin* (see footnote 10)
14   *Ex parte Gorenkin and others*, QBD 13 May 1997, *Times*, 9 June 1997
15   *R v SSH ex parte London Borough of Hammersmith*, the *Independent,* 15 July 1997; *R v Secretary of State for Health ex parte Hammersmith & Fulham LBC and others*, CA, 27 July 1998, *Times* 9 September 1998
16   *R v Camden LBC ex parte Al-Shakarchi* [1996] 20 November 1996
17   SW(S)A 1968; C(S)A 1995

Chapter 19

• •

Collection of charges and enforcement

This chapter explains how your charges are collected and the actions social services can take if you do not pay your charges or if it has been decided that you have deliberately deprived yourself of resources. It covers:

1. How charges are collected

When social services departments arrange for your care, either in one of their own homes or in an independent residential or nursing home, they must establish, under Section 22 National Assistance Act 1948, using the rules described in the previous chapters, how much you should pay. In Scotland, section 87(3) of the Social Work (Scotland) Act 1968 provides that accommodation provided under the 1968 Act and section 7 of the Mental Health (Scotland) Act 1984, shall for charging purposes be regarded as provided under Part III of the National Assistance Act 1948. They must ensure you are given a clear explanation, usually in writing, of how your charge has been calculated and how much it will be each week. They should also inform you of why your charge may fluctuate. This is especially important in the first few weeks, when changes to your benefits will affect how much you have to pay[1] (see Chapter 21). You should also be told of how you will be billed for your charge.

There are two ways to pay if you are in an independent residential or nursing home:
- social services pay the home the full cost and pay social services your assessed contribution;[2]

- you can pay your assessed contribution direct to the home and social services will pay the difference if you, the home owner, and the social services all agree.[3]

The latter method was introduced for administrative efficiency only and *has* to be with the agreement of all parties. If any of you disagree then social services have to pay the full cost and bill you for your contribution.

The guidance makes it clear that social services have the contractual obligation with the home, and are responsible for paying the full fees. If you do not pay your contribution, it is social services' responsibility to recover the charge from you.[4] It should not be the responsibility of the home to ensure that you pay your assessed charge.

In practice, some social services departments use this method of collection without making it clear that it must be with your agreement and do not explain the alternative.

2. If you cannot or will not pay your assessed charge

Social services departments cannot stop providing you with residential or nursing care purely because you are unable or unwilling to pay the assessed charge.[5] They have a variety of methods open to them for pursuing money owed to them which are discussed in this chapter. It is up to each authority to decide what enforcement actions social services departments will take. Auditors who monitor local authority expenditure will query any debts building up. They will also want to know what is being done to avoid such situations and what is being is done to pursue debts which have accrued.

Each social services department will have worked out its own procedures for tracking debts and following them up. Some will have early warning signals built into their systems so that as soon as you have missed a few payments you will be visited to establish the reason. If you pay the home direct it is likely there will be an arrangement for any non-payment to be reported as soon as possible. Some authorities have panels to authorise and monitor debts when they reach a certain level and to decide whether enforcement action should begin.

You do not normally have a contractual relationship with social services when they arrange your accommodation, but the legislation provides that any sum due under the National Assistance Act shall be recoverable as a civil debt.[6] This allows social services to take the same steps as any creditor to enforce payment of your assessed contributions.

You should normally have enough money to pay your assessed contribution, but there may be times when this will not be the case. The most common reasons are:

- you have been assessed to pay the full cost because of your capital, but you are unable to access it because an application for receivership is with the Court of Protection (or in Scotland a curator bonis is being appointed) (see p338) or an application has been made to register an Enduring Power of Attorney in England and Wales (see p337). Social services should be prepared to wait in these circumstances. The person taking over your affairs may be able to get permission from the Public Trust Office to enable you to pay your residential or nursing home fees. They should ring the customer services section of the Public Trust Office for advice (see p338 for provisions in Scotland);

- you have been assessed as paying the full cost because you have a property, the value of which is correctly included in the assessment, but which has not yet been sold. This is one of the most common reasons for not being able to pay your assessed charge (see p324);

- you have been assessed as paying a charge based on the assumption that you receive income support (IS). Because many residents can get IS, and social services finance officers are aware of the amount which is usually paid if you are in a residential or nursing home, the calculation often assumes you receive this amount. You should always check your calculation very carefully and see if it tallies with your income, which includes any IS you get. It may be that you have not applied for IS, or there has been a decision that you are not entitled, but social services is not aware of this. Or the amount that the DSS has paid may be different to what the finance officer thinks should be paid. There can be a number of reasons for this. You should ask social services for a reassessment. You should not be charged as if you have IS if you have not applied for it, unless you have deliberately decided not to apply. In this case it could be considered to be notional income (see p288). If it is necessary to appeal about the level of IS you get, you should ask social services to assess your charge based on what you currently receive and reassess you if you win the appeal.

If you do not wish to pay your assessed charge (eg, because you disagree with the amount calculated or you are in dispute about the value of a jointly owned property) you should seek advice about the subject under dispute and whether you should make any payments and if so how much, while the dispute is resolved.

If there is any other reason you are not willing to pay the charges you have been assessed to pay, it is likely that social services will be prepared to consider remedies to enforce payment of the money due.

Actions to avoid debts building up

There are a number of practical steps social services can take to avoid debts building up. What happens in practice varies considerably.

If you are becoming forgetful and have difficulty in managing your financial affairs

Social services may help you to get a friend or relative to become an appointee (if you do not have much capital and your main income is benefits). If you already have authorised an Enduring Power of Attorney (in Scotland Power of Attorney) and can no longer manage your affairs it may need to be registered, so that your attorney can take over your affairs. Or social services may suggest that someone approaches the Court of Protection to become your receiver (or in Scotland a curator bonis is appointed to manage your financial affairs). For more details on appointees, attorneys and receivers see Chapter 20.

By helping you to arrange for someone to take over your affairs if you are no longer able to manage, social services ensures that your charges are paid regularly and so avoid any debt building up.

If your appointee, attorney or receiver does not pay the charges

If you are unable to manage your affairs and have an appointee, attorney or receiver and s/he is not paying your fees, social services will negotiate with her/him and may inform the DSS in order to get her/him removed from dealing with your affairs. If necessary social services may take over this role.

Giving budgeting advice

Some local authorities have money advisers who could offer you advice about budgeting and ways of making it easier to pay your charge, if this happens to be the problem. If you have other debts, a money adviser may be able to help with negotiating with your creditors. In exceptional circumstances, social services may allow you an extra personal expenses allowance (see Chapter 15). In some cases social services may be prepared to write off your debt to them.

Direct deductions of income support or income-based jobseeker's allowance

If you are not using your IS or income-based JSA for your charges, the Benefits Agency can make direct deductions if it is in your interests. If social services has arranged your accommodation, the deductions can be paid direct to them. If you have arranged your own accommodation, the deduction can be paid to the home. In the case of a home run by a voluntary organisation for people dependent on alcohol or drugs, direct payments can be made even if you are not in debt.[7] Your consent is not needed.[8]

3. **Legal charges on property**

Social services departments cannot force you to sell your property in order to pay the assessed charge (which in most cases will be the full cost). Instead, if you fail to pay your assessed charge they may create a legal charge on your interest in any land that is in England and Wales[9] and a charging order if your land is in Scotland.[10] Note that a legal charge can only be created if you have failed to pay your charge, so unless you have a debt to social services there is no power for them to create a legal charge on your land.

If you have a beneficial interest in land, then a charge may be registered against the legal title, or if the property is unregistered a Class B land charge may be registered.[11] If the land is in Scotland then the charging order is recorded in the Register of Sasines or registered in the Land Register as appropriate.[12] In effect this means that when you come to sell you property, it will have an encumbrance against it which will have to be discharged before it can be sold.

The charge is created by a declaration in writing[13] and guidance in England and Wales says that social services should advise or assist you to consult a solicitor if they are considering creating a legal charge.[14]

Jointly owned property

If you jointly own property your interest is technically in the proceeds of sale of that land and not in the land itself. Local authorities can only create a legal charge on the interest in the land, not on the interest in the proceeds of the sale of that land.[15]

In England and Wales local authorities have therefore been advised in guidance to register a 'caution' in the cases of jointly owned property.[16] A caution affords local authorities less protection than a legal charge, but would alert them if a sale is going through, so that they could take action.

Social services are referred to the guidance about valuing jointly owned property.[17] Before any caution is registered it is important that the value of your interest in the property has been established, as it may have a low or nil value if there is no willing buyer.

Charging interest

Interest on the legal charge or charging order cannot be charged during your lifetime, but will be added from the date you die.[18] The interest has to be at a 'reasonable rate'. How local authorities set the rate varies around the country, but most use formulas which are within average market rates.

As there is a specific provision under HASSASSAA to place a legal charge, social services cannot use any other legislation to create a legal charge and interest therefore can only be charged from the date of the resident's death.[19]

Prior to this guidance issued in England and Wales, some social services had argued that the legal charge was created under section 111 of the Local Government Act 1972 which gives general powers to local authorities.

Costs of creating the charge

The law is silent on whether social services or you should bear the cost of creating the legal charge or charging order. Some authorities will pass the cost on to you. If this happens you should establish under what legislation this is done, as the provision in HASSASSAA only relates to the failure to pay the assessed charge. Some social services departments in England and Wales have sought legal advice which looks to section 111 of the Local Government Act 1972. This has not, as yet, been challenged in the courts.

Calculating the debt accruing

You continue to be charged for the full cost of your residential or nursing home fees, until such time as your debt means that the value of your property and any other capital you have has reached £16,000. From that point charges should be based on your income and tariff income, until the value of your property and other capital is down to £10,000 and from then only based on your income (see pp287 and 293).

In the case of property it can be difficult to calculate the debt, as it is based on a valuation which may or may not reflect the final price you receive. It only becomes a problem if the value of your property after your debt has been taken into account, falls to £16,000. Until that time you have to pay the full fees.

In practice it appears that most social services departments re-adjust the amount you owe when the property is sold, as they can base the calculation of your debt on the actual sale price of your property. In some cases this will mean that you are asked to pay more if your property is sold for more than expected, or you might be charged less or refunded some money if your property sells for less than the amount at which it has been valued.

A rule of thumb is that you should not be left with total capital (other capital and your property sale) of less than £10,000 unless:

- your debt was accrued before 1996 when the capital limits changed from £8,000 to £16,000. If by 1 April 1996 your debt had already taken you below £10,000 then it should have stopped accruing any further at that point and remained at the point it had reached under the old capital limits;
- interest has been charged under the rules explained on p324. As interest is added to the debt, this interest could take capital below £10,000.

4. **Deprivation of assets**

Treating you as if you still have those assets

If social services decides that you have given away your assets or not applied for them, in order to avoid or lessen your liability for charges for your care (see p300 for details of how they come to that decision), then it **will** in the case of income and **may** in the case of capital treat you as if you still possess those assets.[20] This means that your charge will be assessed as if you still have that income or capital using the notional income and capital rules (see below and pp288 and 299). Unless you are able to pay the assessed charge you will accrue a debt which can be enforced as a civil debt, or if you still own any land, a legal charge or charging order on it can be created by the local authority. If you have given away your property then there is no power for a legal charge or charging order to be created on it as you no longer have an interest in land.

Diminishing notional capital

In the case of capital, if social services decide to treat you as having capital you have given away, you will be assessed as notionally having that amount, but it will be reduced each week.[21] The amount of the reduction will be the difference between what you actually pay and the amount you would have paid if you had not been treated as having capital which you have given away.

Example:
You have been assessed as having £6,000 actual capital and £20,000 notional capital which you have given away. Your weekly income means you are assessed as having to pay £150 and the home you are in costs £350. The level of your notional capital will be reduced by £200 per week. This means that after 50 weeks you will be reassessed as having only £16,000 and your assessed charge will be reduced to the level of your income plus tariff income from capital above £10,000.

Transferring the liability to the person who has received your assets

In addition to deciding whether to treat you as if you still have the assets, social services has the legal power to take enforcement proceedings against the person (or persons) who now owns the assets if you have knowingly and with the intention of avoiding charges, transferred it, either for nothing or at less than its value.[22] Even if the person to whom you transferred those assets had no idea that you did this to avoid paying charges, s/he will still have the liability for your fees transferred to them. The question is whether **you** knowingly transferred your assets to avoid charges.

This rule can only be used if you transferred your assets within the six months immediately before you went into residential accommodation. Guidance makes it clear that in this context 'residential accommodation' is where social services have assessed you as needing residential care *and* have arranged it for you in an independent or local authority home. Even if you are already in an independent home when you transfer your assets, if you have not been assessed and not had your placement arranged by social services within six months of the transfer, this rule does not apply. The guidance gives an example of a resident who paid for his own accommodation in full for two years, then the following March gave his daughter £20,000 and continued to self-fund until December, when he approached the local authority for support.[23] In this case the six month rule does not apply, but social services could treat the resident as still possessing the capital (see p326). Time limits only apply to the transfer of liability to pay onto the person who has received the asset. There appear to be no time limits for social services to treat you as still possessing your assets. This was recently confirmed in a Scottish court case.[24]

Calculating the cost for which the owner is liable

Once social services decide that you have transferred your assets to another person within the six months prior to going into care, knowingly to avoid or lessen the charges then the owner *shall* be liable to pay the difference between what you actually pay social services and what you have been assessed as having to pay.[25]

The amount for which the person who has received the asset is liable should be restricted to the benefit accruing from the transfer. If the asset has been transferred to more than one person, each person can only be held liable up to the value of her/his share of the asset.[26]

The asset is valued at the amount that would have been realised on the open market at the time it was transferred, and secured debts and reasonable costs of sale will be taken into account.[27]

5. **Court action that can be used**

It is outside of the scope of this book to give advice about dealing with any debts you have to social services caused by charges for care (see CPAG's *Debt Advice Handbook*). As with any debt it is important to negotiate at an early stage and check carefully that you are actually liable for the debt (this is particularly so if someone else is managing your affairs and they receive the bills) and that you agree with the calculation of the amount owing. As your debt may have built up over several years, and you will probably have been paying some of the cost out of your income, which will have altered over time, mistakes can be made. You should also establish whether the debt can still be collected as there are time limits. These are normally six years, but in the case of money owed for your residential charges, proceedings for its recovery under the National Assistance Act 1948 can only be brought within three years of the sum becoming due.[28] Seek advice if your debt accrued more than three years ago.

Although debt advisers (or money advisers) may have had little experience of dealing with debts for residential charges, they should be very experienced in negotiating and checking whether the debt can be enforced. Your local Citizens Advice Bureau may have a debt adviser, or sometimes local authorities offer money advice, although they may be limited in the amount of advice they can offer if you are in dispute with their employing authority.

This section lists possible action through the courts that social services have at their disposal. Although court action has to date rarely been used and there may be concern about taking frail residents to court, the provisions are there. Where there are debts, local authorities have to justify inaction to their auditors. Often the threat of legal action resolves the problem for local authorities because the debt is settled before going to court.

Civil debt

Where the assessed charges have not been paid, local authorities can seek to recover the sum as a civil debt.[29] Proceedings under this legislation may be brought at any time within three years of the sum becoming due.[30] If the debt being recovered is older than three years seek advice.

If the local authority intends to issue proceedings, it will normally be its legal department that writes giving you notice and a final chance of settling the debt.

In England and Wales your case will be dealt with in the magistrates court, although there is not any rule which would stop a local authority from using county court or bankruptcy proceedings. In Scotland it would be normally the sheriffs court and may be the Court of Session.

In practice, very few cases have gone to court for enforcement of charges owed to the local authority. If the local authority does pursue, most people settle before this stage, which is why it is important to get advice at an early stage from someone experienced in debt advice.

It is more likely that social services would be prepared to pursue the person who now owns your assets if you gave them away or sold them for less than their value within six months of needing social services help with residential or nursing home care. If that person who is now liable to pay part of your fees (see p326) does not do so, the local authority could pursue the debt through the courts.

If you have given false information to avoid or lessen the charge

It is an offence to give information which you know to be false. In England and Wales if you do so, you could be liable to a fine not exceeding £100 or up to three months in prison or both.[31] Proceedings may be started at any time within three months from the date on which, in the opinion of the local authority, sufficient evidence comes to light to justify a prosecution, or within 12 months of the offence, whichever is longer.

Although this provision has existed since 1948 there is no evidence that it has ever been used. It is more likely that social services would use their other enforcement procedures to recover the money owed.

Recovery from a liable relative

If your spouse fails to make maintenance payments, s/he can be forced to do so through the family court[32] (see p311). Guidance points out that, ultimately, only the courts can decide what is an appropriate amount of maintenance to pay.[33]

Using Insolvency Procedures (England and Wales)

The Insolvency Act 1986

If you do not have the money to pay your debts there are particular problems for social services in ensuring that any debt is paid. There are two provisions in the Insolvency Act which social services could consider if you owe more than £750, have transferred your assets and are unable to pay your charge.

- If you have given away your assets at an undervalue and can be declared bankrupt, the local authority can apply to the court for an order to set the 'gift' aside. The time limits are five years before the presentation of the petition, if you were bankrupt at the time of the transaction, or became insolvent because of the transaction, and two years in all other cases.[34] The court may make such an order that it thinks fit for restoring the position to what it would have been before the transaction.
- If it can be proved that the purpose of giving away your assets at an undervalue was to place the assets beyond the reach of a possible creditor, the local authority would have to show that the dominant purpose of the 'gift' was to remove assets from a potential creditor.[35] There are no time limits on these powers and you do not need to be declared bankrupt.

It may be difficult for the local authority to prove, although if you have used a business which specialises in avoiding assets being taken into account, this could be considered to be useful to the local authority in establishing your motive. Normally solicitors' files are confidential but a case has established that in some cases the court could require disclosure.[36]

Bankruptcy (Scotland) Act 1985

If you do not have the money to pay your debts then there are particular problems for Social Services in ensuring that any debts are paid. There is provision in the Bankruptcy (Scotland) Act 1985 which might be considered if you owe more than £1,500, whereby you can be declared bankrupt and have your assets transferred where you are unable to pay your charge.

It is possible that proceedings could be taken by the Local Authority to set aside a transfer which is known under the legislation as a gratuitous alienation. This is where an asset has been transferred, either for no payment or for payment of less than the value of the asset. The time limit for challenging such a transfer is five years before the date f bankruptcy where the person to whom the asset is transferred is an associate and two years, for any other person.[37]

Notes

1 CRAG para 1.015; SWSG para 1.013
2 s22(3) NAA 1948
3 s23(3A) NAA 1948; CRAG 1.023 and 1.024; SWSG 1.015-1.016
4 CRAG 1.024; SWSG 1.016

2. If you cannot or will not pay your assessed charge
5 This is because of the mandatory nature of s21 of the NAA and LAC (93)10 WOC/35/93. In Scotland it is because of the mandatory nature of s59 of the SW(S)A 1968 and ss7 and 8 of the MH(S)A 1984
6 s56 NAA 1948; s87 SW(S)A 1968
7 Sch 9 para 4 SS(C&P) Regs
8 Sch 9 para 8 SS(C&P) Regs

3. Legal charges on property
9 s22(1) HASSASSAA 1983
10 CO(RA)(S)O 1993; SWSG 15/93
11 s22(8) HASSASSAA 1983
12 s23(3) HASSASSAA 1983
13 s22(7) HASSASSAA 1983
14 CRAG Annex D 3.4
15 s22(8) HASSASSAA 1983
16 CRAG Annex D 3.5
17 CRAG 7.012 and 7.014
18 s24 HASSASSAA 1983
19 CRAG Annex D 3A

4. Deprivation of assets
20 Reg 17(1) and 25 (1) AoR Regs 1992; CRAG 8.071 and 6.O57; SWSG 8.071 and 6.056
21 Reg 26 AoR Regs 1992 and CRAG 6.068; SWSG 6.067
22 s21 HASSASSAA 1983
23 CRAG Annex D 2.1
24 *Yule v South Lanarkshire Council* (CCLR) December 1998
25 s21(1) HASSASSAA and CRAG Annex D 2.6; para 9 SWSG 7/97
26 s21(4) and (5) HASSASSAA and CRAG Annex D 2.4 and 2.5; SWSG 15/98 2.4
27 s21(7) HASSASSAA and CRAG Annex D 2.3; SWSG 15/93 2.3

5. Court action that can be used
28 s56(2) NAA 1948
29 s56 NAA 1948
30 s56(2) NAA 1948
31 s52 NAA 1948
32 s43(6) NAA 1948 (applies in Scotland by virtue of s87(3) SW(S)A 1968)
33 CRAG 11.006
34 s339 and 341 IA 1986
35 s423 IA 1986
36 *Barclays Bank v Eustice* 1995
37 s34 Bankruptcy (Scotland) Act 1985

Chapter 20

Administration

This chapter explains all the administrative aspects of how your charge is assessed, and what to do if you have any problems. It covers:
1. The financial assessment (p331)
2. Reviews of your assessment (p333)
3. Dealing with your money in a residential or nursing home (p334)
4. If you cannot manage your financial affairs (p334)
5. If you have a complaint about your charge (p340)

1. The financial assessment

There are no set rules about the way the financial assessment is carried out. Guidance makes it clear that the financial assessment should be carried out after your needs assessment and any decisions about service provision.[1] However, in the case of residential and nursing care, legislation allows social services to calculate your resources to establish whether you need to be provided with residential accommodation by them.[2] If, for instance you have capital of above £16,000, then in some circumstances social services will decide they do not need to make the arrangements for you (see p263).

You should not be asked questions about your finances until you have had a needs assessment and it has been agreed that residential or nursing home care is appropriate. Only at that point should there be any calculation of your finances to see whether you can afford to make your own arrangements. This should be a proper calculation, following the rules in the Assessment of Resources Regulations, not a 'best guess' based on questions such as 'Have you got more than £16,000?' or 'Do you own your house?' If you are asked about your capital early on in your needs assessment or told you will have to make your own arrangements, before a proper calculation of your income or capital is done, you should complain (see p57).

Collecting financial information

The way local authorities collect financial information varies. In some you will be visited by the financial assessment officer, who will go through the assessment with you. In other authorities your care assessor/worker/manager will help you fill in the form. In others you will merely be sent a form to fill in yourself.

However, once the form is completed, it will normally go to the section in the local authority which will use the information to calculate how much you will have to pay. This is normally the finance section in the social services department but sometimes it will go to another department.

Unlike for social security benefits, there is no standard form used throughout the country for the financial assessment. Each local authority has devised its own form. In some cases the same form will cover both domiciliary and residential charges. As these charges are based on different legislation, the form should make it clear which parts you need to fill in if you are going into a residential or nursing home. Guidance states that the forms should not require information about your partner's income and capital as it is only your resources which can be used in the assessment of your charge.[3] If you consider that the form asks questions that are irrelevant to the proper assessment of your charge, you should complain.

Verifying the details you have given

Social services have been told it is good practice to verify information – eg, to look at bank statements or building society account books. They have also been told to make use of information available to them from other departments within the authority (eg, housing benefit and council tax records) to verify details. They have been advised to check, with your permission, with other agencies such as the Benefits Agency, banks and pension firms. It is for authorities themselves to determine the extent to which and circumstances in which they will verify information.[4]

Claiming DSS benefits

Because some benefits are used to pay social services charges, it is in social services departments' interest to ensure that you claim all the benefits to which you are entitled. Social services have been advised to maintain good links with their local benefit office.[5] Many social services departments have developed service level agreements with the Benefits Agency to make it as smooth as possible for you to claim benefits and for details to be transferred from one department to another.

How much help you get from social services in claiming benefits varies around the country. In some areas the person filling in the financial assessment form will also help you complete the income support (IS) claim form at the same time and will undertake to send it to the Benefits Agency. In other areas you will merely be advised to make a claim and told how to get the claim form.

Although social services have no legal obligation to provide direct advice on welfare benefits, where such advice or information is offered staff should have sufficient knowledge and the ability to make correct referrals to sources of advice. There have been a number of Ombudsmen complaints regarding advice or delays caused by social services. One recent case was in relation to an authority failing to inform a family that attendance allowance (AA) would have been payable if they had chosen not to have social services make the arrangements.[6]

Information about how much you have to pay

Social services should give you clear information about how much you should be expected to pay, and how this has been calculated. They should explain the normal weekly assessed charge and of any reasons why the charge may fluctuate.[7] Fluctuation in charges is most likely to occur during the first few weeks of residential care when your AA or disabled living allowance (DLA) will be withdrawn. It can also occur because social services has to reassess your charge because of different benefit pay days.

Social services should also explain how you should pay. If you have agreed to pay your part of the charge directly to the home, you will need to arrange with the home how frequently you will pay (see p281). If you are going to be billed by social services, you should be given some choice about the method you will pay. Most will prefer direct debit, but if you want to choose to pay by some other method you should explore that possibility with them. If you think that social services has limited the range of payment methods too much, you should complain (see p57).

2. Reviews of your assessment

It has been left to each local authority to make its own arrangements about how frequently and when your charge will be reviewed and the policy to adopt if undercharging or overcharging comes to light.[8]

Nearly all social services departments review their charges annually at the time when your benefits are up-rated. This is also the time when the home you are in is most likely to alter its fees.

However, your income or capital could change at anytime – eg, you could be left money, or your occupational or private pension could go up. You should inform social services when you have a change of circumstances, in the same way as you should inform the Benefits Agency.

If you have capital above £10,000 you should inform social services every time it goes down a £250 band. Unless you do this, you are likely to continue to be charged at a higher rate until the annual review of charges. Some local authorities have computer systems to track the tariff income, and will alter it automatically. Others do not and so it is safer to regularly inform them of changes. If they refuse to reassess you when you tell them about a change of circumstances, you should complain as you may be charged too much.

3. **Dealing with your money in a residential or nursing home**

Unless you are unable to manage, you should remain in control of your financial affairs and pay the charges yourself or you may have decided to appoint an attorney to do so for you. In this way you keep in control of being sure the correct charge is paid and that you keep your personal expenses allowance.

Some homes take residents' pension books and collect their benefits on their behalf as an agent. Although this might make it easier for you because you do not need to go to the post office, you might wish to consider other ways of having your benefits paid, so that you keep full control over all your money.

This practice is particularly common in local authority homes, where arrangements can be made for an officer of the local authority to become the 'signing agent'. This means that this officer can collect your benefit by signing for it her/himself, rather than you countersigning each week to allow the agent to collect your benefit. Internal guidance for Benefits Agency staff says that this person is also responsible for informing social services of any change of circumstances. This arrangement should only be made if you agree to it.[9] All your pension should be handed back to you, but in practice what often happens is that the benefit is kept to pay your charge, and you are given your personal expenses allowance.

4. **If you cannot manage your financial affairs**

If you are unable to give social services the information they need to assess your charge because you lack the mental capacity, then they have been told to find out if anyone has power of attorney, receivership (or a curator bonis in Scotland) or appointeeship. If no one has taken on any of these roles, social services cannot properly financially assess you until someone has been duly authorised to act for you. In practice many authorities will make the arrangements for your care and give an estimate of the likely costs to you. They are unlikely not to make the arrangements just because you have no one to give them financial details.

If there is no one suitable to act for you, social services may become your appointee or receiver, depending on your financial circumstances.

There are some very significant legal differences in Scotland regarding the management of another person's affairs, with a wide variety of different legal appointments possible. Some of these measures are made under the Mental Health (Scotland) 1984. The court system is also very different from England and Wales and legal advice should be sought about these matters. The whole field of management and personal decision-making is subject to major change at the moment, due to the Adults with Incapacity Bill being introduced into the Scottish Parliament. See also Appendix 000 for further reading.

In England and Wales changes are also proposed in the White Paper 'Making Decision'. This section only outlines the different methods of dealing with your finances if you can no longer manage.

Appointeeship

The Secretary of State can authorise someone to act on your behalf if you cannot claim for yourself or if you can no longer manage to deal with your financial affairs.[10] Your appointee would take on all your rights and responsibilities as a claimant – eg, notifying the Benefits Agency of any change of circumstances. Your appointee is responsible for making sure the benefits received are spent on your behalf. If you are in a residential or nursing home, this would include ensuring that the benefits are used to pay your assessed charge.

Note: Appointeeship only gives authority to deal with your benefits and any small amount of capital which has accumulated from those benefits. It does not give any authority to deal with your other income or capital. In England and Wales, if you have other income or capital, there would need to be an application to the Court of Protection through the Public Trust Office (see p336). The Public Trust Office has suggested that if you have savings from benefits of no more than one month's accommodation costs and about £500 as a cash float, no other authority would normally be needed. In Scotland a curator bonis should be appointed to deal with all financial affairs if there is no power of attorney (see p339). In practice, many relatives assist people on an informal basis.

The person who agrees to become the appointee has to be over 18 and needs to apply in writing. Benefits Agency staff should visit both you and your prospective appointee. They should be satisfied that:

- you are unable to manage your own financial affairs and if necessary obtain medical evidence;

- there is not already a receiver appointed by the Court of Protection or a valid enduring power of attorney or in Scotland a curator bonis appointed (see p336); *and*
- the person who has applied to become the appointee is a fit person to act for you. This could be the owner of the home, but only as a last resort if there is no one else who will act for you.[11]

If there is an advocacy scheme in your area, an advocate may agree to become your appointee. In some cases an officer of social services can be appointed. Which officer becomes the appointee varies from authority to authority, although often the person will be based in the social services finance department. Some authorities have special officers who deal with appointeeship and receivership.

Cancelling the appointeeship

The appointeeship can be revoked at any time if the person who is your appointee fails to use the benefits for your interests. If your appointee fails to pay your assessed charge to social services they will normally contact the appointee promptly. If matters cannot be resolved, they will ask the Benefits Agency to revoke the appointment. If no one else can be found to take over the responsibility, then it is likely in these circumstances that a member of social services staff will become the appointee or they will arrange for an advocate to take over this role.

Enduring power of attorney (England and Wales)

If you have already appointed an attorney under the Enduring Power of Attorney Act 1985 then the power for them to act for you will continue if you lose the mental capacity to manage your financial affairs. However, the enduring power of attorney will only remain valid if the person or persons you have named register it with the Public Trust Office once they have reason to believe that you have become or are becoming incapable of managing your affairs.

Because the power extends beyond the time you are capable of managing your affairs it is very important that you choose someone that you completely trust. The person must be over 18, and in most cases will be a relative or friend. If your financial affairs are complex you may wish to appoint a professional – eg, a solicitor or accountant. The appointment of a single attorney may offer less security for your assets than a joint or joint and several attorneyship.

Normally you will have made an enduring power of attorney long before you have gone into residential or nursing home, although it can be done at any time as long as at the time of signing the appropriate forms you are capable of understanding what the enduring power of attorney is and what it is intended to do.

The attorney(s) can take over your affairs at once while you are still capable of managing your affairs, or you can specify that you only want the attorney(s) to take over when you are no longer mentally capable to act for yourself.

An attorney can only do the things you have authorised them to do. If you have given your attorney(s) a general power they have complete authority to act on your behalf in relation to financial matters. You can give limited powers, by defining precisely what the attorney can and cannot do, although you will need to consider other arrangements for dealing with those affairs outside of the limited power of attorney.

If you are no longer capable of managing your financial affairs, and have been assessed for your charges by social services, then they will deal with your attorney(s). They should seek proof that the power has been registered in order to establish that they are dealing with a duly authorised person. If it is not yet registered then your attorney should be advised by social services about the need to register it.

Registering the enduring power of attorney

The enduring power of attorney is registered by applying to the Public Trust Office which is the administrative arm of the Court of Protection. No medical evidence is required. As soon as the application is made, the powers of the attorney are suspended until registration has taken place. This can take a while as there are rules about who has to be notified (you and at least three of your nearest relatives in priority). Once all these people have been notified the application should be sent to the Public Trust Office with the fee for registration. The papers are held for 35 days after the last notification. If there are no objections it will be registered.

During this time it may be difficult to pay the homes fees or the social services charges because the attorneyship is suspended. However, the rules allow for your money to be used to provide for your immediate needs. The Public Trust Office will be able to advise your attorney on this.

After registration

Your attorney will be responsible for your income and capital, and for paying your charges. Responsibilities may include selling your former home if you are required to pay the full cost of the home. If there is any question about your charge it will be for your attorney to take this up with social services (see p340).

Revoking an enduring power of attorney

Neither the Public Trust Office nor the Court of Protection normally supervise the actions of an attorney once registration has taken place. You can revoke an enduring power of attorney at any time while you are still mentally capable, but once it is registered it cannot be revoked by you.

If your attorney fails to pay your charges to social services or there are other concerns that the attorney may be abusing her/his power, then social services may ask the Court of Protection to investigate the suitability of the attorney. If necessary the Court will supervise the exercise of the powers and as a last resort could impose a receivership.

Power of attorney (Scotland)

There is no detailed provision in Scotland equivalent to the Enduring Power of Attorney in England and Wales. In Scotland a power of attorney granted on or after 1 January 1991 remains in force not withstanding the granter's subsequent loss of capacity, unless the power of attorney specifies otherwise. There is no formal change required to the power of attorney in connection with the loss of capacity. This is as a result of section 71(1) of the Law Reform (Miscellaneous Provisions) (Scotland) Act 1990. A power of attorney granted prior to 1 January 1991 will lapse if the granter loses capacity.

Receivership, short orders and directions (England and Wales)

If you have lost the capacity to deal with your financial affairs and appointeeship is not appropriate because you have income and capital that is not related to benefits, and you have not made an enduring power of attorney, then the Court of Protection will need to be involved in authorising the management of your financial affairs. The Public Trust Office deals with the administration of the court's decisions.

The Mental Health Act 1983 confers powers to the Court of Protection to make orders and give directions for people who are incapable, by reason of mental disorder of managing their own affairs. If this is the case you will become a 'patient' of the court.

There are three types of order:
- receivership;
- a short order, if your affairs are simple and can be covered by a few directions authorising the way your money or property should be used for your benefit. This may include paying fees to the home or local authority charges;
- a direction of the Public Trustee which can be used if an application for receivership has not already been made and the total value of your assets is less than £5,000 and your gross income from a private pension or annuity is less that £1,200.

Normally the receiver will be a relative, friend, or solicitor. Social services can cause an application to be made when this is needed and there is no one else to make that application. Occasionally the court will appoint the Public

Trustee as receiver. You must be notified of the application (although in rare cases it might be waived if it would cause harm or distress).

The court only has jurisdiction if medical evidence has established that you are suffering from a mental disorder, and it must be satisfied that you are also incapable of managing your financial affairs.

The responsibilities of the receiver

Your receiver should do everything in relation to your property and financial affairs that the court has ordered or authorised. For some actions, the receiver must obtain specific authority from the Public Trust Office. These include:

- using your savings or capital;
- buying or selling property;
- varying your investments;
- taking or defending legal proceedings.

Patients are encouraged to deal with as much of their financial affairs as they can. So although your receiver may be paying your fees on your behalf, you may be able to manage your personal expenses allowance or your pension book.

Your receiver will have to submit accounts of all receipts and payments made on your behalf, when requested to by the Public Trust Office, usually annually.

Social services will arrange for your receiver to pay any charges due and if your receiver fails to pay may ask the court to intervene and if necessary to change the receiver or take on the receivership themselves.

Social services as receiver

Most social services departments are reluctant to take on the role of receiver, but will do so if necessary. Who has the role varies from local authority to local authority. In some areas it will be the director, or a person with specific responsibilities for receivership or appointeeship, or a person in the finance section. Many recognise the conflict of interest when they are the receiver or appointee and yet also collect charges. Until recently the Public Trust Office did not visit patients where the local authority is the receiver. Some visits are now carried out. Some local authorities use advocacy services when they are the receiver to oversee your interests, or the receiver is a person who is separate from the finance section. in order to keep the conflict of interest to a minimum.

Curator bonis in Scotland

In Scotland a person known as a curator bonis (or simply curator) can be appointed to manage a person's financial affairs. An application may be made to the sheriff court or to the Court of Session. Curatories are supervised by the Accountant of Court, who must approve major decisions affecting the person's property. Many curatories are accountants or solicitors, and it can be an expensive form of management. In some cases informal arrangements may be better. In some circumstances the Mental Health (Scotland) Act 1984 allows a local authority or the Mental Welfare Commission to petition the court to appoint a curator.

5. **If you have a complaint about your charge**

If you have a concern about your charge, you have a right to complain about it using the complaints procedure[12] (see p57). As the rules for charging are national, a complaint will normally be to resolve an error in the calculation or in the interpretation of the rules. These are often dealt with in the initial stage by discussing it with the finance officer dealing with your case.

It is important to check the calculation very carefully to make sure that your income and capital used in the calculation are correct. You also need to check that any bills presented on the sale of your former home accurately reflect whether you were a temporary or permanent resident at the start of your stay. You should be clear exactly what period is covered and that increases in fees are correctly recorded, along with what you may have already paid from your income.

Where social services have some discretion includes:
- the way jointly owned property is valued (see p294);
- the use of discretion to disregard your former home (see p296);
- whether you have deprived yourself of capital (see p300);
- whether your personal expenses allowance will be varied (see p304);
- whether a liable relative payment is expected (see p311);
- whether you have to have a third party to top up (see p307);
- whether you count as a temporary or permanent resident (see p391);
- how frequently reviews are carried out (see p333).

it is more likely that you will need to take your complaint through to the formal stage and may be to a complaints panel.

Some social services have a separate procedure of appeals for charges. This should not debar you, however, from using the complaints procedure, and you should not have to go through that appeal procedure before you are allowed to make a formal complaint.

If you have concerns about your charges you can also use the other remedies outlined in Chapter 2. Often it is difficult to decide which route is the best for you to follow so it is important to seek advice.

Notes

1. **The financial assessment**
   1 Community Care in the Next Decade and Beyond – Policy Guidance 1990; para 3.31 Assessment and Care Management SW11/91
   2 CC(RA)A 1998; CRAG para 1.007A
   3 CRAG; SWSG 11.005
   4 Annex H LAC (98)8 WOC 12/98 para 10; SWSG 6/98 para 9
   5 CRAG 1.026; SWSG 1.024
   6 LGOR 98/C/1842
   7 CRAG 1.015; SWSG 1.013

2. **Reviews of your assessment**
   8 CRAG Annex H LAC (94)1 WOC 4/94, SWSG 5/94 para 16

3. **Dealing with your money in a residential or nursing home**
   9 Agents Appointees and Receivers Handbook (not published)

4. **If you cannot manage your financial affairs**
   10 Reg 33 SS(C&P) Regs
   11 Agents, Appointees and Receivers Handbook (not published)

5. **If you have a complaint about your charge**
   12 CRAG 1.027; SWSG 1.025

Part 5

. . . .

Benefits and charges in care homes

This part explains the system of social security benefits in care homes post-April 1993 (see Chapter 21); the preserved rights to benefits if you were in a care home from before April 1993 (see Chapter 22); and the charges in care homes in the post-April 1993 system which will usually involve the local authority (see Chapter 23).

Examples in these chapters demonstrate how the rules explained in these chapters and in the general provisions chapters of Part III and Part IV of this *Handbook* are used in practice to establish your benefit entitlement and your contribution to the accommodation and care costs of your placement in a care home.

This part also attempts to unravel the complexities of the way the two systems (social security benefits and local authority charging) which interact, not always very smoothly, when you are paying for care in a care home. There are problems that commonly occur in both systems and in the interaction of the two systems. These are highlighted in Chapter 21.

Chapter 21

Social security benefits in care homes

This chapter explains the rules from April 1993 for social security benefits for single people and couples in care homes. The pre-April 1993 system is dealt with in Chapter 22. It covers:

1. Social security benefits affected (p345)
2. Types of care homes (p346)
3. Types of stay (p349)
4. How benefits are effected by the type of care home and stay (p350)
5. Example calculations of income support (p359)
6. Self-funding (including loophole cases) (p368)
7. Temporary absences from care homes (including going into hospital) (p371)
8. Other sources of financial assistance in care homes (p372)
9. Effects on carers (p374)

Sections 1 to 3 identify the benefits, types of care home and types of stay, and provide basic information and definitions where appropriate. Section 4 gives details of how the three categories in sections 1 to 3 inter-relate. Section 5 gives examples of how the system works in practice for the main benefit involved – income support (IS). Sections 6 to 9 deal with issues relating to social security benefits in care homes.

Note: All references to IS also apply to income-based jobseeker's allowance (JSA).

---

1. Social security benefits affected

If you go into a care home (see p346) either temporarily or permanently (see p349 for definitions) the following benefits will be affected:

- IS/income-based JSA;
- housing benefit (HB);
- council tax benefit (CTB);

- disability living allowance (DLA) care component;
- attendance allowance (AA) (including constant attendance allowance and exceptionally severe disablement allowance payable with industrial injury disablement benefit or war disablement benefit).

All other social security benefits (eg, DLA mobility component, state retirement pension, widow's pension or incapacity benefit) can be claimed and paid in the normal way when you are in a care home subject to the standard rules (see Chapter 3). 'Care homes' for the purposes of this chapter, means local authority residential accommodation, independent residential care homes and independent nursing homes.

2. Types of care homes

Social services departments have a duty to make arrangements for providing residential care for all those who 'by reason of age, illness, disability, or any other circumstances are in need of care and attention which is not otherwise available to them' (or in Scotland, for 'persons in need').[1] Residential care can be provided in any of the following categories of care homes. See p268 for definitions.

1. local authority residential accommodation (sometimes known as Part III homes or Part IV homes in Scotland);
2. registered independent residential care homes (including registered 'small homes');
3. registered independent nursing homes;
4. dual registered independent residential care and nursing homes;
5. independent or local authority homes not providing board.

For social security benefit purposes the homes in categories 2 to 4 above are treated in the same way.

Abbeyfield Homes

You may receive care in an Abbeyfield Home. In the pre-April 1993 system there were special rules for social security benefits in Abbeyfield Homes which still apply for people who moved in prior to April 1993 (see p379). In the post-April 1993 system there are no special rules. If your Abbeyfield Home is *not* registered, then the ordinary social security benefit rules will apply (see Chapter 3). If your Abbeyfield Home is registered, then the rules that apply for social security benefit purposes are the same as for independent residential care or nursing homes (see p352).

Hospitals or similar institutions

You may receive care as an in-patient in a 'hospital or similar institution'. A 'similar institution' includes a placement in a private nursing home which is funded by the health authority (see p265) rather than by social services. 'Hospital or similar institution' is not defined in social security legislation but it is clear that you will be treated as being in a 'hospital or similar institution' if you are receiving in-patient medical treatment or professional nursing care under specified NHS legislation.[2] In these circumstances, there are different rules to those which apply to people in care homes for the purposes of social security benefits

If you are in a hospital or similar institution your accommodation and care is provided free of charge by the NHS but you are only entitled to the lower hospital rates of social security benefits (see p125). If the responsibility for the funding of your accommodation and care falls to social services (or for placements prior to April 1993, the Department of Social Security (DSS)) you are entitled to higher rates of social security benefits but you are subject to a charge for your accommodation and care based on a financial assessment that will usually leave you with a personal expenses allowance of £14.75 (see Chapter 15 and p393 for information about financial assessments).

It may not always be clear which authority should be responsible for the funding of your accommodation and care and therefore whether or not you should be treated as an in-patient in a 'similar institution' to a hospital. Two cases concerning placements made prior to April 1993 demonstrate this.[3] In both cases the health authority had sought to transfer financial responsibility for placements in private nursing homes to the DSS. However, in the first case the Court of Appeal held that, although the nursing home was not maintained under the NHS Act 1977, the claimant was receiving treatment there pursuant to arrangements made by the health authority on behalf of the Secretary of State under the 1977 Act, which was enough to bring the nursing home within the hospital in-patients legislation.[4] In the second case,[5] the Court of Appeal held that the claimant was receiving care that was to be regarded as 'medical or other treatment', and that the home was a 'similar institution' to a hospital, and therefore she was a 'patient for the purposes of IS.[6]

Hospices

You may receive care in a 'hospice' which is defined as 'a hospital or other institution whose primary function is to provide palliative care for persons resident there who are suffering from a progressive disease in its final stages' (but not an NHS hospital).[7] This is usually arranged via your GP through your health authority. For social security benefit purposes a hospice is a 'hospital or similar institution', and therefore the same rules as for being in a hospital apply (see p125). The only difference is that DLA mobility component will continue in payment beyond 28 days,[8] and the DLA care component or AA will also continue in payment beyond 28 days,[9] except where you are normally living in a care home owned or managed, or owned and managed, by a local authority.[10]

Joint funded placements

You may receive care in a care home which is purchased out of a health authority and social services budget (see p267). In these circumstances, the benefit situation is far from clear. There can be confusion over whether you should be considered as having your accommodation provided by the health authority under the 'similar institution' part of the definition of a 'hospital or similar institution' (see p347), in which case you should receive your care free of charge and the hospital rate of benefits will apply (see p125); or whether you should be considered as having your accommodation provided by social services, in which case the rules for social security benefits in independent residential care and nursing homes will apply (see p352). It is important to find out what the terms of the contract with the home are in respect of your placement. Often the health authority funding for your placement is received by social services rather than by the care home and therefore it is social services who have assessed your need, arranged and contracted with a home for provision of your accommodation and care[11] and they are required[12] to charge you subject to the means tests.[13]

If your benefits have been reduced to hospital in-patient rates, but you are still responsible for paying toward the cost of your accommodation and care, seek advice.

Moving from a local authority care home to an independent residential care or nursing home

If you moved into local authority (Part III) residential accommodation after 31 March 1993 (see below) your applicable amount for IS purposes is set at the basic retirement pension rate (residential accommodation or Part III rate) only (see p351). However, if you subsequently move to an independent residential care or nursing home, the appropriate IS applicable amount including the residential allowance will apply (see p352).

If on 31 March 1993 you were in (or temporarily absent from) local authority residential accommodation and subsequently social services arrange a move to an independent residential care or nursing home, then your IS applicable amount will remain at the Part III rate.[14]

A recent social security commissioner's decision[15] called into question the applicable amount remaining at the residential accommodation (Part III) rate when a person living in (or temporarily absent from) local authority accommodation moves to an independent care home. In brief, the

Commissioner held that the amendment of the definition of 'residential accommodation' in 1995[16] where regulation 21(3C) is applied meant that arrangements made under section 26 of the NAA 1948 could no longer be included.[17] Prior to the amendment the definition of 'residential accommodation' included 'accommodation provided by a local authority in a home owned or managed by that or another local authority[18] *or provided in accordance with arrangements made by a local authority*[19] – (a) under section 21 to 24 **and 26** of the National Assistance Act 1948'.[20] Following the amendment, however, the definition in (a) no longer refers to '**and 26'** as it has been deleted. This means that you should be able to get the appropriate applicable amount including the residential allowance if you move into an independent care home (see p352).

However, if you are in local authority residential accommodation and that accommodation becomes a residential care home (ie, social services transfers the care home to the independent sector) then as an existing resident you will continue to be treated as if you were still in local authority residential accommodation and the Part III rate of IS will continue to apply.[21]

3. **Types of stay**

There are four types of stay in care homes:
- permanent;
- temporary;
- respite;
- trial period.

A **permanent stay** is one which is permanent from the day you enter the care home, or if you enter on a temporary or trial period basis, from any subsequent day on which you make the decision that you do not intend to return to the community to live.

A **temporary stay** is defined in terms of a temporary absence from your normal home in the community. The conditions are that:
- you intend to return to your home in the community; *and*
- the part of your home normally occupied by you has not been let or sub-let in the meantime; *and*
- the period of your absence is unlikely to exceed 52 weeks, or, in exceptional circumstances, is unlikely to substantially exceed that period.[22]

A **respite stay** is not defined in social security benefits legislation. It is a planned programme of temporary stays and therefore the definition of 'temporary' stay above applies.

A **trial period stay** is a stay in residential accommodation 'for the purpose of ascertaining whether the accommodation suits [your] needs' and 'with the intention of returning to the dwelling which [you] normally occupy as [your] home should, in the event, the residential accommodation prove not to suit [your] needs'.

In these circumstances IS housing costs, HB and CTB can continue to be paid for up to 13 weeks in respect of your home in the community, where:

- you intend to return to your home (if the residential accommodation does not suit your needs); *and*
- the part of your home normally occupied by you has not been let or sub-let in the meantime; *and*
- the period of absence is unlikely to exceed 13 weeks.[23]

You will also be entitled to those benefits even if your absence extends beyond 13 weeks as long as your total absence does not exceed 52 weeks.[24] If the type of your stay changes (ie, in social security terms the reason for your absence changes once the absence has begun) it is the latest reason for absence which determines whether the temporary or trial period rules apply. Whether benefit is still payable for any period remaining will depend on whether you still satisfy the general qualifying rules for that period and on how long the absence has already lasted, as the period of absence is always measured from the date that you ceased to occupy your home in the community and not the date that the reason for your absence changed.

Unlike for many other aspects of the social security benefits system, there are no linking rules for periods of absence. Therefore, if you are in residential accommodation for a trial period or temporary stay and you genuinely return home for at least 24 hours, you can subsequently receive benefit for a fresh period of absence of either 13 (trial period) or 52 (temporary) weeks.

There is no definition of 'trial period' for financial assessment or charging purposes. Therefore there can be problems in the inter-relationship of the financial assessment system with the social security benefits system. (For more information see p431.)

In addition to your social security benefits being affected by the type of care home you are in and the type of stay you are having, the means-tested benefits are also effected by your status – ie, whether you are a single person, a person with responsibility for children, or one of a couple (see p350).

4. **How benefits are affected by the type of care home and stay**

This section covers:

- IS/JSA:
  - local authority residential accommodation (board provided);

Chapter 21: Social security benefits in care homes
4. How benefits are affected by the type of care home and stay

21

- – independent residential care and/or nursing homes (registered);
- – independent or local authority homes not providing board;
- HB:
  - – local authority residential accommodation (board provided);
  - – independent residential care and/or nursing homes (registered);
  - – independent or local authority homes not providing board;
- CTB:
- DLA care component/AA:
  - – local authority residential accommodation (board provided);
  - – independent residential care and/or nursing homes (registered);
  - – independent or local authority homes not providing board.

Income support/income-based jobseeker's allowance

Local authority residential accommodation (board provided)

This is accommodation owned and/or managed by the local authority (usually by the social services department). It is sometimes known as Part III accommodation. When there is reference to 'residential accommodation' in the legislation it refers to local authority care homes and not independent sector care homes.

The applicable amount, if you are in local authority residential accommodation where board is provided, is at the residential accommodation rate, previously known as the Part III rate, which is a single amount equivalent to the basic retirement pension.

'Board' is defined as at least some cooked or prepared meals, cooked or prepared by someone other than the resident and eaten in the accommodation and the cost of which is included in the standard rate fixed for the accommodation.[25]

Temporary stays (including respite and trial period)
- **Single person** – your weekly IS applicable amount is £66.75 of which £14.75 is for your personal expenses allowance (PEA) plus housing costs for your normal home in the community if appropriate (see p99).[26]
- **Single parent** – your IS applicable amount is £66.75 of which £14.75 is for your PEA, plus the personal allowance for each child for whom you were receiving benefit before going into care, plus the family premium (see p97) and housing costs for your normal home in the community if appropriate.[27]
- **Couple where both are in residential care** – your IS applicable amount is £133.50 (2 x £66.75) of which £29.50 (2 x £14.75) is for the PEA, plus housing costs for your own home if appropriate.[28]
- **Couple where one member is in residential care** – your IS applicable amount is £66.75 for the person in residential care of which £14.75 is for your PEA, plus a single person's normal applicable amount for the person in the community.[29]

21

Chapter 21: Social security benefits in care homes
4. How benefits are affected by the type of care home and stay

Permanent stays
- **Single person** – as for a temporary stay (see p351), except that housing costs are no longer included in your applicable amount.[30]
- **Single parent** – you are treated as a single person when you become permanent (see p351) unless the child(ren) are living with you in the care home. Housing costs are no longer included in your applicable amount.[31]
- **Couple** – you will no longer be treated as a couple if one of you is in a care home and the other is living in the community or in another care home or, recent case law suggests, even if you are both in the same care home sharing the same room you should not be treated as a couple (see p428).[32] This means that you should each be treated as a single person (see p351). Your IS entitlement will be based on your own resources and will be paid to each of you separately. Housing costs will no longer be included in the applicable amount of the person(s) in care.[33]

You may stop being entitled to IS while you are in local authority residential accommodation. This is because the applicable amount is much lower than either at home in the community or in independent sector care homes. If this occurs while you are a temporary resident you should make a claim for any HB/CTB that you may still be entitled to while you are in the care home. You should also make a fresh claim for IS when you return to your own home. The exception to IS stopping is if you are one of a couple and your partner is remaining in the community. In these circumstances, if you were not entitled to IS in your home in the community you may become entitled for the period of your stay in care. The person who assesses you from social services should be able to advise you.

Independent registered residential care and/or nursing homes
If you are a resident in an independent residential or nursing care home your applicable amount for IS purposes is calculated by adding together:
- your personal allowance;
- any premiums to which you are entitled (including the severe disability premium – see p354);
- any housing costs where appropriate for your home in the community (temporary residents only)[34] (see p99);
- plus a **residential allowance** where you satisfy the following criteria:[35]
  - you require personal care by reason of old age, disablement, past or present dependence on alcohol or drugs, past or present mental disorder or a terminal illness *and* the care is provided in the home;
  - you do not have a preserved right (see Chapter 22);
  - you are aged 16 or over;
  - your accommodation and such meals (if any) are provided for you on a commercial basis;

Chapter 21: Social security benefits in care homes
4. How benefits are affected by the type of care home and stay

21

- no part of the weekly charge for your accommodation is met by housing benefit;
- the care home is registered or deemed to be so.[36]

Temporary stays (including respite and trial period)
- **Single person** – your weekly IS applicable amount is the normal personal allowance plus any appropriate premiums, plus housing costs for your normal home in the community if appropriate, plus the *residential allowance* of £59.40 (£66.10 in Greater London).[37]
- **Single parent** – your IS applicable amount is the normal personal allowances for a single person and for each child for whom you are responsible plus any appropriate premiums, plus housing costs for your normal home in the community if appropriate, plus the *residential allowance* of £59.40 (£66.10 in Greater London).[38]
- **Couple where both are in the same residential care home** (ie, not temporarily separated) – your IS applicable amount is the normal personal allowance for a couple plus any appropriate premiums at the couple rate, plus housing costs for your home in the community where appropriate, plus *two residential allowances* totalling £118.80 (£132.20 in Greater London).[39]
- **Couple where one member is in residential care or where you are both in different residential care homes** (ie, temporarily separated) your IS applicable amount is *either*:
  - the normal personal allowance for a couple, plus any appropriate premiums at the couple rate, plus housing costs for your home in the community where appropriate, plus the *residential allowance(s)* (£59.40 per qualifying person, £66.10 in Greater London); *or*
  - the aggregate of the normal personal allowance for each of you as if you were single people, plus any appropriate premiums for each of you at the single person rate, plus housing costs for your home in the community where appropriate, plus the *residential allowance(s)* (£59.40 per qualifying person, £66.10 in Greater London);

whichever is the greater.[40] Normally, the 'greater' amount will be the applicable amount for each of you as single people.

Note: if your stay in care is temporary, you and your partner will still be assessed as a couple in terms of your resources which will be aggregated and your IS will be paid to the person who claims IS in respect of both of you.

If you enter or are expected to enter a care home for a period of no more than eight weeks, your IS can be paid from the date of admission. If your stay is expected to be more than eight weeks, your IS can only be altered from the start of your benefit week.[41]

21

Chapter 21: Social security benefits in care homes
4. How benefits are affected by the type of care home and stay

Permanent stays
- **Single person** – as for a temporary stay (see p353) except that housing costs are no longer included in your applicable amount.
- **Single parent** – you are treated as a single person when you become permanent (see p353) unless the child(ren) are living with you in the care home. Housing costs are no longer included in your applicable amount.
- **Couple** – you will no longer be treated as a couple if one of you is in a care home and the other is living in the community or in another care home. Recent case law also suggests that even if you are both in the same care home sharing the same room, you should not be treated as a couple (see p428).[42] This means that you should each be treated as a single person (see p353). Your IS entitlement will be based on your own resources and will be paid to each of you separately. Housing costs will no longer be included in the applicable amount of the person(s) in care.

Note: Unlike for local authority care homes[43] there is no amount specified for the PEA for IS in independent care homes. You get your PEA of £14.75 because of the way social services calculate your charge (see p394).

Even if you are not entitled to IS in your own home in the community, you may be entitled to it when you go into residential care due to the residential allowance being included in your applicable amount (or, if you are a permanent resident, due to the increase in the capital limit). The person who assesses you from social services should be able to advise you.

The severe disability premium
Where you are entering an independent care home on a **permanent** basis and you are still in receipt of AA or DLA care component and no one is in receipt of invalid care allowance (ICA) for caring for you, the severe disability premium (SDP) should be included in your applicable amount as a single person or as one of a couple being treated as a single person.

Where you are entering care on a **temporary** basis (including respite and trial period stays), there is often confusion about whether or not the SDP should be included in your applicable amount.

If you are a **single person** in receipt of DLA care component or AA and the SDP is not included in your applicable amount when you are in your home in the community because there is a non-dependant (see p97) living with you, then you will not be entitled to the SDP when you are going temporarily into a care home. If you do receive the SDP in your applicable amount when you are at home in the community then you will continue to receive it in the care home for as long as you are in receipt of DLA care component or AA.

If you are **one of a couple** and your partner is remaining at home or you are both in different care homes, the SDP can be included in the applicable amount for each person in receipt of DLA care component or AA, where you

Chapter 21: Social security benefits in care homes
4. How benefits are affected by the type of care home and stay

21

are joint owners or tenants of your home, even where it was not included in the applicable amounts when you were at home. If ICA is paid to a person who cares for you the SDP will not be included in your applicable amount.

Independent or local authority homes not providing board

If you are **temporarily** or **permanently** in an independent sector home which is not required to be registered, or in local authority accommodation where board is not provided (see p351) then you are a 'less dependent resident' and you will receive the normal rates of IS applicable to a person living in the community.[44] If you are **one of a couple** and only one of you goes into residential care, the same rules apply as for accommodation where board is provided regarding whether you are assessed as a couple or as single for IS purposes. If you are a permanent resident in a local authority home not providing board, then the capital rules that apply to you are the more generous £16,000 limit and £10,000 before tariff income is applied (see p191).

Housing benefit

Local authority residential accommodation (board provided) and independent registered residential care and/or nursing home

You will not be able to get HB (see p102) for the cost of local authority owned and/or managed residential accommodation which provides board, nor for the costs of an independent residential or nursing care home. However, if you go into a care home for a **temporary** (including respite) stay (see p349 for definitions) you can continue to receive HB in respect of your home in the community for up to 52 weeks. If you have entered a care home on a **trial period** basis (see p349 for definition) HB will be paid for up to 13 weeks in respect of your home in the community. You cannot get HB if you are a **permanent** resident in a care home, as it is assumed you no longer have a home in the community.

It is worth noting that, unlike for IS, your applicable amount for HB purposes will not be reduced to the residential accommodation rate of £66.75. Instead it remains at the normal rate that applies to you in the community.

If you lose your entitlement to IS upon entering a local authority residential care home, you will need to complete an HB application form in respect of your home in the community in order to continue receiving HB. Similarly, if you become entitled to IS only while you are in residential care, you will need to re-claim HB upon your return to your home in the community.

If you are **one of a couple** and you are going into care permanently while your partner is remaining at home in the community, you will need to make sure that your partner claims HB if it was previously claimed under your name.

21

Chapter 21: Social security benefits in care homes
4. How benefits are affected by the type of care home and stay

Independent or local authority homes not providing board

If you are a 'less dependent resident' (see p351) you may be able to receive HB to help meet the cost of your rent in the care home. However, you can normally only receive HB in respect of the dwelling that you occupy as your home. Therefore, where you are only a temporary (including respite and trial period) resident, *and* you have HB in payment in respect of your home in the community, you will not be able to receive HB in respect of your stay in the care home. For the calculation of HB for permanent residents, the tariff income rule is only applied to capital over £10,000 and the capital limit is £16,000 (see p191).

However, social services may not be able to grant a license to a 'less dependent resident' in a local authority home because as the direct service provider it might constitute selling a service to a non-public body, which would be in breach of Social Services (Goods and Services) Act 1970.[45]

Council tax benefit

For **any type of care home**, you will only be able to get council tax benefit (CTB) if you are liable to pay council tax in respect of your home in the community.

If your home is unoccupied because you are a **temporary** (including respite and trial period) resident in a care home, you will get a 50 per cent status discount on your council tax. You may be able to get CTB for your 50 per cent council tax (see p111). The rules for getting CTB during a temporary stay in residential care are the same as for HB (see p355).

If you are a **permanent** resident, and therefore the care home has become your 'sole or main' home, *and* your home in the community is left unoccupied, you will be exempt from council tax as a single person and may also qualify for CTB (see p111).

If you are one of a couple and your partner is remaining in the home in the community, s/he will be able to get a 25 per cent status discount on her/his council tax as a single person and may qualify for CTB (see p111).

Disability living allowance care component and attendance allowance

The DLA care component and AA (including constant attendance allowance and exceptionally severe disablement allowance payable with industrial injury disablement or war disablement benefit) is affected by a stay, whether **temporary or permanent**, in 'certain accommodation' (also called 'special accommodation') other than hospitals.

Chapter 21: Social security benefits in care homes
4. How benefits are affected by the type of care home and stay

21

'Certain accommodation'/'special accommodation' is defined as where your accommodation is provided:

- 'in pursuance of Part III of the National Assistance Act 1948, or part IV of the Social Work (Scotland) Act 1968 or section 7 of the Mental Health (Scotland) Act 1984';[46]
- 'in circumstances where the cost of the accommodation is borne wholly or partly out of public or local funds in pursuance of those enactments or any other enactment relating to persons under disability (or to young persons or to education or training – DLA care component only);[47] *or*
- 'in circumstances where the cost of the accommodation *may be borne* [emphasis added] wholly or partly out of public or local funds in pursuance of those enactments or any other enactment relating to persons under disability (or to young persons or to education or training – DLA care component only)'.[48] This is sometimes called the 'may be borne' provision.

The main principle is that DLA care component or AA is not payable in certain accommodation/special accommodation as defined above, unless one of the exceptions listed below applies.

The legislation regarding DLA care component and AA in certain accommodation is complex. There are many inter-related provisions and exceptions. If the Benefits Agency tells you that DLA care component or AA is not payable and you have any doubts (perhaps because you are not in the normal type of care home) you should seek further advice.

The DLA mobility component is not affected by a stay in certain accommodation other than hospitals.

The DLA care component or AA is usually payable for the first four weeks of a stay in certain accommodation[49] (see p359 for when it is payable for longer). However, if you have had a stay in certain accommodation or in hospital within the previous 28 days, that period of stay will be linked to your present stay so that benefit will only be paid for a total of four weeks including the period of your previous stay. The day you enter a care home and the day you leave do not count as days in certain accommodation.[50] If you first claim DLA care component or AA when you are already in certain accommodation it is not payable until you leave. If you go into certain accommodation again (even within 28 days) your four week concession will start from the first day of that stay.

If you are receiving respite care (ie, a planned programme of temporary stays) you may be able to arrange a pattern of stays that allows you to keep your DLA care component or AA. The following example illustrates how the **'linking rule'** works.

21

Chapter 21: Social security benefits in care homes
4. How benefits are affected by the type of care home and stay

Example:

Mr Hammond is in receipt of AA and he has respite care every weekend. He goes into a care home on a Friday and leaves on the following Monday. This is counted as two days of respite care (Saturday and Sunday) because the day of entering (Friday) and the day of leaving (Monday) are not counted.

Mr Hammond continues with this pattern of respite care but he is mindful that each of his weekend stays after his first stay are being linked together because they are within 28 days of the previous stay. This means that after 14 weekend stays of two days each he has reached the end of his 28 days' payment of AA while in care. If Mr Hammond spent a 15th weekend in respite care, his attendance allowance would stop for the two days in care and only start in payment again when he went home until his next respite care stay, when it would stop again.

However, in order to avoid any break in the payment of his AA, Mr Hammond breaks the 'link' by having shorter respite care stays. For four weekends following the 14th weekend stay he doesn't go into the care home until the Saturday and he leaves on Sunday. As there are no days counted as days in care, he has effectively spent 29 days without a stay in care, thus breaking the link. On the 19th weekend, Mr Hammond goes back to going into the care home on a Friday and leaving on a Monday. If he continues to repeat this pattern his AA will be paid without any break for his stays in the care home.

Note: For reasons demonstrated in the above example, it is important to inform the Disability Benefits Unit in Blackpool, as well as your local Benefits Agency office, of any stay in care and, if you have a pattern of respite care planned, to advise them of this in advance. If you cannot arrange your respite care to break the link, you will at some point have to send your order book back. In this situation, it may be better to receive your benefit by way of automatic credit transfer (ACT) payments, as the Unit can adjust each credit transfer payment as necessary. You should contact the Disability Benefits Unit about this.

Local authority residential accommodation (board provided)

If you are a **temporary** (including respite and trial period) or **permanent** resident in local authority residential accommodation you will not be able to get DLA care component or AA after the first four weeks of your stay (or after a shorter period if the linking rule applies – see p357).

Unlike for independent sector care homes (see p359), this applies even if you are paying the full cost yourself.[51] If you know you will be required to pay the full cost yourself because of the level of your resources, then you may be better off choosing an independent sector care home so that you can continue to receive your DLA care component or AA.

Independent registered residential care and/or nursing homes

As for local authority residential accommodation, if you are a **temporary** (including respite and trial period) or **permanent** resident in a registered independent residential care or nursing home, you will normally not be able to get DLA care component or AA after the first four weeks (or after a shorter period if the linking rule applies – see p357). Unlike for local authority residential accommodation, if you are self-funding (ie, paying the full cost yourself[52]) or, you are receiving IS to help pay for the cost of your care but you are not receiving funding from social services (ie, a 'loophole' case – see p369), you can continue to receive DLA care component or AA.

If you have been funded by social services (eg, while your former home is up for sale) but this funding has now stopped, your AA or DLA care component will be put back in payment. It is important to let the Disability Benefits Unit at the Benefits Agency know that the social services funding has stopped so that payment can be re-instated.

Independent or local authority homes (board not provided)

If you are in a **local authority home** where board is not provided, it does not matter whether you are paying the full cost yourself, DLA care component or AA is not payable beyond the maximum four week period because it is Part III, or in Scotland Part IV, accommodation.[53]

If you are in an **independent sector home** which does not provide board and is not required to register, your DLA care component or AA will continue to be payable in the normal way (eg, very sheltered accommodation – see Chapter 5).

5. **Example calculations of income support**

The following are examples of how income support (IS) is calculated for people in different types of care home for different types of stay and in different situations – ie, for a single person and for one member of a couple. These examples cover the IS calculation which, if you are reliant on social security benefits to make a contribution to social services for the cost of your accommodation and care, is the first step to determine the amount of your contribution. The second part is the contribution calculation undertaken by social services using the information from your financial assessment. Each of the examples below continue with the contribution calculation in Chapter 23 (see p394).

These examples deal with the most common situations:

- a single person in local authority residential accommodation for a temporary stay;

- a single person in local authority residential accommodation for a permanent stay;
- one of a couple in local authority residential accommodation for a temporary stay;
- one of a couple in local authority residential accommodation for a permanent stay;
- a single person in an independent care home for a temporary stay;
- a single person in an independent care home for a permanent stay;
- one of a couple in an independent care home for a temporary stay;
- one of a couple in an independent care home for a permanent stay.

There are examples of more complex situations in the complete benefits and contributions calculations on pp394–404.

A single person in a local authority residential accommodation for a temporary stay

Mr Guest is a single person aged 64 years living in a rented council house. His income, before entering the home, is made up of long term incapacity benefit (IB), IS and DLA care and mobility components. Mr Guest also receives maximum HB and CTB. He has savings of £3,500. He goes into local authority residential accommodation for a temporary stay of two weeks.

Mr Guest's income support is now calculated in the following way:

Income:		
	IB (long term)	£75.65
	Tariff income from savings	£2.00
	Total	**£77.65**

(DLA care component £52.95 disregarded.)
(DLA mobility component £37.00 disregarded.)
Applicable amount: £66.75 (Local authority residential accommodation rate).
Applicable amount (£66.75) minus income (£77.65) = IS (NIL).
Mr Guest is not entitled to IS as he has excess income of £10.90 per week. (His only income will be his IB and DLA).
As Mr Guest will lose his entitlement to IS he will need to make a fresh claim for HB and CTB and with an excess income of £10.90 per week he will be required to pay £7.08 per week towards the rent of his home in the community and £2.18 per week towards his council tax.
For the calculation of Mr Guest's contribution to his accommodation and care costs see p394.

A single person in local authority residential accommodation for a permanent stay

Mrs Gascoigne is a single person aged 80 years living in a rented council house. Her income before entering the home is made up of state retirement pension, a works pension, IS and AA. Mrs Gascoigne also receives maximum HB and CTB. She goes into local authority residential accommodation on a permanent basis.

As she is a permanent resident in the home she gives up her council tenancy and, therefore, she is no longer liable for rent or council tax.

Mrs Gascoigne's income support is now calculated in the following way:

Income:	State retirement pension	£68.20
	Works pension	£3.10
	Total	**£71.30**

(AA £52.95 payable for the first four weeks but disregarded as income.)

Applicable amount: £66.75 (Local authority residential accommodation rate).

Applicable amount (£66.75) minus income (£71.30) = IS (NIL).

Mrs Gascoigne is not entitled to IS as she has excess income of £4.55 per week.

(Her only income will be her retirement pension and AA for the first four weeks.)

For the calculation of Mrs Gascoigne's contribution to her accommodation and care costs see p394.

- -

One of a couple in local authority residential accommodation for a temporary stay.

Mr and Mrs Love, aged 65 and 53 years respectively, are home owners (without a mortgage). Mr Love's weekly income before entering the home is made up of a state retirement pension, IS and DLA care and mobility components. Mrs Love also receives state retirement pension and maximum CTB is in payment. Mr Love goes into a local authority residential accommodation for a temporary stay of three weeks.

The income support in payment to Mr Love for Mrs Love and himself as a couple is reviewed in the following way:

Income:	State retirement pension (Mr Love)	£75.45
	State retirement pension (Mrs Love)	£39.95
	Works pension (Mr Love)	£4.64
	Total	**£120.04**

(DLA mobility component (Mr Love) £37.11 disregarded as income.)

(DLA care component (Mr Love) £35.40 disregarded as income.)

Applicable amount:	Mr Love	£66.75 (local authority residential accommodation)
	Mrs Love	£51.40 (normal single persons allowance)
		£23.60 (normal single pensioner premium)
	Total	**£141.75**

Applicable amount (£141.75) minus income (3120.04) = IS (£21.71) Mr and Mrs Love are entitled to IS of £21.71 per week payable to Mr Love as the claimant (on top of Mr Love's retirement pension, works pension and DLA and Mrs. Love's retirement pension).

IS is paid at a higher rate whilst Mr Love is staying in residential accommodation than it was when they were both in the community. This is because Mr Love is one of a couple and Mrs Love is remaining in the community, therefore, her applicable amount is calculated as if she were a single person. Their income is still added together, because Mr Love is only a temporary resident in the care home. During Mr Love's temporary stay they will continue to receive maximum CTB as they remain entitled to IS.

Note: If Mr Love's works pension was more than £9.91 per week, Mr and Mrs Love would not be entitled to IS whilst claiming as a couple in the community. However, if Mr Love's works pension was more than £9.91 but less than £26.35, then, when Mr Love enters care, they would become entitled to IS because of the new applicable amount that applies.

For the calculation of Mr Love's contribution to his accommodation and care costs see p394.

One of a couple in local authority residential accommodation for a permanent stay.

Mr and Mrs Leal aged 85 and 80 years respectively are home owners (without a mortgage). Mr Leal's weekly income before entering the home is made up of state retirement pension, works pension and AA. Mrs Leal also receives state retirement pension. They have joint savings of £10,000. They are not entitled to IS but they receive some CTB as a couple in the community. Mrs Leal goes into local authority residential accommodation on a permanent basis.

As Mr and Mrs Leal are now permanently separated they will be treated as single people for IS purposes. Therefore, Mr Leal and Mrs Leal each put in a claim for IS. The joint savings are divided equally and £5,000 each is assessed as savings.

Mr Leal

Mr Leal's savings of £5,000 fall below the amount of £10,000 that, for a permanent resident, does not attract any tariff income. His home in the community is not taken into account as capital because Mrs Leal is still living there.

Mr Leal's claim will be calculated in the following way:

Income:		
	State retirement pension	£66.75
	Works pension	£12.88
	Total	**£79.63**

(AA £52.95 payable for the first four weeks but disregarded as income.)

Applicable amount: £66.75 (Local authority residential accommodation rate.)

Applicable amount (£66.75) minus income (£79.63) = IS (NIL).

Mr Leal is not entitled to IS as he has excess income of £12.88 per week. (His only income will be his retirement pension, works pension and attendance allowance for the first four weeks).

Mrs Leal

Mrs Leal's claim will be calculated in the following way:

Income:	State retirement pension	£39.95
	Tariff income from savings	£8.00
	Total	**£47.95**
Applicable amount:	£51.54 (single person allowance)	
	£30.84 (single higher pension premium)	
Total:	**£82.25**	

Applicable amount (£82.25) minus income (£47.95) = IS (£34.30)
Mrs Leal is entitled to £34.30 IS per week (paid on top of her retirement pension).
Mrs Leal will also be entitled to maximum CTB.
For the calculation of Mr Leal's contribution to her accommodation and care costs see p394.

• •

A single person in an independent care home for a temporary stay

Mrs Kaur is a single person aged 70 years living on her own. She is a home owner with a mortgage. Her income before entering the home is made up of state retirement pension, works pension, IS and AA. She also receives maximum CTB and she has savings of £7,000 in the building society. She goes into an independent residential care home for a temporary stay of six weeks.

Mrs Kaur's IS is increased to include a residential allowance and is now calculated in the following way:

Income:	State retirement pension	£74.05
	Works pension	£15.45
	Tariff income from savings	£16.00
	Total	**£105.50**

(AA £52.95 payable for the first four weeks but disregarded as income.)

Applicable amount 1:

(first 4 weeks)	£51.40	(personal allowance)
	£30.85	(higher pensioner premium)
	£39.75	(severe disability premium)
	£6.00	(mortgage interest allowance by DSS)
	£59.40	(residential allowance)
Total:	**£187.40**	

Applicable amount (£187.40) minus income (£105.50) = IS (£81.90)
Mrs Kaur us entitled to IS of £81.90 per week for the first four weeks of her stay (paid on top of her retirement pension, works pension and AA).

Applicable amount 2:

(last 2 weeks)	£51.40	(personal allowance)
	£23.60	(pensioner premium)
	£6.00	(mortgage interest allowance allowed by DSS)
	£59.40	(residential allowance)
Total:	**£140.40**	

The higher pensioner premium and the severe disability premium are only applicable whilst Mrs Kaur continues to receive the qualifying benefit of AA, but this is stopped after 28 days in the care home.

Applicable amount (£140.40) minus income (£105.50) = IS (£34.90).

Mrs Kaur is entitled to IS of £34.90 per week for the last two weeks of her stay (paid on top of her retirement pension and works pension).

Because she continues to receive IS throughout the six weeks of her stay her maximum CTB would not be affected.

For the calculation of Mrs Kaur's contribution to her accommodation and care costs see p394.

* *

A single person in an independent care home for a permanent stay

Mr Hughes is a single person aged 58 years. He is a home owner (without a mortgage) and he lives with his sister who is disabled. His income before entering the home is made up of long-term IB and DLA care and mobility components. He also receives some CTB and has savings of £5,000. Mr Hughes is not entitled to IS whilst he is living in the community. He goes into an independent nursing home on a permanent basis. As he is a permanent resident in the home he is no longer liable for council tax.

Mr Hughes makes a claim for IS. His savings of £5,000 are less than the amount of £10,000 that does not attract a tariff income for a permanent resident. His home in the community is not taken into account as capital because his disabled sister is still living there.

Mr Hughes' claim for IS is calculated in the following way:

Income:	IB (long-term)	£80.80
	Total	**£80.80**

(DLA mobility component £37.00 disregarded as income.)

(DLA care component £52.95 payable for the first four weeks but disregarded as income.)

Applicable amount 1:

(first 4 weeks)	£51.40	(personal allowance)
	£21.90	(disability premium)

£39.72	(severe disability premium)
£59.40	(residential allowance)
Total: £172.45	

Applicable amount (£172.45) minus income (£80.80) = IS (£91.65).
Mr Hughes is entitled to IS of £91.65 per week for the first four weeks of his stay (paid on top of his IB and DLA).
Applicable amount 2:

(after 4 weeks)		
	£51.40	(personal allowance)
	£21.90	(disability premium)
	£59.40	(residential allowance)
Total:	**£132.70**	

The severe disability premium is only applicable whilst Mr Hughes continues to receive the qualifying benefits of DLA care component but this is stopped after 28 days in the care home.
Applicable amount (£132.70) minus income (£80.80) = IS (£51.90).
Mr Hughes is entitled to IS of £51.50 per week after four weeks of his stay (paid on top of his IB and DLA mobility component).
For the calculation of Mr Hughes' contribution to his accommodation and care costs see p394.

. . . .

One of a couple in an independent care home for a temporary stay

Mr and Mrs McEwan, aged 65 and 55 years respectively, are council tenants. Mr McEwan's weekly income is made up of state retirement pension and a works pension. Mrs McEwan's weekly income before entering the home is made up of severe disablement allowance and DLA care and mobility components. They also receive some HB and CTB and they have joint savings of £4,000. They are not entitled to IS as a couple in the community. Mrs McEwan goes into an independent residential care home for 3 weeks.

Mrs McEwan claims IS for Mr McEwan and herself as a couple. The claim is calculated in the following way:

Income:

State retirement pension (Mr McEwan)	£70.60
Works pension (Mr McEwan)	£43.35
Severe disablement allowance (Mrs McEwan)	£54.40
Tariff income from savings	£4.00
Total	**£172.35**

(DLA care component (Mrs McEwan) £52.95 disregarded as income.)
(DLA mobility component (Mrs McEwan) £14.05 disregarded as income.)

Applicable amount:	Mr McEwan	£51.40 (single person allowance)
	Mrs McEwan	£23.60 (single pensioner premium)
		£51.40 (single personal allowance)
		£21.90 (single disability premium)
		£39.75 (severe disability premium)
		£59.40 (residential allowance)
	Total	**£247.45**

If Mrs McEwan's stay was for more than four weeks her DLA care component would normally stop her after the fourth week and the severe disability premium would not be included in the applicable amount, therefore, the amount of IS would reduce accordingly.

Applicable amount (£247.45) minus income (£172.35) = IS (£75.10).

Mr and Mrs McEwan are entitled to IS of £75.10 per week payable to Mrs McEwan as the claimant (paid on top of Mr McEwan's retirement pension and works pension and Mrs McEwan's severe disablement allowance and DLA).

Mr and Mrs McEwan are entitled to IS whilst Mrs McEwan is staying in the residential care home. This is because the applicable amount used in the calculation is based on the appropriate amounts for Mr and Mrs McEwan as single people and Mrs McEwan is entitled to an extra 'residential allowance' due to being in an independent registered care home. Their income is still added together because Mrs McEwan is only a temporary resident in the care home. During Mrs McEwan's temporary stay they will also be entitled to maximum HB and CTB.

For the calculation of Mrs McEwan's contribution to her accommodation and care costs see p394.

Care of a couple in an independent care home for a permanent stay.

Mr and Mrs Spore aged 59 and 65 years respectively are council tenants. Mr Spore's weekly income is made up of long term IB and IS. Mrs Spore's weekly income before entering the home is made up of state retirement pension and DLA care and mobility components. They also receive maximum HB and CTB. Mrs Spore goes into an independent nursing home on a permanent basis.

As Mr and Mrs Spore are now permanently separated they will be treated as single people for IS purposes. Therefore, Mrs Spore makes a claim for income support in her own right and Mr Spore informs the DSS of the change of circumstances so that his claim can be reviewed.

Mr Spore

Mr Spore's claim will be calculated in the following way:

Income:	IB (long-term)	£71.20
	Total	**£172.35**

Applicable amount:

£51.40	(single personal allowance)
21.90	(single disability premium)
Total	**£73.30**

Applicable amount (£73.30) minus income (£71.20) = IS (£2.10).
Mr Spore is entitled to IS of £2.10 per week (paid on top of his IB).
Mr Spore will also be entitled to maximum IS and HB.

Mrs Spore

Mrs Spore's claim will be calculated in the following way:
The claim is calculated in the following way:

Income:	State retirement pension	£47.98
	Total	**£47.98**

(DLA mobility component £37.00 disregarded as income.)
(DLA care component £52.95 payable for first four weeks but disregarded as income.)

Applicable amount 1:

(first 4 weeks)		
	£51.40	(single person allowance)
	£30.85	(single higher pensioner premium)
	£39.75	(severe disability premium)
	£59.40	(residential allowance)
Total	**£181.40**	

Applicable amount (£181.40) minus income (£47.98) = IS (£133.42).
Mrs Spore is entitled to IS of £133.42 per week for the first four weeks of her stay (paid on top of her retirement pension and DLA).

Applicable amount 2:

(after 4 weeks)		
	£51.40	(single person allowance)
	£30.85	(single higher pensioner premium)
	£59.40	(residential allowance)
Total	**£141.65**	

The severe disability allowance was only applicable whilst Mrs Spore continued to receive the qualifying benefit of DLA care component.
Applicable amount (£141.65) minus income (£47.98) = IS (£93.67).
Mrs Spore is entitled to IS of £93.67 per week after four weeks of her stay (paid on top of her retirement pension and DLA).
For the calculation of Mrs Spore's contribution to her accommodation and care costs see section p394.

6. **Self-funding (including loophole cases)**

You are described as self-funding if can meet the whole cost of your accommodation and care in an **independent sector care home** from your own resources (or with help from relatives, friends or charity), without any financial help from social services, and without claiming IS/income-based jobseeker's allowance (JSA) and/or HB.[54] If you are in local authority residential accommodation you can never be treated as self-funding for social security benefit purposes even if you are paying the whole cost.[55]

You may be required to meet the cost of your accommodation and care because of your income or capital (see Chapters 13 and 14). In most cases it is the level of a person's capital that determines whether they will be required to fund themselves.

If you are making your own arrangements to go into an independent care home but it is likely that your capital will eventually fall to £16,000 or less, it would be sensible to talk to social services first and perhaps have an assessment of your needs carried out so that there will not be a problem in the future if you ask for financial help from social services.

There are a number of issues surrounding the extent to which social services can become involved (see p369) in your placement in different situations in order for you to receive DLA care component or AA.

Income support

You may be able to claim IS to help you continue to meet the costs of your accommodation and care when your capital reduces to £16,000 or less if you are a permanent resident, or to £8,000 or less if you are a temporary resident, and your income is below your applicable amount (see p353).

Social services funding

If you are entitled to IS you will qualify for financial help from social services as long as you are assessed as needing the type of care home you are in.

Even if you are not entitled to IS (eg, because your income is above your applicable amount (see p353) or because you are a temporary resident and you have capital in excess of £8,000 (see Chapter 14)) you are still likely to qualify for financial help from social services to meet the costs of your accommodation and care. However, if your income is of a high enough level to meet the whole cost of the care home and the personal expenses allowance (see Chapter 15) you will not qualify for financial help from social services.

Disability living allowance care component/attendance allowance

If you are self-funding (ie, not receiving financial help from social services or IS and/or HB) you will be able to continue receiving any DLA care component or AA to which you are entitled beyond the first four weeks in the care home. Even if social services have helped you find the placement or contracted with the home to provide your accommodation and care, you will still be able to get DLA care component or attendance allowance *as long as you are meeting the whole cost yourself* (or with help from relatives, friends or charity) without IS or funding from social services.[56]

'Loophole' cases

In England and Wales only, under the 'may be borne' provision (see p356), DLA care component and AA are not payable where your 'accommodation may be funded wholly or partly out of public funds which includes local authority funding'.[57] However, it has been shown that this provision has no real function because if you have made your own arrangements, social services do not have the power to intervene (as accommodation and care are 'otherwise available'[58]) unless the home is not suitable for your needs.[59]

This situation is known as a 'loophole' in the law, meaning that as long as social services do not have a current contract with the care home for the provision and funding of your accommodation and care, you can continue to receive DLA care component or AA after the first four weeks, *even if you receive IS.*

However, depending on the level of the fee for the care home, there is still likely to be a shortfall between the fee and the total amount of IS you receive (either on its own or as a top-up of other income such as state retirement pension) and DLA care component or AA.

In these circumstances you may still prefer to make your own arrangements. This may be particularly preferable if you have a property to sell and can meet the shortfall until it is sold because, once your house is sold, any IS and DLA care component or AA paid to you is not repayable to the Benefits Agency. If you were funded by social services, however, you would lose your DLA care component or AA and, when your home was sold, you would have to repay social services all the money they had paid on your behalf.

Social services departments are advised by guidance[60] that, as part of the whole assessment process, they should provide full information about the financial consequences of different options. An Ombudsman case reported that a council had met the full costs of a placement in a care home in the period before the financial assessment was complete, on the assumption that the family could not do so until the resident's home was sold. It was accepted by the council that it should have put the option of paying the full cost to the family, given its knowledge of the rules governing the payment of attendance allowance. In this case the Benefits Agency decided that because social services had made payments wrongly, it could backdate attendance allowance for that period.[61]

Also in a recent social security commissioner's case,[62] social services had become involved in a person's placement by contracting with the care home but the person was able to, and did, make the payments for their accommodation and care to the home out of their own resources, albeit that a claim for IS had been made (also the subject of an appeal). The case was remitted to a tribunal for re-hearing with the direction that the question for determination by the freshly constituted tribunal was not whether social services *did act* under the National Assistance Act 1948,[63] but whether it had *the power to act* – ie, whether the care and attention was 'otherwise available' and if it was there was no power to act, and therefore the 'loophole' provision could become effective and AA would be payable.

In Scotland the Benefits Agency has interpreted the same regulations as meaning that DLA care component/AA cannot be paid to people who make their own arrangements. This is because the Scottish legislation gives social work departments wider powers to provide accommodation. This interpretation has been questioned and you should seek advice if you are affected.

Retrospective self-funding

If you are required to meet the whole cost of your accommodation and care because you have a property worth more than £16,000, but you have not sold the property yet, and you do not have additional resources with which to pay the full cost, social services may make payments to the care home for your placement until your property is sold and you can repay them from the proceeds of the sale.

It has been argued that because the full cost has to be refunded to social services once you have sold your property you are actually self-funding and therefore DLA care component or AA should be payable in arrears when you have fully repaid social services. There are a number of conflicting social security commissioners decisions about this issue.[64] Some of the Northern Ireland decisions are being appealed to the Court of Appeal.

If you have been refused DLA care component or AA for a period when social services were making payments to the care home on your behalf and you have now repaid the amount, you should seek advice.

Chapter 21: Social security benefits in care homes
7. Temporary absences from care homes (including going into hospital)

21

7. Temporary absences from care homes (including going into hospital)

Local authority residential accommodation

If you are temporarily absent from a local authority care home for any reason other than being admitted to hospital, your IS will need to be reviewed to take account of your temporary situation – ie, if you are staying with friends or relatives the normal IS applicable amount will apply (see p96). If you do not receive IS because you receive another benefit such as a state retirement pension which is more than the residential accommodation applicable amount (£66.75), you may be able to claim IS for your temporary situation. DLA care component or AA may also be payable while you are temporarily in the community.

If your temporary absence is due to being admitted to hospital your IS applicable amount is immediately reduced to £14.75.[65] If you are not paying the full cost of the care home placement yourself and you are in receipt of any of the following benefits:

- retirement pension;
- widow's pension;
- widowed mother's allowance;
- incapacity benefit;
- severe disablement allowance;
- unemployability supplement and industrial death benefit,

and you are a permanent resident in the care home, then your benefit is reduced to £13.35 (or less) from the first day you become an in-patient, as if you had been an in-patient for 52 weeks under the normal hospital in-patient rules (see p125). In these circumstances you may be able to claim £1.40 IS to make your income up to the £14.75 applicable amount.

If you are only a temporary resident in the care home, the period you have spent there counts towards the periods of 6 and 52 weeks, after which your benefit is reduced under the normal rules for in-patients (see p125).[66]

Any DLA mobility component payable to you will remain in payment for the first 28 days of your stay in hospital. Periods of absence because you are in hospital that are separated by less than 28 days are linked together and treated as one long period of absence.

Independent registered residential care or nursing homes

If you are temporarily absent from an independent sector home in which you are a permanent resident for any other reason than being admitted to hospital, your IS residential allowance will continue for three weeks as long as you

21

Chapter 21: Social security benefits in care homes
7. Temporary absences from care homes (including going into hospital)

intend to return to the care home.[67] Each period of absence is treated separately – ie, there are no linking rules. If you are temporarily absent from the care home and staying in the community (eg, with friends or relatives) then DLA care component or AA may also be payable during your temporary absence.

If your temporary absence is due to being in hospital, you will continue to be entitled to your normal rate of IS for the first six weeks, including the residential allowance, as long as you intend to return to the care home.[68] After six weeks your IS is calculated under the normal rules for in-patients (see p125).

Other benefits (see p371) will be affected after six weeks when they will be reduced to £13.35 or less.[69]

Periods of absence because you are in hospital that are separated by less than 28 days are linked together and treated as one long period of absence.

8. **Other sources of financial assistance in care homes**

Health benefits

If you are a permanent resident in a care home and your placement is being wholly or partly funded by social services you can obtain an HC2 certificate from the NHS health benefits division for full exemption from NHS charges (eg, prescriptions, dental treatment, wigs, fabric supports and eye tests), vouchers for glasses or contact lens, and fares to hospital. You must complete a special short application form HC1(RC). The capital limit is £16,000 and your certificate will last for 12 months. You should make a repeat claim about four weeks before the end of the period on your certificate.

If you do not receive any funding for your placement from social services you may still be able to get a full or partial exemption for the same charges under the normal rules that apply for health benefits in the community – ie, automatic exemption because of your age or particular personal circumstances, passporting to full exemption if you are in receipt of IS, income-based JSA, working families tax credit or disabled person's tax credit, or on low income grounds (see p137).

Special help for war pensioners

If you get a war disablement pension or you have had a gratuity for your disability, you can apply to the War Pensions Agency for free medical treatment and services that you need wholly or mainly because of that disability. You are not means-tested for these services (ie, it does not matter how much income or capital you have), but you must apply before arranging for them.

You may be able to get help for nursing home fees where you are provided with skilled nursing care if you need permanent care in a care home or if you need a short break for convalescence or if you need a respite break in order to give your carer a break.

For a permanent stay in a nursing home you must need 24-hour nursing care because of your pensioned disability. The War Pensions Agency can pay up to a maximum of £411 (£467 in London) a week for nursing home fees provided that social services have not been involved in assessing your nursing needs or arranging a placement. A higher rate can be paid if there is no other nursing home that is suitable for your needs. The nursing home must be approved by the War Pensions Agency which may send a doctor to visit you to assess your needs. In this situation your basic war disablement pension will continue to be paid in full while you are in the nursing home but any constant attendance allowance payable will stop after four weeks. Some other extra allowances such as unemployability supplement are reduced or withdrawn after eight weeks.

For a short-term break for convalescence you can claim nursing home fees for a maximum of four weeks a year. However, if you have recently been discharged from hospital or are recovering from an operation, the War Pensions Agency is unlikely to pay as it considers this is an NHS responsibility.

For a respite break you may be able to claim nursing home fees if your carer needs a break from caring for you for medical reasons (medical evidence is required).

Other expenses for medical treatment and services may also be available. You can ask your local war pensioners' welfare officer to visit you to discuss your needs and help you apply for any services.

Help from charities

A charity may be able to help you with some of the costs of a stay in a care home if your benefits and/or social services funding cannot meet the full charges of the home. This may happen where the charge for a care home is more expensive than the amount usually allowed by social services and you cannot meet the shortfall.

There are many charities which provide help to people in need. The social services department may know of appropriate charities that you could contact. There are also publications (eg, *Guide to Grants for Individuals in Need* or the *Charities Digest*) available from your local library.

The organisations Counsel and Care for the Elderly[70] or the Elderly Accommodation Council[71] or the Royal United Kingdom Beneficent Association[72] may be able to help you find an appropriate charity.

9. **Effects on carers**

If you are the carer of a person who goes into a care home on a temporary (including respite or trial periods) or permanent stay, the following benefits you receive will be affected:

* invalid care allowance (ICA) (see p88);
* IS/income-based JSA (see p93).

If the person you are caring for receives DLA care component or AA, you may be claiming ICA for caring for them. The ICA rules allow breaks in care of up to 12 weeks within a 26-week period. Up to four weeks of the 12-week period are allowed for any temporary breaks in care – eg, holidays or if the person you care for goes into a care home for a temporary or respite stay. The remaining eight weeks of the 12-week period allow for either you, as the carer, or the person you care for, to undergo medical or other treatment as an in-patient in hospital. However, if the person you care for goes into hospital or into a care home, their DLA care component or AA will stop after four weeks, or sooner if they have had a previous stay in hospital or a care home within the previous 28 days (see p369). This means your ICA will also stop.

The person you care for may be able to arrange a pattern of respite care that allows them to keep their DLA care component or AA (see example on p358) thus allowing you to keep your ICA. All changes of circumstances (yours or the person you care for) must be reported to the ICA unit. The main rule to remember is that you can be paid ICA for any week (Sunday through to Saturday) in which you are caring for the disabled person for at least 35 hours, so odd days or weekends away are unlikely to affect your entitlement.

If your ICA stops, you continue to be eligible for IS with the carer's premium (£13.95) for eight weeks. After this you may need to claim income-based JSA instead. The carer's premium is also included in any calculation for HB, CTB, income-based JSA and health benefits for eight weeks after your ICA stops (see p99).

If, as a carer, you are also responsible for the disabled person's benefits because they cannot manage their financial affairs (ie, you are their appointee – see p226) you may wish to continue in this role when the disabled person is living in a care home. However, in addition to being responsible for their benefits, you will have the added responsibility of forwarding the contribution to social services for the disabled person's accommodation and care costs and of providing information for the social services financial assessment. If you do not wish to have this responsibility you could choose to relinquish the appointeeship in favour of social services.

Notes

2. Types of care homes

1 s21(1)(a) of part III NAA 1948 as amended by the NHS & CCA 1990; ss13B and 59 of SW(S)A 1968 and s7 MH(S)A 1984
2 Reg 2(2) SS(HIP) Regs 1975.
3 *White and Others v Chief Adjudication Officer*, *The Times*, 2 August 1993; *Botchett v Chief Adjudication Officer*, *The Times*, 8 May 1996
4 Reg 2(2) SS(HIP) Regs 1975
5 *Botchett v Chief Adjudication Officer*, *The Times*, 8 May 1996
6 Reg 2(2) SS(HIP) Regs 1975
7 Reg 10(7), SS(DLA) Regs 1991; reg 8(5) Reg SS(AA) Regs 1991
8 Reg 12B(9A) SS(DLA) Regs 1991
9 Reg 10(6) SS(DLA) Regs 1991; reg 8(4) SS(AA) Regs 1991
10 Reg 10(9) SS(DLA) Regs 1991; reg 8(7) SS(AA) Regs 1991
11 s26 NAA 1948
12 s22 NAA 1948
13 Under NA(AR) Regs 1992
14 Reg 21(3B) and (3C) ISG Regs 1987
15 CIS/16440/1996
16 Reg 21 ISG Regs 1987
17 Reg 21(3C) ISG Regs 1987 amended by S1 1995 No 516 from 10.4.95
18 Reg 21 ISG Regs 1987
19 Reg 21(3C) ISG Regs 1987
20 Reg 21 ISG Regs 1987
21 Reg 21(3A) ISG Regs 1987 introduced by SI 1991 No 1656 on 12 August 1991

3. Types of stay

22 Sch 3 para 3(11) ISG Regs 1987; reg 5(8B) HBG Regs 1987 and reg 4C(4) CTB Regs 1992
23 Sch 3 paras 3(8) – 3(10) ISG Regs 1987 and Regs 5(7B) -(8) HB; regs 1987 and Regs 4(1) to (3) CTB Regs 1987
24 CIS/613/1997

4. How benefits are effected by the type of care home and stay

25 Reg 2(1) ISG Regs 1987; reg 1(3) JSA Regs 1996
26 Reg 21 and Sch 7 para 10A ISG Regs 1987
27 Reg 21 and Sch 7 para 10C ISG Regs 1987
28 Reg 21 and Sch 7 para 10B(3) ISG Regs 1987
29 Reg 21 and Sch 7 para 10B(1) ISG Regs 1987
30 Reg 21 and Sch 7 para 13 ISG Regs 1987
31 Reg 21 and Sch 7 para 13 ISG Regs 1987
32 CIS/4934/97; CIS/4935/97; CIS/5232/97; CIS/5237/97 and CIS/3767/97 and common appendix to these decisions
33 Reg 21 and Sch 7 para 13 ISG Regs 1987
34 Reg 17 and Sch 3 ISG Regs 1987
35 Reg 17(1)(bb) and Sch 2 para 2A ISG Regs 1987
36 Sch 2 para 2A(3) ISG Regs 1987
37 Reg 17(1) and Sch 2 paras 1(1) and 2A ISG Regs 1987
38 Reg 17(1) and Sch 2 paras 1(2) and 2A ISG Regs 1987
39 Reg 17(1) and Sch 2 paras 1(3) and 2A ISG Regs 1987
40 Sch 7 para 9 ISG Regs 1987
41 Reg 26 and Sch 7 para 7(2)(C) SS(C&P) Regs 1987
42 CIS/4935/97
43 Sch 7 ISG Regs 1987
44 Reg 21(4) ISG Regs 1987
45 p12 Issue 1 *Community Care News* (Rowe & Maw) February 1999
46 Reg 9(1)(a) SS(DLA) Regs 1992 and reg 7(1)(a) SS(AA) Regs 1992
47 Reg 9(1)(b) SS(DLA) Regs 1992 and reg 7(1)(b) SS(AA) Regs 1992
48 Reg 9(1)(c) SS(DLA) Regs 1992 and reg 7(1)(c) SS(AA) Regs 1992
49 Reg 10(1) SS(DLA) Regs 1992 and reg 8(1) SS(AA) Regs 1992

50 Reg 10(2) SS(DLA) Regs 1992 and reg
    8(2) SS(AA) Regs 1992
51 Reg 10(9) SS(DLA) Regs 1992 and reg
    8(7) SS(AA) Regs 1992
52 Reg 10(8) SS(DLA) Regs 1992 and reg
    8(6) SS(AA) Regs 1992
53 Reg 9(1)(a) SS(DLA) Regs 1992 and
    reg 7(1)(a) SS(AA) Regs 1992

6. Self-funding (including loophole cases)

54 Reg 10(8) SS(DLA) Regs 1992 and reg
    8(6) SS(AA) Regs 1992
55 Reg 10(9) SS(DLA) Regs 1992 and reg
    8(7) SS(AA) Regs 1992
56 para 7 of CAS circular 7/17 December
    1993 and para 77721 AOG
57 Reg 9(1)(c) SS(DLA) Regs 1992 and
    reg 7(1)(c) SS(AA) Regs 1992
58 s21(1)(a) NAA 1948
59 *Steane v. CAO* 1996; para 77723 AOG
60 Part 1D of letter to Directors of Social
    Services dated 12 September 1994
    from ACC and AMA
61 Complaint No.98/C/1842 against
    Stockport MBC 30 March 1999
62 CA/2985/1997
63 s21(1)(a) NAA 1948
64 Those against payment are CA/7126/
    1995, CA/11185/1995, CA/84/1996;
    those for are CA/4723/1995, C3/
    95(AA), C4/95(AA), C2/96(AA), C3/
    96(AA) and C15/96(AA)

7. Temporary absences from care homes

65 Sch 7 para 13(2) ISG Regs 1987
66 Reg 17(2) SS(HIP) Regs 1975
67 Sch 2 para 2A(4A)(b) ISG Regs 1987
68 Sch 2 para 2A(4A)(a) ISG Regs 1987
69 Reg 17(3) SS(HIP) Regs 1975

8. Other sources of financial assistance in care homes

70 Twyman House, 16 Bonny Street,
    London NW1 9PG; tel: 0845 300
    7585
71 46A Chiswick High Road, London W4
    1SZ; tel: 020 8742 1182
72 Tel: 020 7602 6274

Chapter 22

....

Preserved rights

In April 1993 there were radical changes to the public funding of placements in residential and nursing care homes. This chapter explains the rules for the pre-April 1993 system of paying for care and how it continues to apply for those residents in independent sector care homes. This system was largely dependent on higher levels of income support (IS) to fund residential and nursing care placements.[1]

The main conditions of entitlement to IS are explained on p93 and (except for two differences – see p381 below) apply to preserved rights.

This chapter covers:
1. Who has preserved rights to income support? (p377)
2. Protection for disability living allowance care component or attendance allowance and housing benefit (p381)
3. The income support personal expenses allowance (p381)
4. The income support accommodation allowance (p382)
5. Payments to meet shortfalls ('topping up' payments) (p386)
6. Temporary absences from the care home (including going into hospital) (p387)

---

1. Who has preserved rights to income support?

Local authority homes

If you were in a local authority residential home on 31 March 1993 you do not have preserved rights to the higher levels of income support (IS) from April 1993, when the new system came into force. Until April 1996 you would have received some protection from financial loss but this would not have been under the preserved rights system. From April 1996 you are treated in the same way as if you had moved into a local authority residential care home after 31 March 1993 (see Chapters 21 and 23).

22

Chapter 22: Preserved rights
1. Who has preserved rights to income support?

Independent residential care and nursing homes

If you were in or temporarily absent from (see below) a registered independent residential care or nursing home on 31 March 1993 you have preserved rights to higher levels of IS (see p381) under the pre-April 1993 system to help meet the costs of the home if:

- you were living in, or only temporarily absent (see below) from a residential or nursing care home on 31 March 1993; *and*
- you were entitled to IS at the higher level (see p381); *or*
- you were paying for the costs of the home without IS (ie, you were self-funding) but now you want to claim IS because your capital is less than £16,000.[2]

There are special rules that apply if you were living in a 'small home' (see below) or an Abbeyfield home or a home provided by a close relative (see p379).

A '**temporary absence**' for the purpose of establishing whether you have preserved rights is defined as:

- up to 52 weeks if you are a patient in hospital throughout the period of absence; *or*
- up to 4 weeks if you are a temporary resident in the home; *or*
- up to 13 weeks if you are a permanent resident in the home.[3]

Once you have acquired preserved rights, a subsequent temporary absence (see p387) from a residential or nursing care home will not remove those rights. Even if you move to a new home or a different type of home – eg, from a residential care home to a nursing home (but not a home owned or managed by the local authority) – you will maintain your preserved rights and will receive IS at the appropriate rate for the type of care you receive in the new home. You will only lose your preserve rights if you are absent from the residential or nursing care home for longer than a temporary absence (see p387). In these circumstances the funding of your stay will be under the new system (see Chapters 21 and 23).

'Small homes'

A '**small home**' is defined as one with fewer than four residents. These homes were required to register with the local authority from 1 April 1993 in England and Wales. Such homes had already had to register in Scotland. If you were in a small home on 31 March 1999 you will have preserved rights to the higher levels of IS if:

- you were living in, or only temporarily absent (see above) from the home on 31 March 1993; *and*
- you were in receipt of the higher levels of IS on that date (see p381); *and*
- the home was either registered or in the process of being so; *or*

Chapter 22: Preserved rights
1. Who has preserved rights to income support?

22

- you were resident on 31 March 1993 in a small home which was exempt from registration (due to one or more residents being treated as close relatives for registration purposes); *and*
- you were continuously resident (apart from 'temporary absences' see p378) between 1 April 1993 and 4 October 1993.[4]

Note: If you were self-funding on 31 March 1993 you do not have preserved rights.

Homes provided by close relatives

If you were living with, or later move to a home that is provided in whole or part by a 'close relative', or other than on a commercial basis, you will not have preserved rights (unless it is provided via a limited company).[5] However, if the ownership changes or you move to a new home which is not provided by a 'close relative', you will be entitled to the preserved rights levels of IS.[6]

A 'close relative' means a parent, parent-in-law, step-parent, son, daughter, son/daughter-in-law, step-son/daughter, sister, brother or the married or unmarried partner of any of these.

Abbeyfield Homes

If you were a resident in an Abbeyfield Home (very sheltered accommodation), you also have preserved rights, but since April 1996 if you are in an unregistered Abbeyfield home your preserved rights are suspended if you have to buy in care over and above that provided by Abbeyfield. You then claim IS at the ordinary rates and housing benefit. Your preserved rights are reinstated if any of the conditions giving rise to the suspension cease to apply.[7]

Couples

If you are one of a couple permanently in a care home and your partner is remaining in the community, you will each be assessed as separate individuals according to individual resources. However, there may be a requirement for the non-resident spouse to pay maintenance (see Chapter 8). This also applies where you both live permanently in different care homes.

Normally for IS purposes, couples who move into a home and share a room are still treated as a couple and their resources aggregated, as they are considered to be part of the same household. However, recent social security commissioners' decisions[8] suggest that in most cases you should still be treated as separate individuals. This is especially important when your capital is considered as if you are treated as one of a couple in permanent care, the capital limit for IS purposes is £16,000 for both of you, whereas if you were treated as separate individuals the joint capital limit would be £32,000 (see also p428).

22

Chapter 22: Preserved rights
1. Who has preserved rights to income support?

If you are one of a couple permanently in a care home with preserved rights and you are later joined by your partner, you will continue to be entitled to the preserved rights to higher levels of IS but your partner will not have preserved rights. S/he will be entitled to the ordinary rate of IS including the residential allowance, and social services rather then the DSS will be responsible for helping to meet the cost of her/his placement under the new system (see Chapters 21 and 23).

If you were residing with your partner (ie, treated as a couple) on 31 March 1993 and your partner had a preserved right, but now *you* need to claim IS yourself (eg, because your partner has died) *you* now have the preserved right.[9]

When you will not be entitled to preserved rights

Even if you were living in an independent residential care or nursing home on 31 March 1993 (or were temporarily absent) you will not be entitled to preserved rights to higher levels of IS if:

- the home is not registered (unless it is a 'small home' which is exempt – see p378);[10] *or*
- the home is not provided on a commercial basis; *or*
- the home is run wholly or partly by a close relative (see p379); *or*
- your placement was sponsored by a local authority before April 1993 and you were only entitled to the Part III residential accommodation rate of IS; *or*
- you move permanently to residential accommodation which is owned or managed by a local authority; *or*
- you were living in local authority residential accommodation which, while you were living there, but after 12 August 1991, was changed to become an independent residential care home[11] (see p348); *or*
- you are absent from the home for a period that exceeds the specified periods that can be treated as a temporary absence (see p387).

If you were living in a local authority owned or managed home on 31 March 1993 and now want to move to an independent care home you may continue to get the Part III residential accommodation rate of IS only.[12] However, a recent social security commissioner's decision suggests that from 10 April 1995 this no longer applies and the normal IS applicable amount including the residential allowance should be applied[13] (also see p348).

2. Protection for disability living allowance care component or attendance allowance and housing benefit

If you have a preserved right to the higher levels of IS and social services does not make any top-up payment for your care (see p386), you will be entitled to receive **disability living allowance (DLA) care component or attendance allowance (AA)** (where you satisfy the conditions for these benefits) under the rules of the pre-April 1993 system. However, these benefits will be treated as income for IS purposes, thus reducing the amount of IS that would otherwise be payable.[14] The advantage of receiving DLA care component or AA is that if you qualify for the highest rate of either of these benefits, it will enable you to qualify for the higher 'very dependent elderly' rate of IS accommodation allowance[15] (see p383).

In England and Wales only, if you have been living in, or temporarily absent from, adult placement scheme accommodation and receiving normal levels of IS and, if the accommodation was then required to register because it provided both board and personal care,[16] you will continue to be entitled to DLA care component or AA.

If you were in receipt of **protected housing benefit (HB)** in respect of an independent care home on 31 March 1993, this will continue. However, if you have preserved rights to IS and subsequently claim the higher levels of IS, your HB will stop permanently after four weeks.

If you were entitled to HB in respect of a registered home on 29 October 1990 you are eligible for life unless you make a claim for the higher levels of IS. However, if you are:

- in registered accommodation and are in remunerative work; *or*
- in a home run by a 'close relative'; *or*
- in a small home which was not required to register until 1 April 1993,

protection will only remain while you live (or are temporarily absent for up to 52 weeks) at the same address.

If you have protected rights to HB (or you are in an unregistered Abbeyfield home – see p379), the tariff income on your capital will only start at more than £10,000 (see p191).

3. The income support personal expenses allowance

The main conditions of entitlement for income support (IS) and the way your income and capital are treated also apply to people with preserved rights in residential care and nursing homes (see Chapters 3, 6 and 7). However, there are two important differences:

- the capital limit is £16,000 rather than £8,000, so you can claim IS when your capital is £16,000 or less. The tariff income starts at more than £10,000 rather than at more than at £3,000. The higher capital limits will continue to apply if you are absent from the home for up to 52 weeks if you are over pensionable age or up to 13 weeks in other cases;[17]
- if you have a spouse who is not living with you and you are giving her/him at least 50 per cent of your occupational pension or personal pension or payment from a retirement annuity, then half your pension is disregarded as income.[18]

If you are in a residential care or nursing home and you have a preserved right, your IS applicable amount is worked out differently. Instead of a personal allowance and premiums, you will get a weekly allowance for personal expenses called a personal expenses allowance (PEA)[19] and an accommodation allowance[20] (see p382).

The personal expenses allowances are:

single person		£14.75
couple		£29.50
dependent child	aged 18+	£14.75
	aged 16–17	£10.25
	aged 11–15	£8.85
	aged 0–10	£6.05

4. **The income support accommodation allowance**

The weekly amount of IS you receive will depend on the type of home you are in and the type of care you receive. It will cover meals and services where these are provided but only up to a maximum national limit (see below).[21] In all categories, in Greater London, the limit for a nursing home is £50 higher and the limit for a residential care home is £45 higher.[22]

If your residential or nursing care home charge does not cover all your meals, your accommodation allowance will include either an amount to cover the actual cost of the meals if they can be purchased in the home, or if they cannot, the following standard amounts for each person:

- £1.10 for breakfast;
- £1.55 for midday meal;
- £1.55 for evening meal.

The above amounts are reduced if meals are provided free or at a lower cost.[23]

If you pay additional charges for heating, attendance needs, extra baths, laundry or a special diet needed for medical reasons, these will be allowed for in your accommodation allowance as long as they are provided by the home and not by an outside agency.[24]

Even if you pay additional charges and/or meals are not included, you cannot get more than the appropriate maximum national limit of accommodation allowance for the type of home you are in and the type of care you receive.

If you receive HB towards part of your accommodation charge, this will be deducted from the charge and reduces your IS accordingly.[25]

Residential care homes

If you are in a residential home, the maximum accommodation allowance varies according to the type of care the home is registered to provide, or if the home is not registered, according to the type of care you receive.[26] The type of care depends on your health condition and/or age (see p384 for definitions used in the tables). If more than one category could apply to you, the amount you will get is decided as follows:

- where the home is registered with the local authority to provide the type of care you get, you will receive the amount that is allowed for that type of care;
- if the care you receive is different from the type that the home is registered to provide, you will receive the allowance for the lower or lowest of the categories of care which the home is registered to provide;
- in any other case you receive the amount most consistent with the care you receive.[27]

Health condition/age	Maximum payable
Old age	£218
Past or present mental disorder (but not mental handicap)	£230
Past or present drug or alcohol dependence	£230
Mental handicap	£262
Physical disablement under pension age, or, if over pension age, physical disablement occurring before reaching 60 years of age (65 if a man)	£298
Physical disablement over pension age	£218
Very dependent elderly	£252
Any other condition	£218

Note: The above amounts are increased by £45 for homes in the Greater London area.

Nursing homes

If you are in a nursing home registered by the health authority the maximum accommodation allowance varies according to the type of care you actually receive, as a nursing home is not registered for particular categories of care. The type of care depends on your health condition and/or age (see p384 for definitions used in the tables). If more than one category could apply to you, you receive the amount most consistent with the care you receive.[28] You could, for example, get the terminal illness rate if that is the type of care you receive, even though you are not, in fact, terminally ill.[29]

Health condition/age	Maximum payable
Past or present mental disorder (but not mental handicap)	£326
Mental handicap	£332
Past or present drug or alcohol dependence	£326
Physical disablement' under pension age, or, if over pension age, physical disablement occurring before reaching 60 (65 if a man)	£367
Physical disablement' over pension age	£325
Terminal illness	£325
Any other condition (including elderly)	£325

Note: The above amounts are increased by £50 for homes in the Greater London area.

Residential care and nursing homes

Some homes may be registered as both a residential care and nursing home (dual registration). In these cases your maximum AA is determined according to whether you are receiving residential or nursing care.

Definitions for health conditions listed in tables

- **'Mental disorder'** means 'mental illness, arrested or incomplete development of mind, psychopathic disorder, and any other disorder or disability of mind'.[30]
- **'Mental handicap'** means 'a stage of arrested or incomplete development of mind which includes impairment of intelligence and social functioning.[31]

Note: 'Senility' is not 'mental handicap' but can amount to a 'mental disorder'.[32]

- **'Physical Disablement'** means 'blind, deaf or dumb or substantially and permanently handicapped by illness, injury or congenital deformity or any other disability prescribed by the Secretary of State'.[33]
- **'Very dependent elderly'** means you are over pension age and either:
  - registered or certified as blind; or

 – entitled to AA or DLA care component at the highest rate; *or*
 – getting war or industrial injury constant attendance allowance.[34]

When you can get more than the maximum accommodation allowance

You can get more than the maximum accommodation allowance if one of the following applies:

- you have lived in the same accommodation for over 12 months and you could afford it without IS when you moved in. In these circumstances you will get the full accommodation charge for up to 13 weeks after you claim IS if you are trying to move but you need time to find suitable alternative accommodation. However, income which is normally disregarded for IS may be taken into account during the 13 weeks;[35] *or*

- you have been living in the same residential care or nursing home since 28 April 1985 and your accommodation allowance under the present rules is lower than the actual weekly charge you were paying immediately before 29 April 1985, plus £10.[36]

- -

Example:

Mr Hill is aged 80 years and has been living in an independent residential care home since 23 February 1993. The home charges £252 a week inclusive of meals and services. He has a state retirement pension of £66.75 a week, an occupational pension of £53.00 a week and attendance allowance at the higher rate of £52.95 a week.

Mr Hill's IS will be calculated in the following way:

Income:

State retirement pension	£66.75
Occupational pension	£53.00
Attendance allowance	£52.95
Total	**£172.70**

Applicable amount:

Personal expenses allowance	£14.75
Accommodation allowance	£252.00
Total applicable amount	£266.75

Applicable amount (£266.75) minus income (£172.70) = IS (£94.05)

Mr Hill is entitled to IS of £94.05 a week. This will top up his income from his retirement pension, occupational pension and attendance allowance so that he can pay the costs of his home (£252) and be left with a personal expenses allowance of £14.75.

- -

5. **Payments to meet shortfalls ('topping up' payments)**

The amount of IS you receive may not meet the full cost of your residential or nursing care home. In these circumstances you may need to seek help from relatives or charities (any payment of this nature is ignored for IS purposes – see Chapter 6). Often residents find that they have to use their PEA or run down their capital. Sometimes it is possible to negotiate your fee with the care home so that you only pay the IS national limit.

In limited circumstances (see below) social services can help. Even where social services cannot provide financial help, they are expected to provide 'advice and guidance' to help people in difficulty to find alternative accommodation using their preserved rights and 'any other resources available to them'.[37]

Legislation prevents social services from helping fund a place in an independent home for a person with a preserved right,[38] unless in specific circumstances they can fund that person under special exemptions.[39]

Social services can only help you in the following circumstances:
- if you were already receiving a topping up payment on 31 March 1993;[40]
- if you are under pension age in either a residential or nursing home;[41]
- if you are over pension age in a residential care home only (see below for nursing homes) and you face eviction or the home is about to close.[42]

Note: If you are faced with eviction, the local authority can only place you in a home which is not owned or managed by the person or organisation which owns or manages the current home.

Health authorities may be able to make arrangements for you if you are over pensionable age and in a nursing home with continuing nursing needs and you face eviction or the home is about to close. If your placement is funded by the health authority it will become a 'health' placement and therefore you will be entitled to the hospital rate of IS (see p128).[43]

In the past when social services contributed towards the costs of accommodation charges above the national limits the payments were called topping-up payments. There are no longer such payments because social services now take on all the arrangements and become responsible for the full fee rather than just the top-up. However, IS is still paid at the higher rates from which social services assess the relevant contribution leaving you with no less than the PEA of £14.75.

If you do not have preserved rights or you lose them (eg, because you are absent from the home for longer than a temporary absence – see p387), social services can make arrangements to provide your residential accommodation and care.[44]

In some circumstances where there is a shortfall between your income and the cost of the care home and there is no payment that can be obtained to meet the shortfall, then the only other option (if it is a viable one) may be to lose your preserved rights so that social services can make arrangements to provide your accommodation and care.

6. Temporary absences from the care home (including going into hospital)

For the purposes of keeping your preserved rights entitlements, a 'temporary absence' is defined as:
- up to 52 weeks if you are a patient in a hospital throughout the period of absence; *or*
- up to 4 weeks if you are a temporary resident in the home; *or*
- up to 13 weeks if you are a permanent resident in the home.[45]

However, for the purposes of IS payment:
- if you are away from the home for up to a week, no alteration is made to the amount of the accommodation allowance payable in your IS;
- if you are away for more than a week (other than in local authority accommodation or hospital) and you are not required to be available for work, a retaining fee of 80 per cent of your accommodation allowance can be paid for up to 4 weeks;
- if you are absent from the home because you are in hospital or temporarily admitted to local authority accommodation, an 80 per cent retaining fee can be paid for up to 52 weeks.[46]

Note: If IS is paid as a retainer to the home, IS can also be paid for you in your current situation. There are conflicting commissioner's decisions about your entitlement to a retaining fee if you are temporarily living in another independent residential care or nursing home.[47]

Going into hospital
- **Up to six weeks:** you remain entitled to preserved rights to the higher levels of IS (taking into account any reduction in the charge payable), while you, or a member of your family, have been an in-patient for up to six weeks.[48] If you are a single claimant and you do not have to pay an accommodation charge while you are an in-patient, your applicable amount is reduced to your personal expenses and meals allowances, as long as you are likely to return to the home.[49] If you are unlikely to return, your IS is calculated under the normal rules for a person not in a care home (see p128).[50]

- **After six weeks:** you are entitled to an IS personal allowance of £16.70. If a member of your family remains in the care home, their personal expenses and accommodation allowance (less any amount included for your meals) remain payable (taking into account any reduction in the charge). Otherwise, an amount to cover any retaining fee of up to 80 per cent that you, as the in-patient, are liable for, is payable for up to 52 weeks.[51] A child or young person who has been an in-patient for more than 12 weeks is entitled to a personal allowance of £13.35.[52]

Notes

1 All references to IS include I-JSA.

1. **Who has preserved rights to IS?**
2 Reg 19(1ZB)(a) ISG Regs 1987
3 Reg 19 (IZB)(b) ISG Regs 1987
4 Reg 19(1ZE) and (1ZEA) ISG Regs 1987
5 R(SB)9/89
6 Reg 19(IZC) ISG Regs 1987
7 Reg 19(IZR) ISG Regs 1987
8 CIS/4934/97, CIS/4935/97, CIS/5232/97, CIS/5237/97 and CIS/3767/97 and common appendix
9 Reg 19(IZB)(a)(iii), (IZN) and (IZO) ISG Regs 1987
10 Reg 19(3) ISG Regs 1987
11 Reg 21(3A) ISG Regs 1987
12 Reg 21 (3C) ISG Regs 1987
13 CIS/16440/1996

2. **Protection for DLA component or AA and HB**
14 Sch 9 para 9 ISG Regs 1987
15 Sch 4 para 6(2)(b) ISG Regs 1987
16 Under the RHA (Amdt) 1991

3. **The IS personal expenses allowance**
17 Reg 45(b) ISG Regs 1987
18 Sch 9 para 15B ISG Regs 1987
19 Sch 4 para 13 ISG Regs 1987
20 Sch 4 para 1(1)(a) ISG Regs 1987

4. **Accommodation allowance**
21 Sch 4 para 5 ISG Regs 1987
22 Sch 4 para 11 ISG Regs 1987
23 Sch 4 para 2(2) ISG Regs 1987
24 Sch 4 para 2(1) ISG Regs 1987
25 Sch 4 para 3 ISG Regs 1987
26 Sch 4 para 9 ISG Regs 1987
27 Sch 4 para 10 ISG Regs 1987
28 paras 9(6) and 10(4) ISG Regs 1987
29 CIS/263/1991
30 s55 RHA 1984
31 Reg 1(2) RCH Regs 1984
32 CSB/1171/1986
33 s20(1) RHA 1984
34 Sch 4 para 6(2) ISG Regs 1987
35 Sch 4 paras 12(1) and (2) ISG Regs1987
36 Sch 4 paras 12(3) and (4) ISG Regs 1987

5. **Payments to meet shortfalls**
37 LAC (93) 6; WOC 12/93
38 s26A(1) NAA 1948; s86A SW(S)A 1968
39 RA(RPORE) Regs 1993
40 Reg 4 RA(RPORE) Regs 1993
41 Regs 6 and 7 RA(RPORE) Regs 1993
42 Regs 8 and 9 RA(RPORE) Regs 1993
43 *White v CAO* 1993, *The Times*, 2 August 1993
44 Reg 5 RA(RPORE) Regs 1993

6. **Temporary absences from the care home**
45 Reg 19 (IZF) ISG Regs 1987
46 Sch 7 para 16 ISG Regs 1987
47 CSIS/833/95 and CIS/5415/95
48 Sch 7 para 18(a)(i) and (ii) ISG Regs 1987
49 Sch 7 para 18(a)(iii) ISG Regs 1987
50 Sch 7 para 18(a)(iv) ISG Regs 1987
51 Sch 7 para 18(b) ISG Regs 1987
52 Sch 7 para 18(c) ISG Regs 1987

Chapter 23

. . . .

Charges in care homes

This chapter explains the rules from April 1993 for the way social services make financial assessments to determine the charge or contribution that a person in a care home is required to pay to social services toward the cost of their accommodation and care. It will cover single people and couples in different types of care home for different types of stay. This chapter will only deal with the post-April 1993 system. Social services departments had a very limited role in the pre-April 1993 system, which is dealt with in Chapter 22. It covers:

1. Types of care home (p390)
2. Types of stay (p391)
3. Financial assessments (p393)
4. Example calculations of contributions (p394)
5. Paying the full cost of your care home (p404)
6. Temporary absences from care homes (including going into hospital) (p405)
7. Benefit and contribution examples – complex cases (p406)

This chapter complements Chapter 21 and, together with the general provisions in Part IV, they provide a comprehensive analysis of benefits and charges in care homes the post-April 1993 system.

---

1. Types of care home

Social services have a duty to make arrangements for providing residential care for all those who 'by reason of age, illness, disability, or any other circumstances are in need of care and attention which is not otherwise available to them' (or, in Scotland, for 'persons in need').[1] Residential care can be provided in any of the following types of care home (see p268 for definitions):

- local authority residential accommodation (sometimes known as Part III homes or Part IV homes in Scotland);
- registered independent residential care homes (including registered 'small homes');
- registered independent nursing homes;
- dual registered independent residential care and nursing homes;

- independent or local authority homes not providing board.

For financial assessment purposes the homes in the first four categories above are subject to the same rules for the calculation of your contribution payable to social services towards the cost of your accommodation and care.

Less dependent residents

If you are a resident in an independent sector home which is not required to be registered, or in local authority residential accommodation where board is not provided, then you are a 'less dependent resident'.[2]

'Board' is defined as 'at least some cooked or prepared meals which are both cooked and prepared, by a person other than the resident or a member of his family, and consumed at those premises or in associated premises, if the cost of those meals is accounted for as part of the standard rate for the accommodation at those premises'.

In these circumstances, social services have complete discretion to ignore the whole of the charging assessment if it is 'reasonable in the circumstances'. This is because it has been recognised that to live as independently as possible, you will need to be left with more than the personal expenses allowance (PEA).[3]

Guidance states that factors to be taken into account in deciding how much it is reasonable to disregard from resources include:

- your commitments – ie, to what extent you are incurring costs directly for necessities such as food, fuel and clothing;
- the degree of your independence – ie, to what extent should you be encouraged to take on expenditure commitments;
- whether you need a greater incentive to become more independent – eg, you may be encouraged to take on paid employment if most or all of your earnings are disregarded.[4]

If you receive care in an unregistered **Abbeyfield Home or as an in-patient in a hospital or similar institution**, you will not be receiving any social services funding and therefore you are not subject to the financial assessment rules explained in this chapter.

2. **Types of stay**

There are four types of stay in a care home:

- permanent;
- temporary;
- respite;
- trial period.

A **permanent** stay for financial assessment purposes is a stay which is permanent from the day that you enter the care home or, if you enter on a temporary or trial period basis, from any subsequent day on which decide that you do not intend to return to the community to live. (This is the same as for social security benefit purposes.)

A **temporary** stay is defined as a stay that is unlikely to exceed 52 weeks or, in exceptional circumstances, unlikely substantially to exceed that period.[5] (This is a similar definition to that for social security benefit purposes except that it is defined in terms of a temporary absence from your normal home and there are also some additional conditions that have to be satisfied – see p349).

A **respite** stay is not defined in the legislation. However, it is merely a stay that is part of a planned programme of *temporary* stays and therefore (as for social security benefit purposes) the definition of 'temporary' stay applies.

A **trial period** stay is not defined in the legislation. However, it is defined in social security legislation (see p349), and the 13 week rule for trial period stays is referred to in the guidance as 'applying to people who enter residential accommodation initially on a temporary basis during which it is decided whether they need to stay in residential accommodation or can return home. Their stay in residential accommodation is generally a conditional one with a number of factors influencing whether or not they will return home or eventually stay permanently in residential accommodation'.[6]

This clearly means that a 'trial period' stay should be treated as a temporary stay by social services until a decision is made with regard to whether the stay is to become 'permanent'. However, some social services departments treat a 'trial period' stay (sometimes called 'temporary with a view to permanent') as a 'permanent' stay. This can be challenged using the complaints procedure (see p340) if you are disadvantaged in the financial assessment by having your stay treated as permanent – eg, if the value of your home in the community is taken into account as capital or the disregard on your income for outgoings is not being allowed.

Some social services departments only use the 'permanent' or 'temporary' definitions of types of stay, which can then cause problems for social security benefits in terms of whether the 52 week temporary rule or the 13 week trial period rule should be applied. In these circumstances, further information would need to be provided to the housing benefits department and/or Benefits Agency.

It is recognised that a stay which was initially expected to be permanent may turn out to be temporary, and a stay initially expected to be temporary may turn out to be permanent. In these circumstances, social services are advised to assess you according to your actual circumstances at the time – ie, not to continue to treat your home in the community as capital in the case of a permanent stay becoming temporary or not to treat your own home in the community as capital from the outset in the case of a temporary stay becoming permanent.[7] Similarly, in the case of a trial period stay, if it is decided during the course of your stay that you will either definitely return home at a future date or that you will not be returning home (ie, your stay changes to temporary or permanent) then the financial assessment will be reviewed accordingly. In these circumstances it will be important to advise the housing benefits department and/or Benefits Agency of the change in the status of your stay.

3. **Financial assessments**

Legislation requires that if you are placed in a residential care home (local authority or independent sector, residential or nursing) by social services, you repay to them the cost of the accommodation if you are capable of doing so.[8] A standard rate is fixed for the accommodation and if you have sufficient income or capital you will be required to pay the full cost – ie, the standard rate.[9]

The 'standard rate' for local authority homes is the full cost to social services of your placement.[10] The 'standard rate' for independent homes is the gross cost to social services of providing or paying for your placement under the contract with the home.[11]

If you are unable to meet the cost in full, and you provide the necessary financial information for an assessment to be carried out, social services will only charge the amount determined by the assessment.[12]

Note: If you are a resident who helps in the running of your residential accommodation and it is managed by the local authority, part of your charges may be waived in recognition of this.[13]

Legislation provides for the assessment of resources that is required by social services (for placements made after 31 March 1993) in order to establish the amount that you will be required to contribute to the cost of your placement in a local authority or an independent care home (see Chapters 13 and 14).[14]

For the first eight weeks of any placement, social services do not have to carry out a financial assessment (although many choose to do so). Instead they can charge what they consider to be reasonable.[15] Many local authorities charge what is commonly referred to as the Part III rate, which is the basic retirement pension (£66.75) minus the personal expenses allowance (£14.75) – ie, £52.00. If you do not consider that the charge is reasonable for your circumstances you can ask social services to undertake a full financial assessment.

The financial assessment should be an assessment of your (as the resident) income and capital only. Social services have no power to assess a couple according to their joint resources. Each person entering care should be assessed according to their individual means although the liability of a married person to maintain their spouse can be considered[16] (see Chapter 17).

The amount you are assessed to pay as your contribution should be reviewed and revised as and when the amount of your income and/or capital changes. For most people this will probably be once a year in April when social security benefits are uprated. Most social services departments send out a letter asking you to state the new amounts of your benefits. As for social security benefit purposes, you have a duty to disclose any change in your circumstances to social services including any changes in your income and/or capital.

The calculation that is undertaken by social services in the financial assessment to determine the amount you will be required to contribute to the cost of your accommodation and care is:

> **Total assessable income** (including any tariff income from your capital) (see Chapters 13 and 14)
> *minus*
> **Outgoings** (for a temporary resident who has outgoings for their home in the community – see Chapter 15)
> *minus*
> **Personal expenses allowance** *(PEA)* (see Chapter 15)
> *equals*
> **Contribution to accommodation and care costs (charge)**

If you disagree with any part of your financial assessment you can use the complaints procedure (a copy of which should be available from social services) to ask for it to be reviewed (see p340).

It is important to remember that if social services make arrangements to provide your accommodation and care under the National Assistance Act 1948 or, in Scotland, the Social Work (Scotland) Act 1968, they have responsibility for payment of the care home fees and for the collection of your contributions and any third party payments (see Chapter 16). The placement itself must be maintained even if payments are not made or made late.

4. **Example calculations of contributions**

The following are examples of how your contribution to the cost of your accommodation and care is calculated for different types of home, for different types of stay, and for different personal situations – eg, for a single person or for one member of a couple.

These examples cover the contribution calculation which, if you are reliant on social security benefits to make a contribution for the cost of your accommodation and care, is the second part of the process. The first part of the process is the determination of the amount of income support (IS) payable. Each of the examples below is continued from the IS calculations in Chapter 21.

If you are not entitled to IS because you have income in excess of your applicable amount, but you are not self-funding as social services help with the cost of your placement, then the contribution calculations can still be appropriate as examples if you substitute your type of income for the IS amounts stated.

These examples deal with the most common situations:
- a single person in local authority residential accommodation for a temporary stay;
- a single person in local authority residential accommodation for a permanent stay;
- one of a couple in local authority residential accommodation for a temporary stay;
- one of a couple in local authority residential accommodation for a permanent stay;
- a single person in an independent care home for a temporary stay;
- a single person in an independent care home for a permanent stay;
- one of a couple in an independent care home for a temporary stay;
- one of a couple in an independent care home for a permanent stay.

There are examples of more complex situations in the complete benefits and contributions calculations – see p406.

A single person in local authority residential accommodation for a temporary stay

Mr Guest is a single person aged 64 years living in a rented council house. His income before entering the home is made up of long-term incapacity benefit (IB), IS and disability living allowance (DLA) care and mobility components. Mr Guest also receives maximum housing benefit (HB) and council tax benefit (CTB). He has savings of £3,500. He goes into local authority residential accommodation for a temporary stay of two weeks.

Following a review, IS is stopped (see Chapter 21 for benefit calculation).

After Mr Guest's benefits have been reviewed by the Benefits Agency, he informs social services, and they amend his financial assessment. There are different capital rules that apply for financial assessment purposes. Any capital/savings of £10,000 or less do not attract a tariff income. Therefore, Mr Guest's savings of £3,500 are not taken into account in the financial assessment.

His contribution to the cost of his accommodation and care will be calculated in the following way:

Income:	Incapacity benefit (long-term)	£75.65
	Total	**£75.65**

(DLA care component £52.95 disregarded as income)
(DLA mobility component £37.00 disregarded as income)

Outgoings:	Water rates	£3.00
	Standing charges for fuel	£1.90
	Total	**£4.90**
	Personal expenses allowance (PEA):	**£14.75**

Income (£75.65) minus outgoings (£4.90), minus (PEA) (£14.75) = contribution (£56.00)

Mr Guest's contribution to the cost is £56.00 a week.
Mr Guest will be left with £109.60 a week (DLA care and mobility components, outgoings and PEA).
The full cost of local authority residential accommodation is £252 a week.
Social services' contribution to the cost is £196.00 a week.

A single person in local authority residential accommodation for a permanent stay

Mrs Gascoigne is a single person aged 80 years living in a rented council house. Her income, before entering the home, is made up of state retirement pension, a works pension, IS and attendance allowance (AA). Mrs Gascoigne also receives maximum HB and CTB. She goes into local authority residential accommodation on a permanent basis.

Following a review, IS is stopped (see Chapter 21 for benefit calculations).

After Mrs Gascoigne's benefits have been reviewed by the Benefits Agency, she informs social services and they amend her financial assessment. There are no disregards on her income for outgoings as she no longer has a home in the community. (If Mrs Gascoigne was serving a notice period on her tenancy and was still required to pay rent, an increase in her PEA could be allowed to cover the rent for the notice period.)

Her contribution to the cost of her accommodation and care will be calculated in the following way:

Income 1:	State retirement pension	£68.20
(first 4 weeks)	Works pension	£3.10
	AA	£52.95
	Total	**£124.25**
	PEA	£14.75

Income (£124.25) minus PEA (£14.75) = contribution (£109.50)

Mrs Gascoigne's contribution to the cost is £109.50 a week.
Mrs Gascoigne will be left with £14.75 a week (PEA).
The full cost of local authority residential accommodation is £252 a week.
Social services' contribution to the cost for the first 4 weeks is £142.50 a week.

Income 2:	State retirement pension	£68.20
(after 4 weeks)	Works pension	£3.10
	Total	**£71.30**
	PEA	£14.75

Income (£71.30) minus PEA (£14.75) = contribution (£56.55)

Mrs Gascoigne's contribution to the cost after 4 weeks is £56.55 a week.
Mrs Gascoigne will be left with £14.75 a week (PEA).
The full cost of local authority residential accommodation is £252 a week.
Social services' contribution to the cost after 4 weeks is £195.45 a week.

One of a couple in local authority residential accommodation for a temporary stay

Mr and Mrs Love, aged 65 and 63 years respectively, are home owners (without a mortgage). Mr Love's weekly income, before entering the home, is made up of state retirement pension, IS and DLA and care mobility components. Mrs Love also receives state retirement pension and maximum CTB is in payment. Mr Love goes into local authority residential accommodation for a temporary stay of three weeks.
Following a review, IS of £21.71 a week is awarded to Mr Love in respect of himself and Mrs Love (see Chapter 21 for benefit calculation).
After Mr and Mrs Love's IS has been reviewed by the Benefits Agency, they inform social services and Mr Love's financial assessment is amended. Although Mr and Mrs Love are a couple, for financial assessment purposes Mr Love, as the person going into care, will be assessed according to his income only. However, as Mr Love receives IS for himself and for Mrs Love based on a calculation of their joint income, social services will consider increasing his PEA in order to allow enough for Mrs Love to meet her living expenses in the community. If the PEA is increased, so that Mr Love can give Mrs Love an appropriate amount to meet her living expenses, then the outgoings can be shared equally and only half of the total amount disregarded from Mr Love's income. As there are no rules about how social services should divide the IS this may vary around the country.

Note: If there were any other adults living with Mr and Mrs Love, the outgoings would be shared equally between the total number of people sharing the home and only Mr Love's appropriate share allowed as a disregard on his income.

Mr Love's contribution to the cost of his accommodation and care will be calculated in the following way:

Income:		
	State retirement pension	£75.45
	Works pension	£4.64
	Income support	£21.71
	Total	**£101.80**

(DLA mobility component £37.00 disregarded as income)
(DLA care component £35.40 disregarded as income)

Outgoings:

Water rates	£3.50	÷ by 2 = £1.75
Standing charges for fuel	£1.90	÷ by 2 = .95
Buildings and contents insurance premium	£8.80	÷ by 2 = 4.40
Total	£7.10	
PEA	(normal rate for Mr Love) £14.75	
	(amount for Mrs Love*) £35.05	
Total	**£49.80**	

* The amount for Mrs Love is calculated on the basis of her IS applicable amount of £75.00 minus her income of £39.95 state retirement pension.

Income (£101.80) minus outgoings (£7.10), minus PEA (£48.80) = contribution (£44.90)

Mr Love's contribution to the cost is £44.90 a week.
Mr Love will be left with £129.30 a week (£35.05 of which he will give to Mrs Love to top up her retirement pension of £39.95 a week; the remainder will be DLA care and mobility components, outgoings and PEA).
The full cost of local authority residential accommodation is £252 a week.
Social services' contribution to the cost is £207.10 a week.

One of a couple in local authority residential accommodation for a permanent stay

Mr and Mrs Leal, aged 85 and 80 years respectively, are home owners (without a mortgage). Mr Leal's weekly income before entering the home is made up of state retirement pension, works pension and AA. Mrs Leal also receives state retirement pension. They have joint savings of £10,000. They are not entitled to IS, but they receive some CTB as a couple in the community. Mr Leal goes into local authority residential accommodation on a permanent basis.

Following their claims for IS, Mr Leal is not entitled but Mrs Leal is entitled to £34.30 a week (see Chapter 21 for benefit calculation).

Social services undertake a financial assessment for Mr Leal. Mr Leal's savings of £5,000 are not taken into account as they fall below the amount of £10,000 allowed for a person in care. His home in the community is not taken into account as capital because Mrs Leal is still living there. There are no disregards on Mr Leal's income for outgoings as he is permanently away from his home in the community.

Mr Leal's contribution to the cost of his accommodation and care will be calculated in the following way:

Income 1:	State retirement pension	£66.75
(first 4 weeks)	Works pension	£12.88
	AA	£52.95
	Total	**£132.58**
	PEA	£14.75

Income (£132.58) minus PEA (£14.75) = contribution (£117.83)

Mr Leal's contribution to the cost for the first 4 weeks is £117.83 a week.
Mr Leal will be left with £14.75 a week PEA.

The full cost of local authority residential accommodation is £252 a week.

Social services' contribution to the cost for the first 4 weeks is £134.17.

Income 2:	State retirement pension	£66.75
(after 4 weeks)	Works pension	£12.88
	Total	**£79.63**
	PEA	£14.75

Income (£79.63) minus PEA (£14.75) = contribution (£64.88)

Mr Leal's contribution to the cost after 4 weeks is £64.88 a week.
Mr Leal will be left with £14.75 a week PEA

The full cost of local authority residential accommodation is £252 a week.

Social services' contribution to the cost after four weeks is £187.12.

A single person in an independent care home for a temporary stay

Mrs Kaur is a single person aged 70 years, living on her own. She is a home owner with a mortgage. Her income, before entering the home, is made up of state retirement pension, works pension, IS and AA. She also receives maximum CTB and she has savings of £7,000 in a building society. She goes into an independent residential care home for a temporary stay of 6 weeks.

Following a review, IS of £81.90 a week is awarded for the first four weeks of Mrs Kaur's stay. £34.90 a week is awarded for the last two weeks of her stay (see Chapter 21 for benefit calculation).

After Mrs Kaur's benefits have been reviewed by the Benefits Agency, she informs social services and they amend her financial assessment. Any capital/savings of

£10,000 or less do not attract a tariff income, therefore, Mrs Kaur's savings of £7,000 are not taken into account in the financial assessment.

Mrs Kaur's contribution to the cost of her accommodation and care will be calculated in the following way:

Income 1:

(first 4 weeks)	State retirement pension	£74.05
	Works pension	£15.45
	IS	£81.90
	Total	**£171.40**

(AA £52.95 disregarded as income)

Outgoings:

	Water rates	£4.00
	Mortgage payments	£22.00
	Buildings and contents insurance premium	£8.80
	Standing charge for fuel	£1.90
	Total	**£36.70**

PEA   £14.75

Income (£171.40) minus outgoings (£36.70), minus PEA (£14.75) = contribution (£111.95)

Mrs Kaur's contribution to the cost for the first four weeks is £119.95 a week.

Mrs Kaur will be left with £104.40 a week (AA, outgoings and PEA).

The full cost of the independent residential accommodation is £252 a week.

Social services' contribution to the cost for the first four weeks is £132.05 a week.

Income 2:

(after 4 weeks)	State retirement pension	£74.05
	Works pension	£15.45
	IS	£34.90
	Total	**£124.40**

Outgoings:

	Water rates	£4.00
	Mortgage payments	£22.00
	Buildings and contents insurance premium	£8.80
	Standing charges for fuel	£1.90
	Total	**£36.70**

PEA £14.75

Income (£124.40) minus outgoings (£36.70) minus PEA (£14.75) = contribution (£72.95)

Mrs Kaur's contribution to the cost of the last two weeks is £72.95 a week.

Mrs Kaur will be left with £51.45 a week (outgoings and PEA).

The full cost of the independent residential accommodation is £252 a week.

Social services' contribution to the cost for the last 2 weeks is £179.05 a week.

A single person in an independent care home for a permanent stay

Mr Hughes is a single person aged 58 years. He is a home owner (without a mortgage) and he lives with his sister who is disabled. His income before entering the home is made up of incapacity benefits (IB) and DLA care and mobility components. He also receives some CTB and has savings of £5,000. Mr Hughes is not entitled to IS whilst he is living in the community. He goes into an independent nursing home on a permanent basis. As he is a permanent resident in the home he is no longer liable for council tax.

Following a claim for IS, Mr Hughes is awarded £91.65 a week for the first 4 weeks of his stay and £51.90 a week after four weeks (see Chapter 21 for benefit calculation). After Mr Hughes' IS claim has been decided by the Benefits Agency, he informs social services and they amend his financial assessment. Mr Hughes' savings of £5,000 do not attract a tariff income as they are less than the amount of £10,000 allowed for a person in care. His home in the community is not taken into account as capital as his disabled sister lives there. There are no disregards on Mr Hughes' income for outgoings as he is permanently away from his home in the community.

Mr Hughes' contribution to the cost of his accommodation and care will be calculated in the following way:

Income 1:

(first 4 weeks)		
	IB (long term)	£80.80
	IS	£91.65
	DLA care component	£52.95
	Total	**£225.40**

(DLA mobility component £37.00 disregarded as income)

PEA £14.75

Income (£225.40) minus PEA (£14.75) = contribution (£210.65)

Mr Hughes' contribution to the cost for the first 3 weeks is £210.65 a week.

Mr Hughes will be left with £51.75 a week (DLA mobility component and PEA).

The full cost of the independent nursing home is £367 a week.

Social Services' contribution to the cost for the first 4 weeks is £156.35 a week.

Income 2
(after 4 weeks)

	IB (long term)	£80.80
	IS	£51.90
	Total	**£132.70**

(DLA mobility component £37.00 disregarded as income)

PEA £14.75

Income (£132.70) minus PEA (£14.75) = contribution (£117.95).
Mr Hughes' contribution to the cost after four weeks is £117.95 a week.
Mr Hughes will be left with £51.75 a week (DLA mobility component and PEA).
The full cost of the independent nursing home is £367 a week.
Social services' contribution to the cost after four weeks is £249.05 a week.

One of a couple in an independent care home for a temporary stay

Mr and Mrs McEwan, aged 65 and 55 years respectively, are council tenants. Mr McEwan's weekly income is made up of state retirement pension and a works pension. Mrs McEwan's weekly income, before entering the home, is made up of severe disablement allowance and DLA care and mobility components. They also receive some HB and CTB and they have joint savings of £4,000. They are not entitled to IS as a couple in the community. Mrs McEwan goes into a private residential care home for three weeks.

Following the claim for IS, Mrs McEwan, as the claimant, is awarded £75.10 a week for herself and Mr McEwan (see Chapter 21 for benefit calculation).

After Mr and Mrs McEwan's IS claim has been decided by the Benefits Agency, they inform social services and Mr McEwan's financial assessment is amended. Although Mr and Mrs McEwan are a couple, for financial assessment purposes Mrs McEwan, as the person going into care, will be assessed according to her income and capital only. However, as Mrs McEwan receives IS for herself and Mr McEwan based on a calculation of their joint income, social services will consider increasing her PEA if necessary in order to allow enough for Mr McEwan to meet his living expenses. In this case, though, Mr McEwan's income is above his individual applicable amount, so it may not be considered necessary to increase Mrs McEwan's PEA. In fact, in these circumstances, it could be considered appropriate for social services to ask Mr McEwan for a reasonable contribution towards the cost of Mrs McEwan's care under the liable relative provisions (see Chapter 17).

Mr and Mrs McEwan's joint savings are divided equally. There are different capital rules that apply for financial assessment purposes. Any capital/savings of £10,000 or less do not attract a tariff income. Therefore, Mrs McEwan's share of the savings of £2,000 are not taken into account in the financial assessment.

Mrs McEwan's contribution to the cost of her accommodation and care will be calculated in the following way:

Income:

Severe disablement allowance		£54.40
IS		£75.10
Total		**£129.50**

(DLA care component £52.95
disregarded as income)
(DLA mobility component £37.00
disregarded as income)

Outgoings:

Water rates £4.00 ÷ by 2 =	£2.00
Standing charges for fuel 1.90 ÷ by 2 =	£0.95
Building and contents insurance premiums 8.80 ÷ by 2 =	£4.40
Total	**£7.35**
PEA	**£14.75**

Income (£129.50) minus outgoings (£7.35), minus PEA (£14.75) = contribution (£107.40)
Mrs McEwan's contribution to the cost is £107.40 a week.
Mrs McEwan will be left with £89.10 a week (DLA care and mobility components, outgoings and PEA).
Mr McEwan will be left with £113.95 a week (retirement pension and works pension).
The full cost of the independent residential care home is £252 a week.
Social services' contribution to the cost is £144.60 a week.

One of a couple in an independent care home for a permanent stay

Mr and Mrs Spore, aged 59 and 65 respectively, are council tenants. Mr Spore's weekly income is made up of long term IB and IS. Mrs Spore's weekly income before entering the home is made up of state retirement pension and DLA care and mobility components. They also receive maximum HB and CTB. Mrs Spore goes into an independent nursing home on a permanent basis.

Following Mrs Spore's claim for IS, she is awarded £133.42 a week for the first four weeks of her stay. After four weeks £93.67 a week is awarded. Mr Spore's IS entitlement is reviewed and £2.10 a week is awarded (see Chapter 21 for benefit calculation).

After Mrs Spore's IS claim has been decided by the Benefits Agency, she informs social services and her financial assessment is amended. There are no disregards on Mrs Spore's income for outgoings as she is permanently away from her home in the community.

Mrs Spore's contribution to the cost of her accommodation and care will be calculated in the following way:

Income 1

(first 4 weeks)	State retirement pension	£47.98
	IS	£133.42
	DLA care component	£52.95
	Total	**£234.35**

(DLA mobility component £37.00
disregarded as income)

PEA £14.75

Income (£234.35) minus PEA (£14.75) = contribution (£219.60)

Mrs Spore's contribution to the cost for the first 4 weeks is £219.60 a week.

Mrs Spore will be left with £51.75 a week (DLA mobility component and PEA).

The full cost of the independent nursing home is £326 a week.

Social services contribution to the cost for the first four weeks is £106.40 a week.

Income 2

(after 4 weeks)	State retirement pension	£47.98
	IS	£93.67
	Total	**£141.65**

(DLA mobility component £37.00
disregarded as income)

PEA £14.75

Income (£141.65) minus PEA (£14.75) = contribution (£126.90)

Mrs Spore's contribution to the cost after four weeks is £126.90 a week.

Mrs Spore will be left with £51.75 a week (DLA mobility component and PEA).

The full cost of the independent nursing home is £326 a week.

Social services contribution to the cost after four weeks is £199.10 a week.

---

5. **Paying the full cost of your care home**

You may be able to meet the full cost of your accommodation and care in an independent care home from your own resources without any financial help from social services and with (loophole cases) or without (self-funding cases) IS/income-based jobseeker's allowance (JSA) and/or HB from the DSS (see p359). If you are in local authority accommodation you may also be able to meet the full cost of your accommodation and care, although you will not be regarded as self-funding.

If you have capital in excess of £16,000 you will be required to pay the full cost of your accommodation and care (see Chapter 14). However, this does not mean you cannot receive help from social services in terms of an assessment of your needs to establish what services you require and help to find a suitable care home[17] (see p263). Contacting social services for this type of help will benefit you if or when your capital reduces to £16,000, because at that point social services will help with funding your placement in the care home that you are in because they have previously agreed that it meets your assessed needs.

Even if you are self-funding (ie, in an independent care home without IS and/or housing benefit) you could still benefit from social services arranging your placement and contracting with the care home if you cannot do it yourself or if you prefer it is done for you. This will not affect your entitlement to DLA care component or AA (see p356).

If you are required to meet the full cost of your accommodation and care because you are a permanent resident and you have a property in the community which is valued at more than £16,000, you may not actually be able to pay the full cost until your house is sold (but see p369 to find out if the 'loophole' could apply). In these cases, social services can help meet the cost of your accommodation and care and claim the amount back from you when your property is sold (see p324).

6. Temporary absences from care homes (including going into hospital)

Payment of care home fees

There are no rules or guidance governing the payment of care home fees during a temporary absence. If your placement is funded wholly or partly by social services, the arrangement for the payment of fees during any temporary absence you have from the care home will usually be covered in their contract or service agreement with the care home (including temporary absence due to admission to hospital).

Many social services departments have adopted or adapted the pre-1993 rules on preserved rights to higher levels of IS for the cost of care homes during a resident's temporary absence (see p387). However, in cases of preserved rights to IS, the 80 per cent payment can be made for up to 52 weeks if you are in hospital or temporarily admitted to local authority accommodation, and for up to four weeks for any other absence. Many social services departments operate a significantly shorter period for which the 80 per cent payment can be made, at least until a review of the situation is undertaken.

Variation of your contribution to the local authority

If you are away from the care home and as a result the amount of your social security benefits has changed (eg, if you are admitted to hospital – see p125), you should advise social services accordingly. Social services should then review your financial assessment in order to establish a level of contribution to care costs which reflects your new level of benefits.

Variation of personal expenses allowance (PEA)

If you are away from the care home because you are on holiday or visiting family or friends, social services can use their discretion to vary your PEA upwards to enable you to have more money.[18]

7. Benefits and contribution examples – complex cases

The following examples illustrate benefits and contribution calculations in some of the most common complex types of situations. The examples assume that social services undertake a financial assessment for any length of stay in a care home. Some social services departments do not assess for the first eight weeks of a stay in a care home but charge a 'reasonable amount'. Even where social services do not assess, the Benefits Agency still pay the residential allowance where appropriate. From the ninth week, the normal charging rules apply.

The examples are as follows:
* Occupational pension
* Liable relative payment
* IS claimed by partner in the community
* Couple with dependent children
* Couple – both going into a shared room in the same care home
* Loophole/self-funding case (England and Wales only)
* Third party contribution.

Occupational pension

Mr and Mrs Lucas, both aged 76 years, are home owners (without a mortgage). Mr Lucas' weekly income is made up of state retirement pension, an occupational pension and AA. Mrs Lucas' weekly income is made up of state retirement pension and industrial injury disablement benefit. They do not receive any CTB and they are not entitled to IS as a couple in the community. **Mr Lucas goes into an independent nursing care home on a permanent basis.**

Mr Lucas is advised by social services that 50 per cent of his occupational pension can be disregarded by social services if he passes at least 50 per cent to his wife. He decides to do this, as social services have told him that Mrs Lucas would not be entitled to IS in her own right with the level of her existing income and, although no amount of CTB would be payable if Mrs Lucas received half of Mr Lucas' occupational pension, they decide that, as she would have a 25 per cent status discount as the only occupant of their home anyway, it would be more advantageous for her to have the extra income.

Benefits

As Mr and Mrs Lucas are now permanently separated, they will be treated as single people for IS purposes. Therefore, Mr Lucas claims IS in his own right. His claim will be calculated in the following way:

Income

State retirement pension	£66.75
Occupational pension	£65.50
Total	**£132.25**

(AA £52.95 payable for first four weeks but disregarded as income)

Applicable amount 1: (first 4 weeks)

Single personal allowance	£51.40
Single higher pensioner allowance	£30.85
Single severe disability premium	£39.75
Residential allowance	£59.40
Total	**£181.40**

(total amount £65.50 but 50 per cent disregarded as passed to his wife.)

Applicable amount (£181.40) minus income (£132.25) = IS (£49.15).

Mr Lucas is entitled to IS of £49.15 a week for the first four weeks of his stay (paid on top of his state retirement pension, his occupational pension and his AA).

After four weeks, Mr Lucas' AA stops and his IS is re-calculated in the following way:

Applicable amount 2: (after 4 weeks)

Single personal allowance	£51.40
Single enhanced pensioner premium	£25.90
Residential allowance	£59.40
Total	**£136.70**

The higher pensioner premium and the severe disability premium are no longer applicable as Mr Lucas is no longer getting AA.

Applicable amount (£136.70) minus income (£132.25) = IS (£4.45).

Mr Lucas is entitled to IS of £4.45 a week after four weeks of his stay (paid on top of his state retirement pension and his occupational pension).

Contributions

After Mr Lucas' IS claim has been decided by the Benefits Agency, he informs social services and his financial assessment is amended. There are no disregards on Mr Lucas' income for outgoings as he is permanently away from his home in the community. Mr Lucas' contribution to the cost of his accommodation and care costs will be calculated in the following way:

Income 1: (first 4 weeks)

State retirement pension	£66.75
Occupational pension (total amount £65.50 but 50 per cent disregarded as passed to his wife)	£32.75
IS	£49.15
AA	£52.95
Total	**£201.60**

Note: AA is taken into account as Mr Lucas is a permanent resident.
PEA £14.75
Income (£201.60) minus PEA (£14.75) = contribution (£186.85).
Mr Lucas' contribution to the cost for the first four weeks is £186.85 a week.
Mr Lucas will be left with £14.75 a week (PEA).
The full cost of the independent nursing home is £326 a week.
Social services' contribution to the cost for the first four weeks is £139.15 a week.

Income 2: (after 4 weeks)

State retirement pension	£66.75
Occupational pension (total amount £65.50 but 50 per cent disregarded as passed to his wife)	£32.75
IS	£4.45
Total	**£103.95**
PEA	£14.75

Income (£103.95) minus PEA (£14.75) = contribution (£89.20)
Mr Lucas' contribution to the cost after four weeks is £89.20 a week.
Mr Lucas will be left with £14.75 a week (PEA).
The full cost of the independent nursing home is £326 a week.
Social services' contribution to the cost after four weeks is £236.80 a week.

Liable relative payment

Mr and Mrs Lawlor, aged 62 and 58 respectively, are home owners (without a mortgage). Mr Lawlor is in full-time employment. Mrs Lawlor is in receipt of long-term IB, DLA care component and DLA mobility component. They do not receive any means-tested benefits. **Mrs Lawlor goes into a local authority care home for a four week temporary stay whilst adaptations are made to their home.**

Benefits

As Mrs Lawlor's stay in a care home is only temporary, they will continue to be treated as a couple by the Benefits Agency and therefore they will not be entitled to IS because Mr Lawlor is in full-time employment. Mrs Lawlor will continue to receive her long-term IB, DLA care component and DLA mobility component.

Contributions
Although the DSS will still treat Mr and Mrs Lawlor as a couple, social services can only undertake a financial assessment of Mrs Lawlor's resources. Mrs Lawlor's contribution to her accommodation and care costs will be calculated in the following way:

Income:

Long term incapacity benefit	£66.75
Total	**£66.75**

(DLA care component £35.40 disregarded as income as temporary stay)
(DLA mobility component £37.00 disregarded as income).

Outgoings:

Water rates	£4.00 ÷ by 2 =	£2.00
Standing charge for fuel	£1.90 ÷ by 2 =	£0.95
Building and contents insurance premiums	£8.80 ÷ by 2 =	£4.40
Council tax	£9.40 ÷ by 2 =	£4.70
Total		**£12.05**
PEA		**£14.75**

Income (£66.75) minus outgoings (£12.05) minus PEA = contribution (£39.95)
Mrs Lawlor's contribution to the cost is £39.95 a week.
Mrs Lawlor will be left with £99.20 a week (PEA outgoings, DLA care and mobility components).
The full cost of the local authority care home is £252 a week.
As Mrs Lawlor's contribution does not cover the full cost and she has a liable relative (ie, her husband) living in the community who is in full-time employment, social services consider that it is appropriate to ask him for a contribution to Mrs Lawlor's care costs.
If Mrs Lawlor had been able to claim IS as a single person social services would have had a contribution of £86.25 a week from Mrs Lawlor. They ask Mr Lawlor for a contribution of £46.30 a week (the difference between £86.25 and £39.95, Mrs Lawlor's actual contribution). Mr Lawlor says he cannot afford this amount due to his financial commitments and he offers to pay £40 a week. Social services accept this amount. However, if they had considered it was not a reasonable amount they could ask Mr Lawlor to provide financial details in order to consider what would be an appropriate amount, although Mr Lawlor would not be obliged to provide such information. Social services may consider referring the case to the magistrates court.

Income support claimed by partner in the community
Mr and Mrs Lloyd, aged 75 and 70 years respectively, are council tenants. Mr Lloyd's weekly income is made up of state retirement pension, works pension, IS and AA. Mrs Lloyd's weekly income is made up of state retirement pension and AA. They also

receive maximum housing and CTB. **Mrs Lloyd enters an independent residential
care home for a two week temporary stay whilst Mr Lloyd is in hospital.**

Benefits

As Mr and Mrs Lloyd are only temporarily separated, the Benefits Agency will continue
to treat them as a couple for the purposes of calculating their resources, although the
single person's applicable amounts will be used. Mr Lloyd applies for a review of the IS
paid to him in respect of both of them, to include the residential allowance for Mrs
Lloyd It will be calculated in the following way:

Income:

State retirement pension (Mr Lloyd)	£79.20
Works pension (Mr Lloyd)	£15.50
State retirement pension (Mrs Lloyd)	£39.95
Total	**£134.65**

(AA (Mrs Lloyd) disregarded as income)
(AA (Mr Lloyd) disregarded as income)

Applicable amount:

Mr Lloyd (single personal allowance)	**£51.40**
(single higher pensioner premium)	£30.85
(severe disability premium)	£39.75
Mrs Lloyd (single personal allowance)	**£51.40**
(single higher pensioner premium)	£30.85
(severe disability premium)	£39.75
(residential allowance)	£59.40
Total	**£303.40**

Applicable amount (£303.40) minus income (£134.65) = IS (£168.75)
Mr and Mrs Lloyd are entitled to IS of £168.75 a week, payable to Mr Lloyd as the
claimant (paid on top of Mr Lloyd's state retirement pension, works pension and AA).

Contributions

Although the Benefits Agency will still treat Mr and Mrs Lloyd as a couple for the
purposes of calculating their resources, social services can only undertake a financial
assessment of Mrs Lloyd's resources.

However, social services are aware that IS is paid to Mr Lloyd in respect of both of
them as they drafted the letter for Mr Lloyd asking for a review to include the
residential allowance.

Mrs Lloyd's contribution to her accommodation and care costs will be calculated in
the following way:

Income:

State retirement pension	£39.95
Total	**£39.95**

(AA £52.95 disregarded as income as
temporary)

Outgoings:

Water rates £5.00 ÷ by 2 =	£2.50
Standing charge for fuel £1.90 ÷ by 2 =	**£0.95**
Total	**£3.45**
PEA	£14.75

Income (£39.95) minus outgoings (£3.45) minus PEA (£14.75) = contribution (£21.75)

Mrs Lloyd's contribution to the cost is £21.75 a week.

The local authority asks Mr Lloyd for an amount a week that they consider would be being paid by way of IS to Mr Lloyd in respect of Mrs Lloyd. They calculate this in the following way:

Applicable amount in respect of Mrs Lloyd:

(personal allowance)	£51.40
(higher pensioner premium)	£30.85
(severe disability premium)	£39.75
(residential allowance)	£59.40
Total	**£181.40**

Mrs Lloyd's income: State retirement pension   £39.95.

Applicable amount (£181.40) minus income (£39.85) = IS in respect of Mrs Lloyd (£141.45).

Social services ask Mr Lloyd for £141.45 a week of the IS payment toward the cost of Mrs Lloyd's accommodation and care.

The total contribution to the cost from Mr and Mrs Lloyd is £163.20 a week.

Mrs Lloyd will be left with £14.75 a week (PEA).

The full cost of the independent residential care home is £252 a week.

Social services' contribution to the cost is £88.88 a week.

Mr Lloyd would be left with IS for himself calculated by the Benefits Agency in the following way:

Applicable amount in respect of Mr Lloyd:

(personal allowance)	£51.40
(higher pensioner premium)	£30.85
(severe disability premium)	£39.75
Total	**£122.00**

Mr Lloyd's income:

State retirement pension	£79.20
Work's pension	£15.50
Total	**£94.70**

Applicable amount (£122.00) minus income (£94.70) = IS in respect of Mr Lloyd (£27.30).

Mr Lloyd will be left with £27.30 IS for himself (paid on top of his state retirement pension and works pension).

If Mr Lloyd does not receive the amount of IS that is assumed by social services then he will need to advise them accordingly.

Couple with dependent children

Mr and Mrs Patel, aged 65 and 55 years respectively, are home owners (without a mortgage). They have two children aged 15 and 16 for whom they receive child benefit. Mr Patel's weekly income is made up of state retirement pension and a works pension. He also has an entitlement to invalid care allowance (ICA), although it is not payable due to the amount of state retirement pension already in payment.

Mrs Patel's weekly income before entering the care home is made up of IS severe disablement allowance, DLA care component and DLA mobility component. They receive maximum CTB. **Mrs Patel goes into an independent residential care home for a temporary stay of 13 weeks. The children are remaining with Mr Patel.**

Benefits

As Mr and Mrs Patel are only temporarily separated, the Benefits Agency will continue to treat them as a couple for the purposes of calculating their resources although the single person's applicable amounts will be used. Mrs Patel applies for a review of the IS, paid to her in respect of both of them, to include the residential allowance. It will be calculated in the following way:

Income:

State retirement pension (Mr Patel)	£70.55
Works pension (Mr Patel)	£45.00
Severe disablement allowance (Mrs Patel)	£54.40
Child benefit (Mrs Patel)	£24.00
Total	**£193.95**

(DLA care component (Mrs Patel) £52.95 payable for first four weeks but disregarded as income)

(DLA mobility component (Mrs Patel) £37.00 disregarded as income)

Applicable amount 1: (first 4 weeks)

Mr Patel (single personal allowance)	£51.40
(child allowance for 15 year old)	£25.90
(child allowance for 16 year old)	£30.95
(family premium)	£13.90
(single pensioner premium)	£23.60
Mrs Patel (single personal allowance)	£51.40
(single disability premium)	£21.90
(severe disability premium)	£39.75
(residential allowance)	£59.40
Total	**£318.20**

Applicable amount (£318.20) minus income (£193.95) = IS (£124.25)

Mr and Mrs Patel are entitled to IS of £124.25 a week for the first four weeks of her stay, payable to Mrs Patel as the claimant (paid on top of Mr Patel's state retirement pension and works pension and Mrs Patel's severe disablement allowance, child benefit and DLA care and mobility components).

After four weeks Mrs Patel's DLA care component stops and the IS is re-calculated in the following way:

Applicable amount 2: (after 4 weeks)

Mr Patel (single personal allowance)	£51.40
(child allowance for 15-year-old)	£25.90
(child allowance for 16-year-old)	£30.95
(family premium)	£13.90
(single pensioner premium)	£23.60
Mrs Patel (single personal allowance)	£51.40
(single disability premium)	£21.90
(residential allowance)	£59.40
Total	**£278.45**

The severe disability premium is no longer applicable as Mrs Patel is no longer getting DLA care component.

Applicable amount (£278.45) minus income (£193.95) = IS (£84.85).

Mr and Mrs Patel are entitled to IS of £84.50 a week after four weeks of her stay, payable to Mrs Patel as the claimant (paid on top of Mr Patel's state retirement pension and works pension and Mrs Patel's severe disablement allowance, child benefit and DLA mobility components).

Contributions

Although the Benefits Agency will still treat Mr and Mrs Patel as a couple, social services can only undertake a financial assessment of Mrs Patel's resources. However, because Mrs Patel is the IS claimant for herself *and* her family, the PEA can be raised to allow her to give a 'reasonable' amount to her family in the community to help them meet their financial commitments. The 'reasonable' amount could be calculated on the basis of the appropriate applicable amount as allowed for in the IS calculation. In order for this calculation to be undertaken social services would need to ask Mr Patel for details of his resources. Mr Patel would not be obliged to provide this information but, by doing so, social services can vary Mrs Patel's PEA to an appropriate amount. Mrs Patel's contribution to her accommodation and care costs is calculated in the following way:

Income 1: (first 4 weeks)

Severe disablement allowance		£54.40
IS		£124.25
Total		**£178.65**

(DLA care component £52.95 disregarded as income).
(DLA mobility component £37.00 disregarded as income).
(Child benefit £24.00 disregarded as income as children not accommodated with her).

Outgoings:

Water rates	£6.00 ÷ by 2 =	£3.00
Standing charge for fuel	£1.90 ÷ by 2 =	£0.95
Building and contents insurance premiums	£8.50 ÷ by 2 =	£4.25
Total		**£8.20**
PEA (Mrs Patel)		£14.75
(Mr Patel and family - see below for how this amount is calculated)		£30.20
Total		**£44.95**

Income (£178.65) minus outgoings (£8.20) minus PEA (£44.95) = contribution (£125.50).
Mrs Patel's contribution to the cost for the first 4 weeks is £125.50 a week.
Mrs Patel will be left with £167.10 a week (PEA - £30.20 of which she will pass to her family, child benefit, DLA care and mobility components).
The full cost of the independent residential care home is £252 a week.

Social services' contribution for the first 4 week is £126.50 a week.

Income 2: (after 4 weeks)

Severe disablement allowance		£54.40
IS		£84.50
Total		**£138.90**

(DLA mobility component £37.00 disregarded as income)

(Child benefit £24.00 disregarded as income as children not accommodated with her).

Outgoings:

Water rates	£6.00 ÷ by 2 =	£3.00
Standing charge for fuel	£1.90 ÷ by 2 =	£0.95
Building and contents insurance premiums	£8.50 ÷ by 2 =	£4.25
Total		**£8.20**
PEA (Mrs Patel)		£14.75
(Mr Patel and children)		£30.20
(see above for how this amount is calculated)		
Total		**£44.95**

Income (£138.90) minus outgoings (£8.20) minus PEA (£44.95) = contribution (£85.75).

Mrs Patel's contribution to the cost after four weeks is £85.75 a week.

Mrs Patel will be left with £114.15 a week (PEA - £30.20 of which she will pass to her family, child benefit, DLA care and mobility components).

The full cost of the independent residential care home is £252 a week.

Social services' contribution after four weeks is £166.25 a week.

The amount allowed in Mrs Patel's PEA for Mr Patel and the children is calculated in the following way:

Income (Mr Patel):

State retirement pension	£70.55
Works pension	£45.00
Total	**£115.55**

Applicable amount (Mr Patel and children):

(single personal allowance)	£51.40
(child allowance for 15-year- old)	£25.90
(child allowance for 16-year-old)	£30.95
(family premium)	£13.90
(single pensioner premium)	£23.60
Total	**£145.75**

Applicable amount (£145.75) minus income (£115.55) = PEA in respect of Mr Patel and children (£30.20).

The amount allowed in Mrs Patel's PEA for Mr Patel and the children is £30.20 a week.

Couple - both going into a shared room in the same care home

Mr and Mrs Devlin, aged 92 and 88 years respectively, are council tenants. Mr Devlin's weekly income, before entering the care home, is made up of state retirement pension, private pension and AA. Mrs Devlin's weekly income before entering the care home is made up of state retirement pension and AA. They have joint savings of £19,000. They do not receive HB or CTB. **They both go into a shared room in an independent nursing home on a permanent basis.**

Benefits

Mr and Mrs Devlin make individual claims for IS. The Benefits Agency decide they should be treated as a couple because, even though they are permanent residents, they are sharing a room and therefore, are maintaining the same household. IS is not allowed as they have savings of more than £16,000. Mr and Mrs Devlin both ask for a revision of the decision within a month of the decision being notified to them. They provide further information about the care home stating: they have a shared bedroom; they do not have their own front door; there is a communal dining room where meals are taken; there is a communal living room; and domestic and personal activities are organised by the staff at the care home. They argue that there cannot be a household unless there is a domestic establishment and there is not a domestic establishment as there is not a sufficient level of independence and self-sufficiency.[19] The Benefits Agency revise their decision and treat them as single people. When they are treated as single people their joint savings are divided equally and it is assumed that Mr Devlin has £9,500 and Mrs Devlin has £9,500 which is not taken into account as it is below £10,000. (A tariff income would be applied to each IS assessment if their savings were between £10,001 and £16,000 each.)

Their IS entitlement is calculated in the following way:

Income: Mr Devlin

State retirement pension	£67.17
Private pension	£35.03
Total	**£102.20**

(AA £52.95 payable for first four weeks but
disregard as income)

Applicable amount 1: (first 4 weeks)

(single personal allowance)	£51.40
(single higher pensioner premium)	£30.85
(severe disability premium)	£39.75
(residential allowance)	£59.40
Total	**£181.40**

Applicable amount (£181.40) minus income (£102.20) = IS (£79.20).

Mr Devlin is entitled to IS of £79.20 a week for the first four weeks of his stay (paid on top of his state retirement pension, private pension and AA).

After four weeks Mr Devlin's AA stops and his IS is recalculated in the following way:

Applicable amount 2: (after 4 weeks)

(single personal allowance)	£51.40
(single higher pensioner premium)	£30.85
(residential allowance)	£59.40
Total	**£141.65**

The severe disability premium is no longer applicable as Mr Devlin is no longer getting AA.

Applicable amount (£141.65) minus income (£102.20) = IS (£39.45).

Mr Devlin is entitled to IS of £39.45 a week after four weeks of his stay (paid on top of his state retirement pension and private pension).

Mrs Devlin

Income: State retirement pension	£40.20
Total	**£40.20**

(AA £52.95 payable for first 4 weeks but disregarded as income)

Applicable amount 1: (first 4 weeks)

(single personal allowance)	£51.40
(single higher pensioner premium)	£30.85
(severe disability premium)	£39.75
(residential allowance)	£59.40
Total	**£181.40**

Applicable amount (£181.40) minus income (£40.20) = IS (£141.20).

Mrs Devlin is entitled to IS of £141.20 a week for the first four weeks of her stay (paid on top of her state retirement pension and AA). After four weeks, Mrs Devlin's AA stops and her IS is recalculated in the following way:

Applicable amount 2: (after 4 weeks)

(single personal allowance)	£51.40
(single higher pensioner premium)	£30.85
(residential allowance)	£59.40
Total	**£141.65**

The severe disability premium is no longer applicable as Mrs Devlin is no longer getting AA.

Applicable amount (£141.65) minus income (£40.20) = IS (£101.45).

Mrs Devlin is entitled to IS of £101.45 a week after four weeks of her stay (paid on top of her state retirement pension).

Contributions

For social services financial assessment purposes, Mr and Mrs Devlin are immediately treated as single people and assessed according to their individual resources. The contributions to their accommodation and care costs are calculated in the following way:

Mr Devlin
Income 1: (first 4 weeks)

State retirement pension	£67.17
Private pension	£35.03
Income support	£79.20
Attendance allowance	£52.95
Total	**£234.35**
PEA	£14.75

Income (£234.35) minus PEA (£14.75) = contribution (£219.60).
Mr Devlin's contribution to the cost for the first 4 weeks is £219.60 a week.
Mr Devlin will be left with £14.75 (PEA) a week.
The full cost of the nursing home is £326 a week.
Social services' contribution for the first four weeks is £106.40 a week.

Income 2: (after 4 weeks)

State retirement pension	£67.17
Private pension	£35.03
Income support	£79.20
Total	**£141.65**
PEA	£14.75

Income (£141.65) minus PEA (£14.75) = contribution (£126.90)
Mr Devlin's contribution to the cost after four weeks is £126.90 a week.
Mr Devlin will be left with £14.75 (PEA) a week.
The full cost of the nursing home is £326 a week.
Social services' contribution for the first four weeks is £199.10 a week.

Mrs Devlin
Income 1: (first 4 weeks)

State retirement pension	£40.20
Income support	£141.20
Attendance allowance	£52.95
Total	**£234.35**
PEA	£14.75

Income (£234.35) minus PEA (£14.75) = contribution (£219.60)
Mrs Devlin's contribution to the cost for the first four weeks is £219.60 a week.

Mrs Devlin will be left with £14.75 a week (PEA).

The full cost of the nursing home is £326 a week.

Social services' contribution for the first four weeks is £106.40 a week.

Income 2: (after 4 weeks)

State retirement pension	£40.20
Income support	£101.45
Total	**£141.65**
PEA	£14.75

Income (£141.65) minus PEA (£14.75) = contribution (£126.90)

Mrs Devlin's contribution to the cost after four weeks is £126.90 a week.

Mrs Devlin will be left with £14.75 a week (PEA).

The full cost of the nursing home is £326 a week.

Social services' contribution for the first four weeks is £199.10 a week.

. . . .

Loophole/self-funding case (England and Wales only)

Mrs Burman, aged 80 years, is a home owner (without a mortgage). Her weekly income before entering the care home is made up of state retirement pension, works pension and AA. She has savings of £11,000 and no one receives invalid care allowance for looking after her. **Mrs Burman is due to enter an independent residential care home on a permanent basis and she puts her house, which has been valued at £44,000, up for sale. The full cost of the home is £252 a week.**

Stage 1 - the 'loophole' and claiming benefits

Mrs Burman claims IS. The value of her home is disregarded as she is taking steps to sell it. Mrs Burman's entitlement, until her house is sold, will be calculated in the following way:

Income:

State retirement pension	£76.40
Works pension	£26.00
Tariff income from savings	£4.00
Total	**£106.40**

(AA £52.95 disregarded as income)

Applicable amount:

(personal allowance)	£51.40
(higher pensioner premium)	£30.85
(severe disability premium)	£39.75
(residential allowance)	£59.40
Total	**£181.40**

Applicable amount (£181.40) minus income (£106.40) = IS (£75.00).

Mrs Burman will be entitled to IS of £75.00 a week (paid on top of her state retirement pension, works pension and AA).

If social services do not contract with the care home and instead Mrs Burman contracts directly with the care home, then AA can continue in payment beyond an initial 4 week period. If AA continues to be paid Mrs Burman would also continue to have the severe disability premium included in her applicable amount.

Note: Social services should still assess Mrs Burman to find out what type of care home would be suitable for her needs and advise her on other relevant issues even though they are not contracting with the care home for the provision of her accommodation and care.

Mrs Burman's total income would be:

Income:	
State retirement pension	£76.40
Works pension	£26.00
Income support	£75.00
Attendance allowance	£52.95
Total	**£230.35**

Stage 2 - the 'loophole' and meeting the shortfall

As the full cost of the care home is £252 a week Mrs Burman's total income is £21.65 a week short of meeting the cost. However, Mrs Burman decides that she will be better off if she meets the £21.65 a week shortfall out of her savings so that she can continue to receive her AA and the severe disability premium.

If Mrs Burman did not have any savings from which she could meet the shortfall and she did not have any friends or relatives that could meet the shortfall for her until her home was sold, then Mrs Burman would have to approach social services for help with the cost of the care home until her home was sold. Unfortunately, as there is no provision for the local authority to disregard a property up for sale, the value of Mrs Burman's home (£39,600 after the 10 per cent deduction for potential costs involved in selling it) will be taken into account as Mrs Burman's capital.

With capital in excess of £16,000 Mrs Burman will be required to pay the full cost of the care home. As she cannot meet the full cost until her home is sold, social services agree to pay some of the cost and place a 'charge' on her property accordingly so that they can recoup the monies they have paid for her accommodation and care from the proceeds of the sale of her home.

If Mrs Burman had to, or chose to, take this option involving social services, she would not only lose her AA and the severe disability premium after the initial four weeks of her stay, she would also lose money from the proceeds of the sale in having to refund social services.

Stage 3 - self-funding

Mrs Burman chooses to take the 'loophole' option and meets the shortfall from her savings. After 12 months, her property is sold. The proceeds from the sale (after costs incurred have been deducted) amount to £40,000. The savings she had previously have fallen to £8,000. She will no longer be entitled to IS but as a self-funding person she will continue to be entitled to AA on top of her state retirement pension and her works pension.

Note: If necessary, social services could now become involved and contract with the care home without it making a difference to her entitlement to AA although they would not be able to help with the cost of the home until her savings fell to £16,000.

Stage 4 - benefits and contributions when no longer self-funding

After three years Mrs Burman's total savings have fallen to £16,000 and she approaches social services for help with meeting the cost of her accommodation and care.

Benefits

She is advised to claim IS which is calculated in the following way:

Income:	
State retirement pension	£76.40
Works pension	£26.00
Tariff income from savings	£24.00
Total	**£126.40**

Mrs Burman's AA ceases as she is no longer self-funding.

Applicable amount:	
(personal allowance)	£51.40
(higher pensioner premium)	£30.85
residential allowance)	£59.40
Total	**£141.65**

Applicable amount (£141.65) minus income (£126.40) = IS (£15.25).

Mrs Burman will be entitled to IS of £15.25 a week (paid on top of her state retirement pension and her works pension).

Contributions

Mrs Burman advises social services about her income. They undertake a financial assessment and Mrs Burman's contribution to her accommodation and care costs is calculated in the following way:

Income:	
Works pension	£26.00
State retirement pension	£76.40
Income support	£15.25
Tariff income from savings	£24.00
Total	**£141.65**
PEA	£14.75

Income (£141.65) minus PEA (£14.75) = contribution (£126.90)

Mrs Burman's contribution to the cost is £126.90 a week

Mrs Burman will be left with £14.75 a week (PEA).

The full cost of the independent residential care home is £252 a week.

Social services' contribution of £125.10 a week.

Note: Mrs Burman's contribution will become less as her savings fall and thus her tariff income reduces. Mrs Burman should advise social services when her savings fall to £15,750 and subsequently by every £250.

Third party contribution

Mr Chand, aged 64 years, is a single person living in a housing association property. His weekly income, before entering care, is made up of long-term IB, IS and DLA care and mobility components. He also receives maximum HB and CTB and his son claims ICA for caring for him. **Mr Chand goes into an independent residential care home for a three-week temporary stay**. He has chosen a care home which costs £15 a week more than social services would pay for a person with his needs. There are other homes available within the usual cost that would be suitable but Mr Chand wishes to go to the higher cost home. Mr Chand's son agrees to pay the extra £15 and he enters into a contract (usually called a third party agreement or a third party contribution contract) with social services to make this payment.

Benefits

Mr Chand requests a review of his IS entitlement to include the residential allowance. It is calculated in the following way:

Income:

Long-term incapacity benefit	£80.80
Total	**£80.80**

(DLA care component £52.95, DLA mobility component £37.00 and the third party contribution £15.00 disregarded as income)

Applicable amount:

(personal allowance)	£51.40
(higher pensioner premium)	£30.85
(residential allowance)	£59.40
Total	**£141.65**

The severe disability premium is not included in Mr Chand's applicable amount as his son is in receipt of ICA.

Applicable amount (£141.65) minus income (£80.80) = IS (£60.85)

Mr Chand is entitled to IS of £60.85 a week (paid on top of his long term IB and DLA care and mobility component).

Contributions

After Mr Chand's IS entitlement has been reviewed, he informs social services and they amend his financial assessment. Mr Chand's contribution to the cost of his accommodation and care is calculated in the following way:

Income:

Long-term incapacity benefit	£80.80
Income support	£60.85
Third party contribution	£15.00
Total	**£156.65**

(DLA care component £52.95 and DLA mobility component £37.00 disregarded as income).

Outgoings:

Standing charge for fuel	£1.90
Service charge (not met by housing benefit)	£2.50
Water rates	£4.00
Total	**£8.40**
PEA	£14.75

Income (£156.65) minus outgoings (£8.40) minus PEA (£14.75) = contribution (£133.50).

Mr Chand's and his son's third party contribution to the cost is £133.50 a week (£118.50 from Mr Chand and £15.00 from his son).

The full cost of the independent residential care home is £267.

Social services' contribution to the cost is £133.50 a week (no more than it would have been if the full cost of the care home was £252 a week – ie, the usual cost).

Notes

1. Types of care home

1 s21(1)(a) of part III NAA 1948 as amended by the NHS and CCA 1990; s13B and 59 of SW(S)A 1968

2 Reg 2(1) NA(AR) Regs 1992

3 para 2.007 CRAG; para 2.002 SWSG 8/96 and reg 5 NA(AR) Regs 1992

4 para 2.010 CRAG; para 2.005 SWSG 8/96

2. Types of stay

5 Reg 2(1) NA(AR) regs 1992

6 para 3.002 CRAG and para 8; para 3.002 SWSG 8/96; LAC(95)7, Annex H CRAG; WOC 22/95; para 9 SWSG 13/95(9)

7 paras 3.004 and 3.004A CRAG

3. Financial assessments

8 s22(1) NAA 1948 as amended by NHS and CCA 1990; s87 SW(S)A 1968

9 s22(3) NAA 1948

10 s22(2) NAA 1948

11 s26(2) NAA 1948

12 s22(2) NAA 1948

13 s23(3) NAA 1948

14 Regs NA(AR) Regs 1992 as amended

15 s22(5A) NAA 1948

16 para 4.001 CRAG; para 4.001 SWSG 8/96

5. Paying the full cost of your care home

17 LAC(98)19; WOC 27/98; SWSG 2/99

6. Temporary absences from care homes (including going into hospital)

18 para 8 LA(97)5, Annex H CRAG; para 15 SWSG 7/97

7. Benefits and contribution examples – complex cases

19 CIS/4935/97

Chapter 24

Common problems – benefits and charges

This chapter explains some of the problems that commonly occur for a person entering a care home in the claiming of social security benefits and in the financial assessment being undertaken to establish the charge/contribution to care home costs required by the local authority.

It covers common problems in the following areas:

1. Housing benefit and income support (p425)
2. Disability living allowance care component/attendance allowance (p429)
3. Financial assessments and charging (p430)
4. Social security benefits and social services charges (p434)

1. Housing benefit and income support

Housing benefit and income support claims in respite care

If you are a person for whom respite care is organised (ie, you have a planned programme of temporary stays in a care home) and your income is £66.75 or higher (not including income support (IS)) and your respite care stays are in local authority residential accommodation (where the applicable amount is only the Part III rate of £66.75), you may no longer be entitled to IS. Any housing benefit (HB) you receive will also cease (because it was paid on the basis of being entitled to IS). As it is likely that you will still be entitled to HB, you will need to make a fresh claim from the time that you enter the care home. When you leave the care home, you will need to make a fresh claim for IS in order to receive the same level of benefits that you received before entering the care home. This will mean that HB will also become payable again based on your entitlement to IS.

The problem in this situation is having to complete an HB claim form upon entering the care home and another claim form (IS) upon leaving the care home, both of which are quite lengthy and time-consuming. On top of this you may also have to keep the Disability Benefits Unit in Blackpool informed of your respite care arrangements if you receive disability living allowance

(DLA) care component or attendance allowance (AA). Some HB sections in local authorities will accept a shortened claim form with a catch-all declaration to the effect that there has been no change of circumstances since the date of the last full declaration of circumstances.[1] However, the Department of Social Security (DSS) will not accept such a shortened form, so the only thing you can do to make it a little easier is to photocopy your IS claim form and transfer the information onto your next claim, remembering to make any appropriate changes.

This type of situation could also occur the opposite way around if you become entitled to IS upon entering an independent care home due to the residential allowance of £59.40 being included in your applicable amount – see p352 Chapter 21. You will need to complete an IS claim form when you go in and a HB claim form when you come out.

Housing benefit and notice of termination of tenancy

If your home in the community is rented and you receive HB you may experience a problem if you go into a care home on a trial period or permanent basis (see p349) for definitions of these types of stay).

The problem arises because HB can only be paid on your normal home.[2] Therefore, if you have decided to leave that home permanently (ie, become a permanent resident in a care home) there is no further entitlement to benefit. Of course, in order to give the notice of termination of tenancy required by housing authorities (usually four weeks) you must have decided you are not going to return to your home in the community; then the period of that notice is not covered by HB. The only time this would not happen is where you were able to plan that on a certain date, which was also the date of the end of the notice of termination period, you would enter the care home on a permanent basis. Often, however, going into a care home cannot be planned in this way.

This issue was raised with the HB policy section at the DSS in October 1995 following the introduction of the 'trial period' in April 1995 in an attempt to get a change in HB regulations to allow payment to the end of the contractual liability in these circumstances. The response was that perhaps local authorities might wish to consider a much shorter notice of termination period when people are in residential accommodation on a trial basis and they then decide to stay permanently.[3]

In practice, a number of different solutions have been adopted by housing and social services departments. The most notable of these are:
- some housing authorities have written off the rent for the notice period on a case-by-case basis;
- some social services departments have increased the personal expenses allowance (ie, charged less) during the notice period while full rent is being paid.

Different benefits agency offices

If you are moving permanently to a care home outside the area covered by your current Benefits Agency office your claims will be transferred to the relevant office for the care home you are moving to. There is sometimes a problem with claims being transferred to a different Benefits Agency office when your stay is only temporary. For temporary stays there should be no change from the Benefits Agency for your normal home address.

Pre-April 1993 placements in local authority residential accommodation moving to independent care homes post-April 1993

If you were in (or temporarily absent from) local authority residential accommodation on 31 March 1993 and subsequently you move to an independent care home (eg, a nursing home because your condition deteriorates) then the Benefits Agency will usually treat you as still being in local authority accommodation for IS purposes and therefore award the lower residential accommodation rate (Part III rate).[4] However, a recent social security commissioner's decision[5] held that from 10 April 1995, when there was an amendment to the definition of residential accommodation, arrangements made for placements in independent care homes[6] are no longer included and therefore the normal rates of IS with the residential allowance are appropriate (also see p348).

Claims for income support

From October 1997 new evidence requirement regulations have meant that most people making claims for IS need to supply all the evidence requested on the claim form in order for the claim to be effective. A period of one month to supply all the evidence requested is allowed from the date of any notification of the intention to make a claim or the date on which an incomplete claim form is received by the Benefits Agency and the missing information is requested.[7]

A standard form for the notification of the intention to make a claim has been suggested as good practice by the Local Government Association.[8] If the required information is not submitted within the one month period it is likely that IS will only be paid from any later date on which the information or evidence is provided unless one of five reasons exists for not providing the information or evidence[9] (see p227).

The encouragement of prompt and complete claims is important to social services finances as they can only make an assessment for your contribution to accommodation and care costs on the basis of the capital you have and the income (including IS) you receive (but see 'notional income' p288).

There will usually be no reward for you in making a valid IS claim as your personal expenses allowance (PEA) will remain the same whatever happens to your benefits (see p303)

For these reasons it is in social services' interest to provide help and advice in the claiming of social security benefits. If a claim for IS is made late it can be backdated for up to three months if there is a specified special reason.[10] If you were misled by incorrect advice from social services this is only considered to be a special reason if the advice was in writing. Claims can also be backdated for up to one month for specified administrative reasons[11] (also see p349).

Couples

For IS purposes, the treatment of couples or one member of a couple in care homes has always been more problematic and complex than the treatment of a single person in a care home. Upon a claim or revision, the Benefits Agency needs to establish whether the stay is a temporary, trial period or permanent one. Different rules apply for couples depending on the type of stay (see pp349–50). Often the Benefits Agency fails to apply the single person rate when they calculate the applicable amount for a couple, one of whom is in a care home (see pp350–59).

A common problem which has been the subject of a number of Social Security Commissioners' decisions is where both members of a couple are permanent residents in a shared room in the same care home. It used to be the case that if a couple were in separate rooms in the same care home or one was in a residential wing and the other in a nursing wing of a dual registered care home, they could be treated as single people, but where a couple were sharing a room they would be treated as a couple as they were maintaining a common household. Social security commissioners' decisions have held the view that 'an essential attribute of a household is a domestic establishment' and that 'if the degree of independence and self-sufficiency falls below a certain level, there is no longer a domestic establishment and therefore no longer a household'.[12]

This means that IS may become payable to each member of the couple treated as a single person when it would not have been payable to them as a couple – eg, because they have joint savings of more than £16,000 but when it is divided their individual shares are less than £16,000.

Chapter 24: Common problems – benefits and charges
2. Disability living allowance care component/attendance allowance

24

2. Disability living allowance care component/attendance allowance

Completing enquiry forms

There are two common enquiry forms that are sent out by the Benefits Agency's disability benefits unit to collect information to enable them to make a decision on whether DLA care component/AA (and in some situations of stays in hospital or similar institutions, DLA mobility component) is payable while you are in the care home.

Form DBD 26 is sent to the manager or owner of the care home and is entitled 'We need some information – urgent benefit involved'. This form asks about the type of accommodation you are in, when you moved in, where you were living before, who pays for your care in the home, and whether you have spent any time away from the home.

Form DBD 46 is sent to social services or the health authority, depending on which authority is helping with the cost of your placement. This form asks whether the authority owns or manages the care home, whether any money has been paid toward the cost of your stay, and under which legislation monies have been paid.

Both of these forms need to be completed accurately and carefully, especially if you are trying to establish that DLA care component/AA should continue in payment. Often forms are incorrectly completed for various reasons, not least that authorities are less than sure about what legislation they are making payments under. This can lead to benefits being withdrawn incorrectly (see p356). There can also be delays caused because of the late return of these forms.

Retrospective self-funding

If you are required to pay the full cost of your accommodation and care costs because of the level of your capital but your capital is not yet available (eg, your own home is for sale but not yet sold) you may be unable to meet those costs. In such situations, social services may fund your placement on a temporary refundable basis. Social services will re-claim the monies they have paid when you have access to your capital. It is not clear (due to conflicting Social security commissioners' decisions) whether, when you refund social services, you can receive DLA care component/AA for the period you were retrospectively self-funding (see p369).

It may be the case that the loophole option would be appropriate to consider in these circumstances (see p355). Social services should provide full information about the financial consequences of the different options available to you.[13]

24

Chapter 24: Common problems – benefits and charges
2. Disability living allowance care component/attendance allowance

Overpayments

Overpayments of DLA care component/AA commonly occur because the Benefits Agency has not been informed about your stay in a care home. This is especially the case in a respite care situation where your stays might only be for weekends but are on a regular basis, so there may come a time when the 28 days entitlement period is exceeded (see p356).

Overpayments of benefits may be recoverable from you if you have failed to disclose, or misrepresented, a material fact (see p245).

All the circumstances of your arrangements for care in a care home and any change in those circumstances should be notified to the Benefits Agency in writing.

3. **Financial assessments and charging**

Types of stay

Problems can occur with social services definitions of the types of stay in care homes. A permanent stay is straightforward but trial periods and temporary stays can be more problematic (see p391 for definitions).

A trial period stay is considered to be of a temporary nature by the Benefits Agency but often social services regard trial periods as permanent stays because a permanent resource is being committed from the budget. This means that the value of your home in the community may be taken into account as capital under the rules that apply to permanent stays rather than being disregarded under the rules that apply to temporary stays.

There is no definition of trial period for financial assessment purposes but guidance indicates that this type of stay should be treated as temporary[14] (see p391). Any decision made by social services can be challenged using the complaints procedure (see p57).

Problems can occur for couples if a stay which is actually permanent from the first day is automatically described as a trial period. This is because if one of a couple (or both members of the couple) is in a care home on a trial period basis they will be assessed as a couple for IS purposes and their resources aggregated, whereas if the stay is a permanent stay they will be treated as single people for IS purposes and their resources will not be aggregated. This could mean the difference between IS being payable or not (see pp351).

There can also be problems with temporary stays where social services insist on a definite date when the stay will end for it to be considered as a temporary stay. This is not correct. The definition of temporary stay in the legislation is a stay unlikely to exceed 52 weeks, or in exceptional circumstances unlikely substantially to exceed that period.[15]

Couples (married or unmarried)

Financial assessments for one member of a couple going into a care home on a temporary basis are more complex and therefore problems can occur. The problems involve the need to ensure that, if the person going into care is the main benefit recipient for both of them as a couple, there will be a variation of the resident's PEA so that the resident can continue to support their partner (see p304).

If the person staying in the community is the main benefit recipient for both of them as a couple then social services may ask the person in the community to make a contribution to the costs of the placement (see p310).

Financial assessments before entering a care home

Social services departments can undertake a financial assessment *before* you enter a care home if you are a prospective resident.[16] This means that the income they assess on includes benefits that are only applicable to you in the community. As explained in Chapter 21, some benefits will change when you enter the care home and, therefore, the initial contribution social services calculate will not be the amount that you will actually be required to pay when you enter the care home. This can be confusing, although some social services departments attempt to explain the situation in the letter they send you about your financial assessment.

As soon as your benefits change as a result of entering the care home, social services will need to be advised of the new amounts so they can complete a re-assessment and advise you of the actual amount that you will be required to contribute.

Assuming income support

If social services undertake a financial assessment *before* you enter a care home (see above) they may make an assumption about your entitlement to, and the amount of, IS that will become payable when you enter the care home. This can cause problems because it involves treating IS as notional income (see p288), and also because social services financial assessors are not usually benefit specialists and may make an incorrect assumption. This is particularly a problem with regard to the severe disability premium element of IS which is subject to complex rules (see p350).

If your IS entitlement has been assumed you should check that what you actually receive when your entitlement has been decided is the same amount as social services assumed. If it is not, you should challenge the social services decision using their complaints procedure (see p57). Alternatively, the amount of your IS may be incorrect. In this situation social services may be able to help you challenge the Benefits Agency decision. In any event, social services cannot assess you on an amount of IS that is not in payment. They will have to re-assess you on the basis of your actual income.

The eight-week option

The eight-week option is where social services do not need to undertake a financial assessment for the first eight weeks of your stay in a care home. Instead they can charge what they consider to be reasonable.[17] Many social services departments charge what is commonly referred to as the 'Part III rate', which is basic retirement pension (£66.75) minus personal expense allowance (£14.75) – ie, £52 a week.

This discriminates in favour of those who have resources above the basic retirement pension level, as these are ignored. It also discriminates against those who have resources below the basic retirement pension level.

If you have been charged an amount under the eight-week option which is not based on your actual resources and you do not consider it is reasonable, you can ask social services for a full financial assessment.

More expensive care homes

Social services departments usually have a number of set amounts for what they consider should be the normal total cost of a care home placement in different types of home. These amounts are sometimes similar to the amounts allowed by the Benefits Agency for preserved rights pre-April 1993 placements (see pp382). However, these set amounts are not always the same as the actual cost of a care home, especially since care homes have recently had to take into account additional costs they may have incurred with the introduction of the minimum wage and working time directives legislation.

This situation can cause problems. There are two different aspects to be considered. It may be that the more expensive care home is the only home which can meet your needs as assessed by social services. In this case social services has an obligation to meet the higher cost themselves without any contribution from a third party (see below).

However, *you* may have chosen a care home which costs more than your social services department would usually expect to pay for someone with your needs. In this case social services can still arrange a placement in the care home provided that it satisfies the other specified conditions (see p277) if a third party is able and willing to meet the shortfall, and to continue doing so for as long as you are likely to be in the care home. These types of payments are usually known as third party contributions (see Chapter 16).

You cannot use your PEA of £14.75 to help pay for more expensive care homes.[18] However, until recently it has not been clear whether you can use your own capital or disregarded income to meet the shortfall. The original guidance was that you could,[19] but this was replaced (England and Wales only) by guidance stating that residents cannot use their own resources to pay for more expensive accommodation – ie, act as their own third party. A third party contribution may only be met by another person – eg, a friend or relative, or organisation such as a charity (see Chapter 16).[20]

In practice social services may still have old third party contribution agreements where the resident is the third party, but new agreements should not involve the resident although it seems that some residents have, without the knowledge of social services, given the money from their capital or disregarded income to the named third party for them to make the payment. In this situation it is the third party who remains under the obligation to make the contribution.

Fifty per cent pension disregard

If you pass at least 50 per cent of your occupational or personal pension or payment from a retirement annuity to your spouse with whom you are not residing, 50 per cent will be disregarded from your income. Social services should give you advice about this disregard and the fact that you have a choice of whether to pass 50 per cent to your spouse or not. They should also advise you about whether your spouse would be better off after taking account of the effect of the pension on social security benefits.[21]

In practice, many social services departments do not give this advice. You should seek independent advice if you have been disadvantaged by the lack of social services advice.

Loophole cases (England and Wales only)

Loophole cases are discussed in Chapter 21 (see p369). Often social services do not appreciate the benefit implications of the actions they take or the advice they give. This means you could lose benefits to which you might otherwise have been entitled if a different choice or course of action was taken. Social services departments are in fact advised that as part of the whole assessment process they should provide *full* information about the financial consequences of the different options.[22] This was confirmed by an Ombudsman investigation where it was accepted by the authority that it should have put the option of paying the full cost of the placement in a care home to the family, given its knowledge of the rules governing the payment of attendance allowance.[23]

Deprivation of income or capital

If social services have decided that, or are considering whether, you have deprived yourself of income or capital in order to avoid a charge or reduce the charge payable (see pp289 and 300), there are various courses of action (see Chapter 19) they may be able to take attempt to secure the contribution assessed, taking into account the notional income or capital. However, it is important to remember that the placement you have been assessed as needing should not be delayed or withheld, even if you have deprived yourself of income or capital or, if you have not made the payment of the assessed contribution. Social services departments have a duty to provide residential care where it is needed and not otherwise available to you. In Scotland the same principle applies although the wording of the legislation varies.[24]

4. Social security benefits and social services charges

Benefit and charging pay days

If you are expected to go into a care home for a period of up to eight weeks, your IS can be paid from the day of admission. However, if your stay is expected to be more than eight weeks, your IS can only be altered from the start of your benefit week. Social services charges should be based on what you actually receive, so if there are days when you receive less money, you should be charged less.

Treatment of jointly owned property

Social services and the Benefits Agency may treat property that is jointly owned differently. If you own property with one or more people, the Benefits Agency treats you as owning an equal share, even if your actual share may be more or less than this.[25] The deemed equal share is then valued. The DSS has detailed guidance[26] and a special agency, the Valuation Office Agency, which deals with these more complex valuations.

Social services value your *actual* share in the jointly owned property.[27] Therefore, if you have more or less than an equal share, the valuation amount may differ from that assessed by the Benefits Agency. Unlike the Benefits Agency, social services have little guidance on how to proceed in these cases. However, if you dispute social services valuation, guidance states that a professional valuation should be obtained[28] (see p294). This should not be an expense passed on to you as there is no provision to charge for such an item.

Both the Benefits Agency and social services value the share that they each determine belongs to you in the same way, by establishing the current market or surrender value – ie, the price a willing buyer would pay to a willing seller for the share, less ten per cent if there would be costs involved in selling, and less any mortgage or debt secured on the property (see p294).

Capital limits for temporary stays

If you enter a care home for a temporary stay and you have capital in excess of £8,000 but below £16,000, you will not be able to claim IS because for temporary residents the capital limit is £8,000, the same as for people living in the community.

However, since April 1996, the social services capital limit for temporary residents is £16,000, the same as for permanent residents. This will not be a problem for you but for social services who will be required to fund your placement without any IS to include in the financial assessment to offset some of their costs of your placement.

Notes

1. HB and IS

1. paras 3 & 4 HB and CTB A10/96
2. Reg 5 HB Regs 1987
3. AMA social services circular 104/1995 23 October 1995
4. Reg 21(3B) and (3C) ISG Regs 1987
5. CIS/16440/1996
6. Under s26 NAA 1948
7. Regs 4(1A) to 4(1C); reg 6(1A) SS(C&P) Regs 1987
8. Attached to LGA circular 126/98 dated 26 February 1998
9. Reg 4(1B) SS(C&P) Regs 1987
10. Reg 19(4) and (5) SS(C&P) Regs 1987
11. Reg 19(6) SS(C&P) Regs 1987
12. CIS/4934/97; CIS/4935/97; CIS/5232/97; CIS/5237/97 and CIS/3767/97 and common appendix to these decisions

2. DLA care component/AA

13. Ombudsman investigation against Stockport MBC Complaint No. 98/C.1842 30 March 1999

3. Financial assessments and charging

14. para 8 LAC(95)7, Annex H, CRAG WOC 22/95; para 13 SWSG 13/95
15. Reg 2(1) NA(AR) Regs 1992
16. LAC (98)19 WOC 27/98; SWSG 2/99 and S.I.1998 No. 1730 NA(AR)(Amdt 2) Regs 1998
17. s22(SA) NAA 1948

18. para 13 LAC(94)1, Annex H, CRAG WOC 4/94; para 13 SWSG 5/94
19. para 13 LAC(94)1, Annex H, CRAG WOC 4/94; para 13 SWSG 5/94 and para 11.16 SWSG 5/93 and para 11.14 of the guidance on the statutory direction on choice LAC(92)27 WOC
20. para 6 LAC(98)8, Annex H, CRAG WOC 12/98
21. para 4 LAC(97)5, Annex H, CRAG WOC 29/97; para 2 SWSG 7/97
22. Part 1D of letter to Directors of Social Services dated 12 September 1994 from ACC and AMA
23. Ombudsman investigation against Stockport MBC Complaint No.98/C.1842, 30 March 1999
24. s21(1)(a) NAA 1948; ss12 and 13 SW(S)A 1968

4. Social security benefits and social services charges

25. Reg 52 ISG Regs 1987
26. Memo AOG memo JSA and IS (98)35
27. Reg 27(2) NA(AR) Regs 1992
28. Para 7 LAC(97)5, Annex H, CRAG WOC 29/97; para 8 SWSG 7/97

Part 6

Future trends

Chapter 25

Future trends

This chapter looks at some of the proposals that have been put forward, which could change the way community care is delivered and how much you may have to pay in the future. It covers:

1. Changes to service delivery (p439)
2. Changes to benefits (p444)
3. Changes to charges (p447)
4. The proposals of the Royal Commission (p448)

1. Changes to service delivery

There are currently numerous changes in the pipeline which are likely, directly or indirectly, to affect the services you receive. Some are specific to community care services, but others are changes to the way all public services are delivered, and as such will inevitably affect community care services over time.

Devolution and regionalisation

From July 1999 the Scottish Parliament and Welsh Assembly started to develop their own policies in relation to community care. Social security has not been devolved but remains the responsibility of central government. Although, as can be seen from this *Handbook*, there have always been some differences between Scottish and English law, from now on this is going to increasingly apply to Wales. Each country has it own White Paper on the future of social services, and much of the detail which is in the English White Paper *Modernising Social Services* is absent from those of Scotland and Wales because it will be for the Parliament and Assembly respectively to make their own decisions. The detail of devolved power will emerge gradually as the process develops, but it is likely that future handbooks will need to highlight the differences between three countries rather than just two, as in this book.

A development which will affect services in London is the establishment of the Greater London Assembly from July 2000. The mayor will be given specific responsibility for the promotion of health in the Greater London area. Since April 1999 there has been a new NHS executive for London which is co-terminous with the Greater London area, and work has already started on a London health strategy.

Across the rest of England, new regional development agencies were introduced from April 1999 to co-ordinate economic, social, and physical regeneration in the regions, with a duty to consult new voluntary regional chambers. These are likely to increase the scope for more regional co-ordination and action in relation to many aspects of local government, including community care. Some see the regional development agencies as a possible precursor to regional government.

Local government reform

The White Paper *Modern Local Government – In Touch with the People* (1998) and the Local Government Bill introduced in November 1999, sets an agenda of reforms which will impact on services for older or disabled people. Some of the reforms (such as Best Value, explained below) are already in place following the Local Government Act 1999. In Scotland the Scottish Parliament will make its own proposals in the wake of the Macintosh Commission on local government reform. The following are the main features of the reforms in England and Wales.

A bigger say for local people

There will be a requirement to consult more with local people and to work in partnership with service users. Referendums, citizens juries, panels and forums are options for local authorities to engage with local people.

A duty to promote economic, social and environmental wellbeing

When making any decisions there will be a requirement to take into account the long-term well-being of local people and the local area. It is aimed at more strategic thinking, not only across local government but with the partners involved.

Improving services through Best Value

From April 2000 there will be a duty on local authorities to obtain best value in all the services they provide either directly or indirectly. It requires a corporate approach in establishing authority-wide objectives and performance measures.

Authorities will have to review all their services and functions. This does not have to be on a service basis. It could for instance review a particular geographical area or a group of people with particular needs. The review must challenge why and how services are being provided, compare performance with other authorities, consult with service users, carers and local people before setting new performance targets, and secure efficient and effective services through fair competition.

The Best Value approach requires a culture of continuous improvement which puts an emphasis on quality not just on cost. There will be independent audits and inspections. If there is persistent failure in the delivery of services there are new powers for the appropriate Secretary of State to intervene.

New political structures to improve accountability

It is expected that the present committee structure of local government will disappear, being replaced by a directly elected mayor with a cabinet, or by a cabinet with a leader or a directly elected mayor and a council manager.

Trends towards consistency

At the same time as the moves to greater local decision-making through the reforms mentioned above, and the establishment of locally-based health groups (see p10), there are clear messages from government about the need for greater consistency across the country both in standards and access to services. The following are some of the initiatives in England that could alter your chances of getting the care you need. Although these might not be happening in quite the same way in Wales and Scotland, many initiatives will broadly follow the same principles in these countries.

National objectives and priorities

Both the NHS White Paper *The New NHS Modern, Dependable* (1997) and the Social Services White Paper *Modernising Social Services* (1998) introduce the setting of national objectives and priorities.

Joint guidance has been issued[1] to health and social services, setting out the key priorities over the next three years for both health and social care. They include cutting health inequalities; improving mental health services; promoting independence; and tackling the causes of cancer and heart disease. New national objectives for social services have been issued which fit into the priorities guidance[2] which stress promoting independence, in particular the capacity to remain in or take up work; working with others to avoid unnecessary admission to hospital; supporting carers; and ensuring resources are planned and provided at levels which represent best value for money.

National service frameworks

There are plans for a series of national service frameworks starting with mental health services, which have now been published, and coronary heart disease. The aim is to reduce unacceptable variations in care and standards of treatment.

A national service framework for older people is also being developed to provide standards and principles for the pattern and level of services required, put in place programmes to support implementation, and establish performance measures.

Fair access to care

Alongside national service frameworks, a new 'Fair access to care' initiative is being developed to introduce greater consistency in the system for deciding who qualifies for services on the assessment of risk. Guidance is to be drafted which will set out the principles that local authorities should follow when devising or applying eligibility criteria (see p44) using clear objectives based on the need to promote independence. Regular reviews of people receiving services will be introduced to ensure that the services continue to meet objectives. The guidance is expected to come into operation by 2001.

Long-term care charter

From June 2000 there will be a joint charter setting out more clearly at a national level what you can expect from your local health, housing and social services departments. The charter was published in December 1999.[3]

National regulatory standards

These are to be set across residential and nursing homes in the first instance, so that all care homes will have to meet required standards which apply consistently across the country.[4] There will be a National Care Standards Commission to oversee these standards, some of which will be set out in legislation. Domiciliary care will be brought into regulation although on a voluntary basis. Social services will only be able to contract with those agencies which have opted for regulation. National standards for regulating domiciliary care are being drawn up. None of these changes are likely before April 2002.

National performance indicators and the performance assessment framework

Performance indicators have been set on a national basis and are being incorporated into the Best Value regime. The performance assessment framework uses the indicators to identify where authorities need to improve. It will allow authorities to compare their performance on a consistent basis. There is a similar framework for the NHS. Good practice in local authorities and health authorities or trusts will be rewarded by 'beacon status'.

Joint working

There is much emphasis on joint working, in particular between the NHS and social services. However, as can be seen from the above reforms, joint working is being encouraged across the whole of local government. The health improvement and public health agenda requires co-operation and co-ordination across local government with the NHS in setting targets for improving health and services.

Some joint working initiatives have already been put into practice from April 1999. The Health Act 1999 will allow greater flexibility to enable joint working from April 2000 in the form of pooled budgets, lead commissioning and integrated provision (see p36).

Prevention and rehabilitation

There is a new emphasis away from targeting services solely on those in the greatest need, and focussing instead on prevention and rehabilitation. The programme outlined in *Modernising Social Services* includes:

- greater prevention and rehabilitation through earmarked money for partnership between health and social services and for providing low level intervention to encourage people to do things for themselves at home (see p23);
- the extension of direct payments to people 65 or over in England. The scheme may become mandatory (see p46);
- promoting employment – this is included in the National Priorities Guidance and social services will be involved in the Single Gateway 'One' for benefit claimants of working age (see p27).

People with mental health problems

There is a new strategy for mental health which aims to balance independence with the safety of individuals and the wider community. It will have its own national service framework and more funding has been made available over the next three years.

The Mental Health Act 1983 is currently being reviewed and proposals have been published for consultants in England and Wales. The Millan Committee review of mental health services in Scotland is currently underway. There has recently been a 'White Paper from the Lord Chancellor's Department *Making Decisions* (for England and Wales). This discusses proposals for decision-making when someone lacks capacity. It includes proposals for changing an enduring power of attorney (see p336) so that as well as managing the person's financial affairs the attorney could make decisions about the health and welfare of the person. More recently a review of the Public Trust Office has recommended that it should be disbanded and its functions go to a variety of other agencies. In Scotland the Scottish Executive published a policy statement *Making the Right Moves* and a Bill has been introduced in the Scottish Parliament.

Carers

A new package has been introduced for carers as part of the Carers' Strategy.[5] It has three strategic elements.

- information – including a helpline for carers, and carers are included in the long-term care charter;
- support – including being involved in planning and providing services;

- care – including the right for carers to have their own health needs met, and new powers to provide services (proposals in England include direct payments) directly to carers as well as those being cared for, in particular helping carers take a break from caring. This is likely to require primary legislation. Extra earmarked money for carers has already been given to local authorities in England. Changes are planned for the financial support of working carers (see p446).

Asylum seekers

A new Immigration and Asylum Bill is due to come into force from April 2000. If enacted, the Bill will remove all existing financial and care responsibilities from the DSS and social services, and asylum seekers will normally be the responsibility of the Home Office

2. Changes to benefits

A number of changes to social security benefits are planned by the government. These could radically affect the amount of money you receive, some of which may be used to pay for your care needs or the extra costs your disability causes.

Welfare reform

A number of changes are part of the Welfare Reform and Pensions Act which received Royal Assent in November 1998. The intention is to implement most of them in 2001. There will be a new 'single work-focused gateway' called 'One' for all people of working age claiming benefits, including incapacity benefits. The Act allows for limited exemptions from compulsory work-focused interviews – eg, terminal illness or recovery from a major operation will mean you can defer your interview. Those over pension age will not be required to attend for interview. Compulsory interviews for new claimants will start from April 2000 in pilot areas. The changes to benefits under the Welfare Reform and Pension Act include as follows:

Disability living allowance and attendance allowance

There is a commitment to these benefits remaining universal and national. There will be new powers to amend conditions of entitlement by regulation, which as well as enabling changes to be made swiftly following decisions made in the courts, might also make it easier for the general conditions of entitlement to be changed. The higher rate of mobility component will be extended to children aged 3 and 4 planned for April 2001.

Incapacity benefit

National insurance contribution conditions will be tightened so that a minimum number of contributions must have been paid in one of the last three tax years before the benefit year in which you make your claim.

For new claims, half of any occupational or personal pension above £85 a week will be deducted from your entitlement. If you receive higher rate DLA care component you will be exempt from the occupational and personal pensions means-test. The Personal Capability Assessment (PCA) will replace the 'all-work' test from April 2000. It will be introduced in 'ONE' pilot areas from 13 December 1999. It appears that the new test is largely unchanged but will include questions used to compile a 'capability' or 'employability' report on what you can do with help or support and used for enhancing your prospects of obtaining work. The report will be passed to the Gateway Personal Advisor.

Severe disablement allowance

This benefit will be abolished, possibly from 2001. People aged 16-19 will be able to claim incapacity benefit instead, and will not have to meet the contribution conditions. Some people in full time education will be able to claim until the age of 25. You will keep your severe disablement allowance if you were getting it when the rules change. If you are over 20 (or in some cases 25) when you first become ill and do not have the contributions for incapacity benefit you will need to claim income support and/or DLA.

Income support

A new higher rate of disability premium and disabled child premium ('the disability income guarantee') will be introduced for those on income support who get the higher rate of DLA (care component)

Pensions

The government is planning a new range of second pension schemes called 'stakeholder pensions'. They are not expected to become available until April 2001.

Bereavement benefits

Changes are planned for benefits for those who have been bereaved. The proposals are:
- to double the lump sum payment to £2,000;
- replace the widowed mother's allowance with a widowed parent's allowance;
- allow a £10 disregard on this if you are on income support;
- pay a transitional 'bereavement allowance' for a year for those aged 45 or over who have no dependent children;

- provide a special income support premium after the end of the transitional year for those aged 55 or more at the start of the new arrangements or who are widowed during the subsequent five years. This is expected to happen no earlier than 2001.

Other proposed changes to benefits

In addition to the changes proposed under the Welfare Reform and Pensions Act, there are a number of other changes to benefits which are being considered.

Residential allowance

Possible changes to the residential allowance which at present is paid as part of income support were mentioned in the White Paper *Modernising Social Services*. The residential allowance is seen as offering social services a 'perverse incentive' to place people into residential care, because the payment of residential allowance as part of income support often makes it cheaper for them to place people in residential care rather than provide help at home. The government has suggested that there is a 'strong case' for phasing out the residential allowance and transferring the resources that would have been used by social security to social services. Social services could use this money more flexibly to help people remain at home. It is not known when or if these changes might occur.

Carers' benefits

In the Carers' Strategy *Caring About Carers* the government has said it will keep under review how financial support for carers, including invalid care allowance, can best meet the needs of working carers.

It is proposed that carers who are not able to work because of their caring responsibilities (or have insufficient earnings to pay NI contributions) will receive credits towards a second pension. It is estimated that by the year 2050 carers could receive up to £50 in today's terms in extra pension, payable in addition to the basic state retirement pension.

Housing benefit

Proposals have been put forward[6] to alter housing benefit for supported housing. A new transitional scheme will be introduced from April 2000 until April 2003 when the new scheme comes into place. The new scheme will replace the current funding arrangements (including housing benefit paid for support services) with a single budget specifically for support services for vulnerable people. It will be administered by local authorities. Local housing, social services and probation authorities will have to agree how the resources will be applied at a local level.

From 2003 housing benefit will not include any payments for support services such as supervision, general counselling, managing behavioural problems, advocacy, community alarms and assistance with paying bills. Instead, the local authority will have powers to provide these services and will use the new budget to do so. The money will go to the scheme or the provider rather than to the individual and may be paid to assist homeowners in addition to tenants.

3. **Changes to charges**

At present little is known about any plans the government might have on changes to the charging system, following the Royal Commission's report (see p448). Two possible changes have been suggested which will affect charges.

Domiciliary charges

It was proposed in the English White Paper *Modernising Social Services* that consideration would be given to improving the system of domiciliary charging, in the light of both the Royal Commission's report and the outcome of an Audit Commission survey due to report in March 2000. The Audit Commission carried a survey of all local authority charging procedures in England and Wales to compare the effects of different charging regimes. The wide variations in charges by different local authorities is considered by the government to be unacceptable. It is expected that any changes proposed would be aimed at ensuring greater consistency in the way income and capital are assessed.

Charges affected by the residential allowance

If the proposals for the transfer of the residential allowance (see p446) go ahead there will be a knock-on effect in that the level of income support you receive will be lower. This will mean you will be charged less out of your income and the amount social services pay the home will increase. This will affect you if you have to refund social services – eg, following the sale of your former home. Social services will bill you for the full amount they have paid. The bill will reflect the greater amounts that will be required if you do not receive the residential allowance. It will also mean that using the benefits route instead of social services if you have property to sell will no longer be as attractive (see p370). However, changes to the residential allowance may be part of a package of changes following from the Royal Commission.

4. **The proposals of the Royal Commission**

In March 1999 the Royal Commission on long-term care reported its proposals for the future funding of long-term care (see Chapter 25 p449 for the government's response in December 1999).

The Royal Commission made a large number of recommendations, which can be split between funding and provision of services. There was a note of dissent from two of the Commissioners, who put forward alternative proposals. The government has said it is looking at all the proposals.

Proposals on funding

The main Royal Commission recommendation is that the costs of care for those who need it should be split between living costs, housing costs and personal care. Personal care should be available free after an assessment. Living and housing costs should be paid by the individual according to means. Personal care would be free at home as well as in residential and nursing care. General living costs would be paid by the individual with help if necessary. The Royal Commission defined personal care as care which directly involves touching another person, although it also includes behaviour management. It excluded services such as cleaning or housework, laundry, shopping, or sitting services (when this was just for companionship) even though these costs are caused by disability.

The two commissioners who dissented from this proposal did so on the grounds that making personal care free would merely help the better off (or specifically, their beneficiaries) and that the money should be used to improve current services. Their top priority was to put an extra £300 million to deal with the present shortfall in funding. They looked towards a more genuine public-private partnership with proposals to remove obstacles in relation to long-term care insurance.

In addition to their main proposal that personal care should be free, the Royal Commission put forward a number of alternative proposals that could either stand alone or be subsumed in the main proposal.

- The value of the former home should be disregarded for three months after going into residential or nursing care to allow the opportunity for rehabilitation.
- The capital rules should be changed, raising the upper limit to £60,000 with no changes to the lower limit or tariff income. The note of dissent suggested the upper limit should be £30,000 and tariff income changed to £1 a week for each £500 above £10,000.
- Nursing care should be free in nursing homes as it is everywhere else. The dissenting Commissioners agreed with this but suggested a detailed examination of the costs of nursing care in nursing homes.

- The dissenting Commissioners also suggested that there should be a loan scheme to ensure that no one had to sell their property if they did not want to in their lifetime, and that personal care should be free to those who had been in residential or nursing homes for more than four years (one commissioner only).
- The residential allowance should be transferred to local authorities (see p446).
- A solution should be found to address the shortfall in funding experienced by those with preserved rights.
- Budgets for aids and adaptations should be in a single budget and local authorities should be able to make loans for aids and adaptations for those with housing assets.
- Direct payments should be extended to those over 65 years.

Proposals to improve service delivery

The main proposal from the Royal Commission was that there should be a National Care Commission to monitor trends, ensure transparency and accountability, represent the interests of consumers, encourage innovations and set national benchmarks now and in the future.

Various other proposals were made, including:
- further research into the cost effectiveness of rehabilitation and the outcomes of preventative interventions;
- a national survey to provide reliable data and monitor trends in health expectancy;
- development of the role of advocacy;
- improved cultural awareness in services to black and ethnic minority elders;
- better services should be offered to people who have carers

The Government's response to the proposals

The Government issued a response to the proposals of the Royal Commission on 2 December 1999. It broadly accepted the recommendation of a National Care Commission by announcing the National Care Standards Commission. In addition to its regulatory role the National Care Standards Commission will act as a single independent national watchdog responsible for ensuring high standards of care. It will investigate complaints and report on them, ensure the provision of clear accurate information, report on service performance against standards, and run its own helplines to guide people to registered providers. It is planned that it will be in operation by the spring 2002.

There have been no final decisions on the funding of long term care which have been left until the conclusions of the next comprehensive spending review in July 2000. However, the Government announced that it will be examining in detail the following:

- the recommendation that consideration should be given to providing nursing care free whether delivered in the NHS or in a private nursing home. It will be looking at ways of overcoming the problems of defining nursing care;
- the financial services industry to see if long term care insurance and other financial products could be made more attractive;
- possible changes to the residential charging rules including the treatment of the former home where a former carer remains in it and measures to avoid immediate house sales;
- the possible transfer of the residential allowance to social services;
- the possible transfer of responsibility to social services for people with preserved rights; and
- ways of reducing the scale of variations in local authority charges for domiciliary care following the Audit Commission report due in March 2000.

There will be a White Paper in the summer of 2000.

What next?

Although the proposals described above give some indication of possible changes, many questions remain unanswered. Some changes are already in the pipeline, others may well require primary legislation. Decisions made in the courts could also influence the future trends.

The one certainty about paying for care and receiving benefits is that the system is constantly evolving and up to date information is essential. A new edition of this Handbook will be produced each year to keep up with the changes.

Notes

1. **Changes to service delivery**
   1 Modernising Health and Social Services the National Priorities Guidance 1998
   2 A New Approach to Social Services Performance DoH 1999

   3 Long-term care charter 'Better Care, Higher Standards', 1999
   4 DoH Consultation 'Fit for the Future', 1999
   5 *Caring About Carers* 1999

2. **Changes to benefits**
   6 *Supporting People* DETR 1998

Appendices

Appendix 1

Key legislation

Reproduced in this appendix is some of the key legislation governing some of the powers and duties of social services departments (and health authorities) relevant to this Handbook. It contains the following legislation which applies in England and Wales:

1. ss21-26A and s29 National Assistance Act 1948 (p453)
2. ss45 and 65 Health Services and Public Health Act 1968 (p462)
3. ss1 and 2 Chronically Sick and Disabled Persons Act 1970 (p463)
4. ss4, 8 and 16 Disabled Persons (Services, Consultation and Representation) Act 1986 (p464)
5. ss46 and 47 National Health Service and Community Care Act 1990 (p465)
6. ss17, 21, 22 and 24 Health and Social Services and Social Security Adjudications Act 1983 (p467)
7. s117 Mental Health Act 1983 (p471)
8. s1 Carers (Recognition and Services) Act 1995 (p471)
9. ss6-7E Local Authority Social Services Act 1970 (p472)
10. ss1-3, 21 and Schedule 8 paras 1-3 National Health Service Act 1977 (p474)

It also reproduces the following legislation which applies in Scotland:
11. ss3-5B, 12-14 and 86-87 Social Work (Scotland) Act 1968 (p477)
12. ss7-8 Mental Health (Scotland) Act 1984 (p487)
13. ss1, 36 and 37 NHS (Scotland) Act 1978 (p487)
14. s117 Scotland Act 1998 (p488)

National Assistance Act 1948

Duty of local authorities to provide accommodation

21.–(1) Subject to and in accordance with the provisions of this Part of this Act, a local authority may with the approval of the Secretary of State, and to such extent as he may direct shall, make arrangements for providing:
  (a) residential accommodation for persons aged eighteen or over who by reason of age, illness, disability or any other circumstances are in need of care and attention which is not otherwise available to them; and

(aa) residential accommodation for expectant and nursing mothers who are in need of care and attention which is not otherwise available to them.

(2) In making any such arrangements a local authority shall have regard to the welfare of all persons for whom accommodation is provided, and in particular to the need for providing accommodation of different descriptions suited to different descriptions of such persons as are mentioned in the last foregoing subsection.

(2A) In determining for the purposes of paragraph (a) or (aa) of subsection (1) of this section whether care and attention are otherwise available to a person, a local authority shall disregard so much of the person's capital as does not exceed the capital limit for the purposes of section 22 of this Act.

(2B) For the purposes of subsection (2A) of this section—

(a) a person's capital shall be calculated in accordance with assessment regulations in the same way as if he were a person for whom accommodation is proposed to be provided as mentioned in subsection (3) of section 22 of this Act and whose ability to pay for the accommodation falls to be assessed for the purposes of that subsection; and

(b) "the capital limit for the purposes of section 22 of this Act" means the amount for the time being prescribed in assessment regulations as the amount which a resident's capital (calculated in accordance with such regulations) must not exceed if he is to be assessed as unable to pay for his accommodation at the standard rate; and in this subsection "assessment regulations" means regulations made for the purposes of section 22(5) of this Act.

(3) [*repealed*]

(4) Subject to section 26 of this Act, accommodation provided by a local authority in the exercise of their functions under this section shall be provided in premises managed by the authority or, to such extent as may be determined in accordance with the arrangements under this section, in such premises managed by another local authority as may be agreed between the two authorities and on such terms as to the reimbursement of expenditure incurred by the said other authority, as may be so agreed.

(5) References in this Act to accommodation provided under this Part thereof shall be construed as references to accommodation provided in accordance with this and the five next following sections, and as including references to board and other services, amenities and requisites provided in connection with the accommodation except where in the opinion of the authority managing the premises their provision is unnecessary.

(6) References in this Act to a local authority providing accommodation shall be construed, in any case where a local authority agree with another local

authority for the provision of accommodation in premises managed by the said authority, as references to the first-mentioned local authority.

(7) Without prejudice to the generality of the foregoing provisions of this section, a local authority may–

(a) provide, in such cases as they may consider appropriate, for the conveyance of persons to and from premises in which accommodation is provided for them under this Part of the Act;

(b) make arrangements for the provision on the premises in which accommodation is being provided of such other services as appear to the authority to be required.

(8) Nothing in this section shall authorise or require a local authority to make any provision authorised or required to be made (whether by that or by any other authority) by or under any enactment not contained in this Part of this Act, or authorised or required to be provided under the National Health Service Act 1977.

Charges to be made for accommodation

22.—(1) Subject to section 26 of this Act, where a person is provided, with accommodation under this Part of this Act the local authority providing the accommodation shall recover from him the amount of the payment which he is liable to make.

(2) Subject to the following provisions of this section, the payment which a person is liable to make for any such accommodation shall be in accordance with a standard rate fixed for that accommodation by the authority managing the premises in which it is provided and that standard rate shall represent the full cost to the authority of providing that accommodation.

(3) Where a person for whom accommodation in premises managed by any local authority is provided, or proposed to be provided, under this Part of this Act satisfies the local authority that he is unable to pay therefor at the standard rate, the authority shall assess his ability to pay, and accordingly determine at what lower rate he shall be liable to pay for the accommodation.

(4) In assessing for the purposes of the last foregoing subsection a person's ability to pay, a local authority shall assume that he will need for his personal requirements such sum per week as may be prescribed by the Minister, or such other sum as in special circumstances the authority may consider appropriate.

(4A) Regulations made for the purposes of subsection (4) of this section may prescribe different sums for different circumstances.

(5) In assessing as aforesaid a person's ability to pay, a local authority shall give effect to regulations made by the Secretary of State for the purposes of this subsection except that, until the first such regulations come into force, a local authority shall give effect to Part III of Schedule 1 to the Supplementary Benefits Act 1976, as it had effect immediately before the amendments made by Schedule 2 to the Social Security Act 1980.

(5A) If they think fit, an authority managing premises in which accommodation is provided for a person shall have power on each occasion when they provide accommodation for him, irrespective of his means, to limit to such amount as appears to them reasonable for him to pay the payments required from him for his accommodation during a period commencing when they begin to provide the accommodation for him and ending not more than eight weeks after that.

(6) [*repealed*]

(7) [*repealed*]

(8) Where accommodation is provided by a local authority in premises managed by another local authority, the payment therefor under this section shall be made to the authority managing the premises and not to the authority providing the accommodation, but the authority managing the premises shall account for the payment to the authority providing the accommodation.

(9)[*repealed*]

Management of premises in which accommodation provided

23.—(1) Subject to the provisions of this Part of this Act, a local authority may make rules as to the conduct of premises under their management in which accommodation is provided under this Part of this Act and as to the preservation of order in the premises.

(2) Rules under this section may provide that where by reason of any change in a person's circumstances he is no longer qualified to receive accommodation under this Part of this Act or where a person has otherwise become unsuitable therefor, he may be required by the local authority managing the premises to leave the premises in which the accommodation is provided.

(3) Rules under this section may provide for the waiving of part of the payments due under the last foregoing section where in compliance with the rules persons for whom accommodation is provided assist in the running of the premises.

Authority liable for provision of accommodation

24.—(1) The local authority empowered under this Part of this Act to provide residential accommodation for any person shall subject to the following provisions of this Part of this Act be the authority in whose area the person is ordinarily resident.

(2) [*repealed*]

(3) Where a person in the area of a local authority—

(a) is a person with no settled residence, or—

(b) not being ordinarily resident in the area of the local authority, is in urgent need of residential accommodation under this Part of this Act,

the authority shall have the like power to provide residential accommodation for him as if he were ordinarily resident in their area.

(4) Subject to and in accordance with the arrangements under section twenty-one of this Act, a local authority shall have power, as respects a person ordinarily resident in the area of another local authority, with the consent of that other local authority to provide residential accommodation for him in any case where the authority would have a duty to provide such accommodation if he were ordinarily resident in their area.

(5) Where a person is provided with residential accommodation under this Part of this Act, he shall be deemed for the purposes of this Act to continue to be ordinarily resident in the area in which he was ordinarily resident immediately before the residential accommodation was provided for him.

(6) For the purposes of the provision of residential accommodation under this Part of this Act, a patient in a hospital vested in the Secretary of State or an NHS trust shall be deemed to be ordinarily resident in the area, if any, in which he was ordinarily resident immediately before he was admitted as a patient to the hospital, whether or not he in fact continues to be ordinarily resident in that area.

(7) In subsection (6) above 'NHS trust' means a National Health Service trust established under Part 1 of the National Health Service and Community Care Act 1990 or under the National Health Service (Scotland) Act 1978.

s25 [*repealed*]

Provision of accommodation in premises maintained by voluntary organisations

26.—(1) Subject to subsections (1A) and (1B) below, arrangements under section 21 of this Act may include arrangements made with a voluntary organisation or with any other person who is not a local authority where—

(a) that organisation or person manages premises which provide for reward accommodation falling within subsection (1)(a) or (aa) of that section, and

(b) the arrangements are for the provision of such accommodation in those premises.

(1A) Subject to subsection (1B) below, arrangements made with any voluntary organisation or other person by virtue of this section must, if they are for the provision of residential accommodation with both board and personal care for such persons as are mentioned in section 1(1) of the Registered Homes Act 1984 (requirement for registration), be arrangements for the provision of such accommodation in a residential care home which is managed by the organisation or person in question, being such a home in respect of which that organisation or person—

(a) is registered under Part 1 of that Act, or

(b) is not required to be so registered by virtue of section 1(4)(a) or (b) of that Act (certain small homes) or by virtue of the home being managed or provided by an exempt body;

and for this purpose 'personal care' and 'residential care home' have the same meaning as in that Part of that Act.

(1B) Arrangements made with any voluntary organisation or other person by virtue of this section must, if they are for the provision of residential accommodation where nursing care is provided, be arrangements for the provision of such accommodation in premises which are managed by the organisation or persons in question, being premises—

(a) in respect of which that organisation or person is registered under Part 11 of the Registered Homes Act 1984, or

(b) which, by reason only of being maintained or controlled by an exempt body, do not fall within the definition of a nursing home in section 21 of that Act.

(1C) Subject to subsection (1D) below, no such arrangements as are mentioned in subsection (1B) above may be made by an authority for the accommodation of any person without the consent of such Health Authority as may be determined in accordance with regulations.

(1D) Subsection (1C) above does not apply to the making by an authority of temporary arrangements for the accommodation of any person as a matter of urgency; but, as soon as practicable after any such temporary arrangements have been made, the authority shall seek the consent required by subsection (1C) above to the making of appropriate arrangements for the accommodation of the person concerned.

(1E) No arrangements may be made by virtue of this section with a person who has been convicted of an offence under any provision of—

(a) the Registered Homes Act 1948 (or any enactment replaced by that Act); or

(b) regulations made under section 16 or section 26 of that Act (or under any corresponding provisions of any such enactment).

(2) Any arrangements made by virtue of this section shall provide for the making by the local authority to the other party thereto of payments in respect of the accommodation provided at such rates as may be determined by or under the arrangements and subject to subsection (3A) below the local authority shall recover from each person for whom accommodation is provided under the arrangements the amount of the refund which he is liable to make in accordance with the following provisions of this section.

(3) Subject to subsection (3A) below, a person for whom accommodation is provided under any such arrangements shall, in lieu of being liable to make payment therefor in accordance with section twenty-two of this Act, refund to the local authority any payments made in respect of him under the last foregoing subsection:

Provided that where a person for whom accommodation is provided, or proposed to be provided, under any such arrangements satisfies the local authority that he is unable to make refund at the full rate determined under that subsection, subsections (3) to (5) of section twenty-two of this Act shall, with the necessary modifications, apply as they apply where a person satisfies the local authority of his inability to pay at the standard rate as mentioned in the said subsection (3).

(3A) Where accommodation in any premises is provided for any person under any arrangements made by virtue of this section and the local authority, the person concerned and the voluntary organisation or the other person managing the premises (in this subsection referred to as 'the provider') agree that this section shall apply—

(a) so long as the person concerned makes the payments for which he is liable under paragraph (b) below, he shall not be liable to make any refund under subsection (3) above and the local authority shall not be liable to make any payment under subsection (2) above in respect of the accommodation provided for him;

(b) the person concerned shall be liable to pay to the provider such sums as he would otherwise (under subsection (3) above) be liable to pay by way of refund to the local authority; and

(c) the local authority shall be liable to pay to the provider the difference between the sums paid by virtue of paragraph (b) above and the payments which, but for paragraph (a) above, the authority would be liable to pay under subsection (2) above.

(4) Subsections (5A), (7) and (9) of the said section twenty-two shall, with the necessary modifications, apply for the purposes of the last foregoing subsection as they apply for the purposes of the said section twenty-two.

(4A) Section 21(5) of this Act shall have effect as respects accommodation provided under arrangements made by virtue of this section with the substitution for the references to the authority managing the premises of a reference to the authority making the arrangements.

(5) Where in any premises accommodation is being provided under this section in accordance with arrangements made by any local authority, any person authorised in that behalf by the authority may at all reasonable times enter and inspect the premises

(6) [*repealed*]

(7) In this section the expression 'voluntary organisation' includes any association which is a housing association for the purposes of the Housing Act 1936, 'small home' means an establishment falling within section 1(4) of the Registered Homes Act 1984 and 'exempt body' means an authority or body constituted by an Act of Parliament or incorporated by Royal Charter.

Exclusion of powers to provide accommodation under this Part in certain cases

26A.—(1) Subject to subsection (3) of this section, no accommodation may be provided under section 21 or 26 of this Act for any person who immediately before the date on which this section comes into force was ordinarily resident in relevant premises.

(2) In subsection (1) 'relevant premises' means—

(a) premises in respect of which any person is registered under the Registered Homes Act 1984;

(b) premises in respect of which such registration is not required by virtue of their being managed or provided by an exempt body;

(c) premises which do not fall within the definition of a nursing home in section 21 of that Act by reason only of their being maintained or controlled by an exempt body; and

(d) such other premises as the Secretary of State may by regulations prescribe;

and in this subsection 'exempt body' has the same meaning as in section 26 of this Act.

(3) The Secretary of State may by regulations provide that, in such cases and subject to such conditions as may be prescribed, subsection (1) of this section shall not apply in relation to such classes of persons as may be prescribed in the regulations.

(4) The Secretary of State shall by regulations prescribe the circumstances in which persons are to be treated as being ordinarily resident in any premises for the purposes of subsection (1) of this section.

(5) This section does not affect the validity of any contract made before the date on which this section comes into force for the provision of accommodation on or after that date or anything done in pursuance of such a contract.

s27 [*repealed*]

s28 [*repealed*]

Welfare arrangements for blind, deaf, dumb and crippled persons, etc

29.—(1) A local authority may, with the approval of the Secretary of State, and to such extent as he may direct in relation to persons ordinarily resident in the area of the local authority shall make arrangements for promoting the welfare of persons to whom this section applies, that is to say persons aged eighteen or over who are blind, deaf or dumb or who suffer from mental disorder of any description, and other persons aged eighteen or over who are substantially and permanently handicapped by illness, injury, or congenital deformity or such other disabilities as may be prescribed by the Minister.

(2) [*repealed*]

(3) [*repealed*]

(4) Without prejudice to the generality of the provisions of subsection (1) of this section, arrangements may be made thereunder-

(a) for informing persons to whom arrangements under that subsection relate of the services available for them thereunder;

(b) for giving such persons instruction in their own homes or elsewhere in methods of overcoming the effects of their disabilities;

(c) for providing workshops where such persons may be engaged (whether under a contract of service or otherwise) in suitable work, and hostels where persons engaged in the workshops, and other persons to whom arrangements under subsection (1) of this section relate and for whom work or training is being provided in pursuance of the Disabled Persons (Employment) Act 1944 or the Employment and Training Act 1973 may live;

(d) for providing persons to whom arrangements under subsection (1) of this section relate with suitable work (whether under a contract of service or otherwise) in their own homes or elsewhere;

(e) for helping such persons in disposing of the produce of their work; for providing such persons with recreational facilities in their own homes or elsewhere;

(f) for providing such persons with recreational facilities in their own homes or elsewhere;

(g) for compiling and maintaining classified registers of the persons to whom arrangements under subsection (1) of this section relate.

(4A)Where accommodation in a hostel is provided under paragraph (c) of subsection (4) of this section—

(a) if the hostel is managed by a local authority, section 22 of this Act shall apply as it applies where accommodation is provided under s21;

(b) if the accommodation is provided in a hostel managed by a person other than a local authority under arrangements made with that person, subsections (2) to (4A) of section 26 of this Act shall apply as they apply where accommodation is provided under arrangements made by virtue of that section; and

(c) sections 32 and 43 of this Act shall apply as they apply where accommodation is provided under sections 21 to 26;

and in this subsection referencs to 'accommodation' include references to board and other services, amenities and requisites provided in connection with the accommodation, except where in the opinion of the authority managing the premises or, in the case mentioned in paragraph (b) above, the authority making the arrangements their provision is unnecessary.

(5) [*repealed*]

(6) Nothing in the foregoing provisions of this section shall authorise or require—

(a) the payment of money to persons to whom this section applies, other than persons for whom work is provided under arrangements made by virtue of paragraph (c) or paragraph (d) of subsection (4) of this section or who are engaged in work which they are enabled to perform in consequence of anything done in pursuance of arrangements made under this section; or

(b) the provision of any accommodation or services required to be provided under the National Health Service Act 1977.

(7) A person engaged in work in a workshop provided under paragraph (c) of subsection (4) of this section, or a person in receipt of a superannuation allowance granted on his retirement from engagement in any such workshop, shall be deemed for the purposes of this Act to continue to be ordinarily resident in the area in which he was ordinarily resident immediately before he was accepted for work in that workshop; and for the purposes of this subsection a course of training in such workshop shall be deemed to be work in that workshop.

Health Services and Public Health Act 1968

Promotion, by local authorities, of the welfare of old people

45.—(1) A local authority may with the approval of the Secretary of State, and to such extent as he may direct shall, make arrangements for promoting the welfare of old people.

(2) [*repealed*]

(3) A local authority may employ as their agent for the purposes of this section any voluntary organisation or any person carrying on, professionally or by way of trade or business, activities which consist of or include the provision of services for old people, being an organisation or person appearing to the authority to be capable of promoting the welfare of old people.

(4) No arrangements under this section shall provide—

(a) for the payment of money to old people except in so far as the arrangements may provide for the remuneration of old people engaged in suitable work in accordance with the arrangements;

(b) for making available any accommodation or services required to be provided under the National Health Service Act 1977.

Financial and other assistance by local authorities to certain voluntary organisations

65.—(1) A local authority may give assistance by way of grant or by way of loan, or partly in the one way and partly in the other, to a voluntary organisation whose activities consist in, or include, the provision of a service similar to a relevant service, the promotion of the provision of a relevant service or a similar one, the publicising of a relevant service or a similar one or the giving of advice with respect to the manner in which a relevant service or a similar one can best be provided, and so may the Greater London Council.

(2) A local authority may also assist any such voluntary organisation as aforesaid by permitting them to use premises belonging to the authority on such terms as may be agreed, and by making available furniture, vehicles or equipment (whether by way of gift, or loan or otherwise) and the services of any staff who are employed by the authority in connection with the premises or other things which they permit the organisation to use.

Chronically Sick and Disabled Persons Act 1970

Information as to need for and existence of welfare services

1.—(1) It shall be the duty of every local authority having functions under section 29 of the National Assistance Act 1948 to inform themselves of the number of persons to whom that section applies within their area and of the need for the making by the authority of arrangements under that section for such persons.

(2) Every such local authority—

(a) shall cause to be published from time to time at such times and in such manner as they consider appropriate general information as to the services provided under arrangements made by the authority under the said section 29 which are for the time being available in the area; and

(b) shall ensure that any such person as aforesaid who uses any of those services is informed of any other service provided by the authority (whether under any such arrangements or not) which in the opinion of the authority is relevant to his needs and of any service provided by any other authority or organisation which in the opinion of the authority is so relevant and of which particulars are in the authorities' possession.

Provision of welfare services

2.—(1) Where a local authority having functions under s29 National Assistance Act 1948 are satisfied in the case of any person to whom that section applies who is ordinarily resident in their area that it is necessary in order to meet the needs of that person for that authority to make arrangements for all or any of the following matters, namely:-

(a) the provision of practical assistance for that person in his home;

(b) the provision for that person of, or assistance to that person in obtaining, wireless, television, library or similar recreational facilities;

(c) the provision for that person of lectures, games, outings or other recreational facilities outside his home or assistance to that person in taking advantage of educational facilities available to him;

(d) the provision for that person of facilities for, or assistance in, travelling to and from his home for the purpose of participating in any services provided under arrangements made by the authority under the said section 29 or, with the approval of the authority, in any services provided otherwise than as aforesaid which are similar to services which could be provided under such arrangements;

(e) the provision of assistance for that person in arranging for the carrying out of any works of adaptation in his home or the provision of any additional facilities designed to secure his greater safety, comfort or convenience;

(f) facilitating the taking of holidays by that person, whether at holiday homes or otherwise and whether provided under arrangements made by the authority or otherwise;

(g) the provision of meals for that person whether in his home or elsewhere;

(h) the provision for that person of, or assistance to that person in obtaining, a telephone and any special equipment necessary to enable him to use a telephone,

then, subject to the provisions of section 7(1) of the Local Authority Social Services Act 1970 (which requires local authorities in the exercise of certain functions, including functions under the said section 29, to act under the general guidance of the Secretary of State) and to the provisions of section 7A of that Act (which requires local authorities to exercise their social services functions in accordance with directions given by the Secretary of State) it shall be the duty of that Authority to make those arrangements in exercise of their functions under the said section 29.

Disabled Persons (Services, Consultation and Representation) Act 1986

4. When requested to do so by—

(a) a disabled person ...

(c) any person who provides care for him in the circumstances mentioned in section 8,

a local authority shall decide whether the needs of the disabled person call for the provision by the authority of any services in accordance with section 2(1) of the 1970 Act (provision for welfare services).

8.—(1) Where—

(a) a disabled person is living at home and receiving a substantial amount of care on a regular basis from another person (who is not a person employed to provide such care by any body in the exercise of its functions under any enactment), and it falls to a local authority to decide whether the disabled person's needs call for the provision by them of any services for him under any of the welfare enactments, the local authority shall, in deciding that question, have regard to the ability of that other person to continue to provide such care on a regular basis.

16. In this Act—

. . .

'disabled person'—

(a) in relation to England and Wales, means

(i) in the case of a person aged 18 or over, a person to whom s29 of the National Assistance Act 1948 applies; and

(ii) in the case of a person under the age of 18, a person who is disabled within the meaning of Part 111 of the Children Act 1989.

National Health Service and Community Care Act 1990

Local authority plans for community care services

46.—(1) Each local authority–

(a) shall, within such period after the day appointed for the coming into force of this section as the Secretary of State may direct, prepare and publish a plan for the provision of community care services in their area;

(b) shall keep the plan prepared by them under paragraph (a) above and any further plans prepared by them under this section under review; and

(c) shall, at such intervals as the Secretary of State may direct, prepare and publish modifications to the current plan, or if the case requires, a new plan.

(2) In carrying out any of their functions under paragraphs (a) to (c) of subsection (1) above, a local authority shall consult—

(a) any Health Authority the whole or any part of whose district lies within the area of the local authority;

(b) [*repealed*]

(c) in so far as any proposed plan, review or modifications of a plan may affect or be affected by the provision or availability of housing and the local authority is not itself a local housing authority, within the meaning of the Housing Act 1985, every such local housing authority whose area is within the area of the local authority;

(d) such voluntary organisations as appear to the authority to represent the interests of persons who use or are likely to use any community care services within the area of the authority or the interests of private carers who, within that area, provide care to persons for whom, in the exercise of their social services functions, the local authority have a power or a duty to provide a service;

(e) such voluntary housing agencies and other bodies as appear to the local authority to provide housing or community care services in their area; and

(f) such other persons as the Secretary of State may direct.

(3) In this section—

'local authority' means the council of a county, a county borough, a metropolitan district or a London borough or the Common Council of the City of London;

'community care services' means services which a local authority may provide or arrange to be provided under any of the following provisions—

(a) Part III of the National Assistance Act 1948;

(b) section 45 of the Health Services and Public Health Act 1968;

(c) section 21 of and Schedule 8 to the National Health Service Act 1977; and

(d) section 117 of the Mental Health Act 1983; and

'private carer' means a person who is not employed to provide the care in question by any body in the exercise of its function under any enactment.

Assessment of needs for community care services

47.—(1) Subject to subsections (5) and (6) below, where it appears to a local authority that any person for whom they may provide or arrange for the provision of community care services may be in need of any such services, the authority—

(a) shall carry out an assessment of his needs for those services; and

(b) having regard to the results of that assessment, shall then decide whether his needs call for the provision by them of any such services.

(2) If at any time during the assessment of the needs of any person under subsection (1)(a) above it appears to a local authority that he is a disabled person, the authority—

(a) shall proceed to make such a decision as to the services he requires as is mentioned in section 4 of the Disabled Persons (Services, Consultation and Representation) Act 1986 without his requesting them to do so under that section; and

(b) shall inform him that they will be doing so and of his rights under that Act.

(3) If at any time during the assessment of the needs of any person under subsection (1)(a) above, it appears to a local authority—

(a) that there may be a need for the provision to that person by such Health Authority as may be determined in accordance with regulations of any services under the National Health Service Act 1977, or

(b) that there may be the need for the provision to him of any services which fall within the functions of a local housing authority (within the meaning of the Housing Act 1985) which is not the local authority carrying out the assessment,

the local authority shall notify that Health Authority or local housing authority and invite them to assist, to such extent as is reasonable in the circumstances, in the making of the assessment; and, in making their decision as to the provision of services needed for the person in question, the local authority shall take into account any services which are likely to be made available for him by that Health Authority or local housing authority.

(4) The Secretary of State may give directions as to the manner in which an assessment under this section is to be carried out or the form it is to take but, subject to any such directions and to subsection (7) below, it shall be carried out in such manner and take such form as the local authority consider appropriate.

(5) Nothing in this section shall prevent a local authority from temporarily providing or arranging for the provision of community care services for any person without carrying out a prior assessment of his needs in accordance with the preceding provisions of this section if, in the opinion of the authority, the condition of that person is such that he requires those services as a matter of urgency.

(6) If, by virtue of subsection (5) above, community care services have been provided temporarily for any person as a matter of urgency, then, as soon as practicable thereafter, an assessment of his needs shall be made in accordance with the preceding provisions of this section.... .

Health and Social Services and Social Security Ajudications Act 1983

Charges for local authority services in England and Wales

17.–(1) Subject to subsection (3) below, an authority providing a service to which this section applies may recover such charge (if any) for it as they consider reasonable.

(2) This section applies to services provided under the following enactments–

(a) section 29 if the National Assistance Act 1948 (welfare arrangements for blind, deaf, dumb, and crippled persons etc.);

(b) section 45(1) of the Health Services and Public Health Act 1968 (welfare of old people);

(c) Schedule 8 to the National Health Service Act 1977 (care of mothers and young children, prevention of illness and care and after-care and home help and laundry facilities);

(d) section 8 of the Residential Homes Act 1980 (meals and recreation for old people); and

(e) paragraph 1 of Part II of Schedule 9 to this Act other than the provision of services for which payment may be required under section 22 or 26 of the National Assistance Act 1948.

(3) If a person—

(a) avails himself of a service to which this section applies, and

(b) satisfies the authority providing the service that his means are insufficient for it to be reasonably practicable for him to pay for the service the amount which he would otherwise be obliged to pay for it,

the authority shall not require him to pay more for it than it appears to them that it is reasonable practicable for him to pay.

(4) Any charge under this section may, without prejudice to any other method of recovery, be recovered summarily as a civil debt.

Recovery of sums due to local authority where persons in residential accommodation have disposed of assets.

21.–(1) Subject to the following provisions of this section, where—

(a) a person avails himself of Part III accommodation; and

(b) that person knowingly and with the intention of avoiding charges for the accommodation—

(i) has transferred any asset to which this section applies to some other person or person not more than six months before the date on which he begins to reside in such accommodation; or

(ii) transfers any such asset to some other person or persons while residing in the accommodation; and

(c) either—

(i) the consideration for the transfer is less than the value of the asset; or

(ii) there is no consideration for the transfer,

the person or persons to whom the asset is transferred by the person availing himself of the accommodation shall be liable to pay to the local authority providing the accommodation or arranging for its provision the difference between the amount assessed as due to be paid for the accommodation by the person availing himself of it and the amount which the local authority receive from him for it.

(2) This section applies to cash and any other asset which falls to be taken into account for the purpose of assessing under section 22 of the National Assistance Act 1948 the ability to pay for the accommodation of the person availing himself of it.

(3) Subsection 1(1) above shall have effect in relation to a transfer by a person who leaves Part III accommodation and subsequently resumes residence in such accommodation as if the period of six months mentioned in paragraph (b)(i) were a period of six months before the date on which he resumed residence in such accommodation.

(3A) If the Secretary of State so directs, subsection (1) above shall not apply in such cases as may be specified in the direction.

(4) Where a person has transferred an asset to which this section applies to more than one person, the liability of each of the persons to whom it was transferred shall be in proportion to the benefit accruing to him from the transfer.

(5) A person's liability under this section shall not exceed the benefit accruing to him from the transfer.

(6) Subject to subsection (7) below, the value of any asset to which this section applies, other than cash, which has been transferred shall be taken to be the amount of the consideration which would have been realised for it if it had been sold on the open market by a willing seller at the time of the transfer.

(7) For the purpose of calculating the value of an asset under subsection (6) above there shall be deducted from the amount of the consideration—

(a) the amount of any incumbrance on the asset; and

(b) a reasonable amount in respect of the expenses of the sale.

(8) In this Part of this Act 'Part III accommodation' means accommodation provided under sections 21 to 26 of the National Assistance Act 1948, and, in the application of this Part of this Act to Scotland, means accommodation provided under the Social Work (Scotland) Act 1968 or section 7 (functions of local authorities) of the Mental Health (Scotland) Act 1984.

Arrears of contributions charged on interest in land in England and Wales

22.—(1) Subject to subsection (2) below, where a person who avails himself of Part III accommodation provided by a local authority in England, Wales or Scotland—

(a) fails to pay any sum assessed as due to be paid by him for the accommodation; and

(b) has a beneficial interest in land in England and Wales, the local authority may create a charge in their favour on his interest in the land.

(2) In the case of a person who has interests in more than one parcel of land the charge under this section shall be upon his interest in such one of the parcels as the local authority may determine.

(2A) In determining whether to exercise their power under subsection (1) above and in making any determination under subsection (2) above, the local authority shall comply with any directions given to them by the Secretary of State as to the exercise of those functions.

(3) Any interest in the proceeds of sale of land held upon trust for sale is to be treated, subject to subsection (8) below, as an interest in land for the purposes of this section.

(4) Subject to subsection (5) below, a charge under this section shall be in respect of any amount assessed as due to be paid which is outstanding from time to time.

(5) The charge on the interest of a joint tenant in the proceeds of sale of land held upon trust for sale shall be in respect of an amount not exceeding the value of the interest that he would enjoy in those proceeds if the joint tenancy were severed but the creation of such a charge shall not sever the joint tenancy.

(6) On the death of a joint tenant in the proceeds of sale of land held upon trust for sale whose interest in the proceeds is subject to a charge under this section—

(a) if there are surviving joint tenants, their interests in the proceeds; and
(b) if the land vests in one person, or one person is entitled to have it vested in him, his interest in it,

shall become subject to a charge for an amount not exceeding the amount of the charge to which the interest of the deceased joint tenant was subject by virtue of subsection (5) above.

(7) A charge under this section shall be created by a declaration in writing made by the local authority.

(8) Any such charge, other than a charge on an interest in the proceeds of sale of land, shall in the case of unregistered land be a land charge of Class B within the meaning of section 2 of the Land Charges Act 1972 and in the case of registered land be a registrable charge taking effect as a charge by way of legal mortgage.

Interest on sums charged on or secured over interest in land

24.—(1) Any sum charged on or secured over an interest in land under this Part of this Act shall bear interest from the day after that on which the person for whom the local authority provided the accommodation dies.

(2) The rate of interest shall be such reasonable rate as the Secretary of State may direct or, if no such direction is given, as the local authority may determine.

Mental Health Act 1983

After-care

117.—(1) This section applies to persons who are detained under section 3 above, or admitted to a hospital in pursuance of a hospital order made under section 37 above, or transferred to a hospital in pursuance of a transfer direction made under section 47 or 48 above, and then cease to be detained and (whether or not immediately after so ceasing) leave hospital.

(2) It shall be the duty of the Health Authority and of the local social services authority to provide, in co-operation with relevant voluntary agencies, after-care services for any person to whom this section applies until such time as the Health Authority and the local social services authority are satisfied that the person concerned is no longer in need of such services but they shall not be so satisfied in the case of a patient who is subject to after-care under supervision at any time while he so remains subject.

(2A) It shall be the duty of the Health Authority to secure that at all times while a patient is subject to after-care under supervision–

(a) a person who is a registered medical practitioner approved for the purposes of section 12 above by the Secretary of State as having special experience in the diagnosis or treatment of mental disorder is in charge of the medical treatment provided for the patient as part of the after-care services provided for him under this section; and

(b) a person professionally concerned with any of the after-care services so provided is supervising him with a view to securing that he receives the after-care services so provided.

(2B) Section 32 above shall apply for the purposes of this section as it applies for the purposes of Part II of this Act.

3) In this section 'the Health Authority' means the Health Authority and 'the local social services authority' means the local social services authority for the area in which the person concerned is resident or to which he is sent on discharge by the hospital in which he was detained.

Carers (Recognition and Services) Act 1995

Assessment of ability of carers to provide care: England and Wales

1.– (1) Subject to subsection (3) below, in any case where—

(a) a local authority carry out an assessment under section 47(1)(a) of the National Health Service and Community Care Act 1990 of the needs of a person ('the relevant person') for community care services, and

(b) an individual ('the carer') provides or intends to provide a substantial amount of care on a regular basis for the relevant person,

the carer may request the local authority, before they make their decision as to whether the needs of the relevant person call for the provision of any services, to carry out an assessment of his ability to provide and continue to provide care for the relevant person; and if he makes such a request, the local authority shall carry out such an assessment and shall take into account the results of that assessment in making that decision.

(2) Subject to subsection (3) below, in any case where—

(a) a local authority assess the needs of a disabled child for the purpose of Part III of the Children Act 1989 or section 2 of the Chronically Sick and Disabled Persons Act 1970, and

(b) an individual ('the carer') provides or intends to provide a substantial amount of care on a regular basis for the disabled child,

the carer may request the local authority, before they make their decision as to whether the needs of the disabled child call for the provision of any services, to carry out an assessment of his ability to provide and continue to provide care for the disabled child; and if he makes such a request, the local authority shall carry out such an assessment and shall take into account the results of that assessment in making that decision.

(3) No request may be made under subsection (1) or (2) above by an individual who provides or will provide the care in question—

(a) by virtue of a contract of employment or other contract with any person; or

(b) as a volunteer for a voluntary organisation. . .

Local Authority Social Services Act 1970

The director of social services

6.—(1) A local authority shall appoint an officer, to be known as the director of social services, for the purposes of their social services functions.

(2) Two or more local authorities may, if they consider that the same person can efficiently discharge, for both or all of them, the functions of director of social services for both or all of those authorities, concur in the appointment of a person as director of social services for both or all of those authorities.

(3) & (4) [repealed]

(5) The director of social services of a local authority shall not, without the approval of the Secretary of State (which may be given either generally or in relation to a particular authority), be employed by that authority in connection with the discharge of any of the authority's functions other than their social services functions.

(6) A local authority which has appointed, or concurred in the appointment of, a director of social services, shall secure the provision of adequate staff for assisting him in the exercise of his functions.

Local authorities to exercise social services functions under guidance of Secretary of State

7.—(1) Local authorities shall, in the exercise of their social services functions, including the exercise of any discretion conferred by any relevant enactment, act under the general guidance of the Secretary of State.

Directions by the Secretary of State as to exercise of social services functions

7A.—(1) Without prejudice to section 7 of this Act, every local authority shall exercise their social services functions in accordance with such directions as may be given to them under this section by the Secretary of State.

(2) Directions under this section—

(a) shall be given in writing; and

(b) may be given to a particular authority, or to authorities of a particular class, or to authorities generally.

Complaints procedure

7B.—(1) The Secretary of State may by order require local authorities to establish a procedure for considering any representations (including any complaints) which are made to them by a qualifying individual, or anyone acting on his behalf, in relation to the discharge of, or any failure to discharge, any of their social services functions in respect of that individual.

(2) In relation to a particular local authority, an individual is a qualifying individual for the purposes of subsection (1) above if—

(a) the authority have a power or a duty to provide, or to secure the provision of, a service for him; and

(b) his need or possible need for such a service has (by whatever means) come to the attention of the authority.

(3) A local authority shall comply with any directions given by the Secretary of State as to the procedure to be adopted in considering representations made as mentioned in subsection (1) above and as to the taking of such action as may be necessary in consequence of such representations.

(4) Local authorities shall give such publicity to any procedure established pursuant to this section as they consider appropriate.

Inquiries

7C.—(1) The Secretary of State may cause an inquiry to be held in any case where, whether on representations made to him or otherwise, he considers it advisable to do so in connection with the exercise by any local authority of any of their social services functions (except in so far as those functions relate to persons under the age of eighteen).

(2) Subsections (2) to (5) of section 250 of the Local Government Act 1972 (powers in relation to local inquiries) shall apply in relation to an inquiry under this section as they apply in relation to an inquiry under that section.

Default powers of Secretary of State as respects social services functions of local authorities

7D.—(1) If the Secretary of State is satisfied that any local authority have failed, without reasonable excuse, to comply with any of their duties which are social services functions (other than a duty imposed by or under the Children Act 1989), he may make an order declaring that authority to be in default with respect to the duty in question.

(2) An order under subsection (1) may contain such directions for the purpose of ensuring that the duty is complied with within such period as may be specified in the order as appear to the Secretary of State to be necessary.

(3) Any such direction shall, on the application of the Secretary of State, be enforceable by mandamus.

Grants to local authorities in respect of certain social services

7E. The Secretary of State may, with the approval of the Treasury, make grants out of money provided by Parliament towards any expenses of local authorities incurred—

(a) in connection with the exercise of their social services functions in relation to persons suffering from mental illness; or

(b) in making payments, in accordance with directions given by the Secretary of State to voluntary organisations which provide care and services for persons who are, have been, or are likely to become dependent upon alcohol or drugs.

National Health Service Act 1977

Secretary of State's duty as to health service

1.—(1) it is the Secretary of State's duty to continue the promotion in England and Wales of a comprehensive health service designed to secure improvement—

(a) in the physical and mental health of the people of those countries; and

(b) in the prevention, diagnosis and treatment of illness, and for that purpose to provide or secure the effective provision of services in accordance with this Act.

(2) The services so provided shall be free of charge except in so far as the making and recovery of charges is expressly provided for by or under any enactment, whenever passed.

Secretary of State's general power as to services

2. Without prejudice to the Secretary of State's powers apart from this section, he has power—

   (a) to provide such services as he considers appropriate for the purpose of discharging any duty imposed on him by this Act; and

   (b) to do any other thing whatsoever which is calculated to facilitate, or is conducive or incidental to, the discharge of such a duty.

This section is subject to section 3(3) below.

Services generally

3.—(1) It is the Secretary of State's duty to provide throughout England and Wales, to such extent as he considers necessary to meet all reasonable requirements—

   (a) hospital accommodation;

   (b) other accommodation for the purpose of any service provided under this Act;

   (c) medical, dental, nursing and ambulance services;

   (d) such other facilities for the care of expectant mothers and young children as he considers are appropriate as part of the health service;

   (e) such facilities for the prevention of illness, the care of persons suffering from illness and the after care of persons who have

suffered from illness as he considers are appropriate as part of the health service;

   (f) such other services as are required for the diagnosis and treatment of illness.

   (2) . . .

   (3) Nothing in section 2 above or in this section affects the provisions of Part 11 of this Act (which relates to arrangements with practitioners for the provision of medical, dental, ophthalmic and pharmaceutical services).

Co-operation and assistance

Local social services authorities

21.—(1) Subject to paragraphs (d) and (e) of section 3(1) above, the services described in Schedule 8 to this Act in relation to—

   (a) care of mothers and young children,

   (b) prevention, care and after care,

   (c) home help and laundry facilities, are functions exercisable by local social services authorities, and that Schedule has effect accordingly.

   (2) A local social services authority who provide premises, furniture or equipment for any of the purposes of this Act may permit the use of the premises, furniture or equipment–

   (a) by any other social services authority, or

(b) by a local education authority. This permission may be on such terms (including terms with respect to the services of any staff employed by the authority giving permission) as may be agreed.

(3) ...

Schedule 8: Local Social Services Authorities

Care of mothers and young children

1.—(1) A local social services authority may, with the Secretary of State's approval, and to such extent as he may direct shall, make arrangements for the care of expectant and nursing mothers (other than for the provision of residential accommodation for them).

Prevention, care and after-care

2.—(1) A local social services authority may, with the Secretary of State's approval, and to such extent as he may direct shall, make arrangements for the purpose of the prevention of illness and for the care of persons suffering, from illness and for the after-care of persons who have been suffering and in particular for—

(a) [repealed]

(b) the provision for persons whose care is undertaken with a view to preventing them from becoming ill, persons suffering from illness and persons who have been so suffering, of centres or other facilities for training them or keeping them suitably occupied and the equipment and maintenance of such centres;

(c) the provision, for the benefit of such persons as are mentioned in paragraph (b) above, of ancillary or supplemental services; and

(d) for the exercise of the functions of the Authority in respect of persons suffering from mental disorder who are received into the guardianship under Part II or III of the Mental Health Act 1983(whether the guardianship of the local social services authority or of other persons).

Such an authority shall neither have the power nor be subject to a duty to make under this paragraph arrangements to provide facilities for any of mentioned in section 15(1) of the Disabled Persons (Employment) Act 1944.

(2) No arrangements under this paragraph shall provide for the payment of money to persons for whose benefit they are made except-

(a) in so far as they may provide for the remuneration of such persons engaged in suitable work in accordance with the arrangements, of such amounts as the local social services authority think fit in respect of their occasional personal expenses where it appears to that authority that no such payment would otherwise be made.

(3) The Secretary of State may make regulations as to the conduct of premises in which, in pursuance of arrangements made under this paragraph, are provided for persons whose care is undertaken with a view to preventing

them from becoming sufferers from mental disorder within the meaning of that Act of 1983 or who are, or have been, so suffering, facilities for training them or keeping them suitably occupied.

(4A) This paragraph does not apply in relation to persons under the age of 18.

(4AA) No authority is authorised or may be required under this paragraph to provide residential accommodation for any person.

(5) A local social services authority may recover from persons availing themselves of services provided in pursuance of arrangements under this paragraph such charges (if any) as the authority consider reasonable, having regard to the means of those persons.

Home help and laundry facilities

3.—(1) It is the duty of every local social services authority to provide on such a scale as is adequate for the needs of their area, or to arrange for the provision on such a scale as is so adequate, of home help for households where such help is required owing to the presence of—

(a) a person who is suffering from illness, lying-in, an expectant mother, aged, handicapped as a result of having suffered from illness or by congenital deformity,

and every such Authority has power to provide or arrange for the provision of laundry facilities for households for which home help is being, or can be, provided under this sub-paragraph.

(2) A local social service authority may recover from persons availing themselves of help or facilities provided under this paragraph such charges (if any) as the authority consider reasonable, having regard to the means of those persons.

Social Work (Scotland) Act 1968

Chief social work officer

3.—(1) For the purposes of their functions under this Act and the enactments mentioned in section 5(1B) of this Act, a local authority shall appoint an officer to be known as the chief social work officer.

Provisions relating to performance of functions by local authorities

4. Where a function is assigned to a local authority under this Act or section 7 (functions of local authorities) or 8 (provision of after-care services) of the Mental Health (Scotland) Act 1984 or Part II of the Children (Scotland) Act 1995 and a voluntary organisation or other person, including another local authority is able to assist in the performance of that function, the local

authority may make arrangements with such an organisation or other person for the provision of such assistance as aforesaid.

Central Authority

Powers of Secretary of State

5.—(1) Local authorities shall perform their functions under this Act. . .under the general guidance of the Secretary of State.

(1A) Without prejudice to subsection (1) above, the Secretary of State may issue directions to local authorities, either individually or collectively, as to the manner in which they are to exercise any of their functions. . .and a local authority shall comply with any direction made under this subsection.

Local authority plans for community care services

5A.—(1) Within such period after the day appointed for the coming into force of this section as the Secretary of State may direct, and in accordance with the provisions of this section, each local authority shall prepare and publish a plan for the provision of community care services in their area.

(2) Each local authority shall from time to time review any plan prepared by them under subsection (1) above, and shall, in the light of any such review, prepare and publish—

(a) any modifications to the plan under review; or

(b) if the case requires, a new plan.

(3) In preparing any plan or carrying out any review under subsection (1) or, as the case may be, subsection (2) above the authority shall consult—

(a) any Health Board providing services under the National Health Service (Scotland) Act 1978 in the area of the authority;

(b) [*repealed*]

(c) such voluntary organisations as appear to the authority to represent the interests of persons who use or are likely to use any community care services within the area of the authority or the interests of private carers who, within that area, provide care to persons for whom, in the exercise of their functions under this Act or any of the enactments mentioned in section 5(1B) of this Act, the local authority have a power or a duty to provide, or to secure the provision of, a service;

(d) such voluntary housing agencies and other bodies as appear to the authority to provide housing or community care services in their area; and

(e) such other persons as the Secretary of State may direct.

(4) In this section—

"community care services" means services, other than services for children, which a local authority are under a duty or have a power to provide, or to secure the provision of, under Part II of this Act or section 7 (functions of local authorities), 8 (provision of after-care services) or 11 (training and occupation of the mentally handicapped) of the Mental Health (Scotland) Act 1984; and

"private carer" means a person who is not employed to provide the care in question by any body in the exercise of its functions under any enactment.

Complaints procedure

5B.—(1) Subject to the provisions of this section, the Secretary of State may by order require local authorities to establish a procedure whereby a person, or anyone acting on his behalf, may make representations (including complaints) in relation to the authority's discharge of, or failure to discharge, any of their functions. . .in respect of that person.

(2) For the purposes of subsection (1) of this section, "person" means any person for whom the local authority have a power or a duty to provide, or to secure the provision of, a service, and whose need or possible need for such a service has (by whatever means) come to the attention of the authority.

(3) An order under subsection (1) of this section may be commenced at different times in respect of such different classes of person as may be specified in the order.

(6) A local authority shall comply with any directions given by the Secretary of State as to the procedure to be adopted in considering representations made as mentioned in subsection (1) of this section and as to the taking of such action as may be necessary in consequence of such representations.

(7) Every local authority shall give such publicity to the procedure established under this section as they consider appropriate.

General social welfare services of local authorities

12.–(1) It shall be the duty of every local authority to promote social welfare by making available advice, guidance and assistance on such a scale as may be appropriate for their area, and in that behalf to make arrangements and to provide or secure the provision of such facilities (including the provision or arranging for the provision of residential and other establishments) as they may consider suitable and adequate, and such assistance may, subject to subsections (3) to (5) of this section, be given in kind or in cash to, or in respect of, any relevant person.

(2) A person is a relevant person for the purposes of this section if, not being less than eighteen years of age, he is in need requiring assistance in kind or, in exceptional circumstances constituting an emergency, in cash, where the giving of assistance in either form would avoid the local authority being caused greater expense in the giving of assistance in another form, or where probable aggravation of the person's need would cause greater expense to the local authority on a later occasion.

(3) Before giving assistance to, or in respect of, a person in cash under subsection (1) of this section a local authority shall have regard to his eligibility

for receiving assistance from any other statutory body and, if he is eligible, to the availability to him of that assistance in his time of need.

(4) Assistance given in kind or in cash to, or in respect of, persons under this section may be given unconditionally or subject to such conditions as to the repayment of the assistance, or of its real value, whether in whole or in part, as the local authority may consider reasonable having regard to the means of the person receiving the assistance and to the eligibility of the person for assistance from any other statutory body.

(5) Nothing in the provisions of this section shall affect the performance by a local authority of their functions under any other enactment

(6) For the purposes of subsection (2) of this section "person in need" includes a person who is in need of care and attention arising out of drug or alcohol dependency or release from prison or other form of detention.

Duty of local authority to assess needs

12A.–(1) Subject to the provisions of this section, where it appears to a local authority that any person for whom they are under a duty or have a power to provide, or to secure the provision of, community care services may be in need of any such services, the authority–

(a) shall make an assessment of the needs of that person for those services; and

(b) having regard to the results of that assessment, shall then decide whether the needs of that person call for the provision of any such services.

(2) Before deciding, under subsection (1)(b) of this section, that the needs of any person call for the provision of nursing care, a local authority shall consult a medical practitioner.

(3) If, while they are carrying out their duty under subsection (1) of this section, it appears to a local authority that there may be a need for the provision to any person to whom that subsection applies–

(a) of any services under the National Health Service (Scotland) Act 1978 by the Health Board–

(i) in whose area he is ordinarily resident; or

(ii) in whose area the services to be supplied by the local authority are, or are likely, to be provided; or

(b) of any services which fall within the functions of a housing authority (within the meaning of section 130 (housing) of the Local Government (Scotland) Act 1973) which is not the local authority carrying out the assessment,

the local authority shall so notify that Health Board or housing authority, and shall request information from them as to what services are likely to be made available to that person by that Health Board or housing authority; and, thereafter, in carrying out their said duty, the local authority shall take unto account any information received by them in response to that request.

(3A) Subject to subsection (3B) below, in any case where–

(a) a local authority make an assessment of the needs of any person ("the relevant person") under subsection (1) (a) above, and

(b) a person ("the carer") provides or intends to provide a substantial amount of care on a regular basis for the relevant person,

the carer may request the local authority, before they make their decision under subsection (1)(b) above, to make an assessment of his ability to provide and to continue to provide care for the relevant person; and if he makes such a request, the local authority shall make such an assessment and shall have regard to the results of that assessment in making that decision.

(3B) No request may be made under subsection (3A) above by a person who provides or will provide the care in question–

(a) by virtue of a contract of employment or other contract; or

(b) as a volunteer for a voluntary organisation.

(3C) Section 8 of the Disabled Persons (Services, Consultation and Representation) Act 1986 (duty of local authority to take into account ability of carers) shall not apply in any case where an assessment is made under subsection (3A) above in respect of a person who provides the care in question for a disabled person.

(4) Where a local authority are making an assessment under this section and it appears to them that the person concerned is a disabled person, they shall—

(a) proceed to make such a decision as to the services he requires as is mentioned in section 4 of the Disabled Persons (Services, Consultation and Representation) Act 1986 without his requesting them to do so under that section; and

(b) inform him that they will be doing so and of his rights under that Act.

(5) Nothing in this section shall prevent a local authority from providing or arranging for the provision of community care services for any person without carrying out a prior assessment of his needs in accordance with the preceding provisions of this section if, in the opinion of the authority, the condition of that person is such that he requires those services as a matter of urgency.

(6) If, by virtue of subsection (5) of this section, community care services have been provided for any person as a matter of urgency, then, as soon as practicable thereafter, an assessment of his needs shall be made in accordance with the preceding provisions of this section.

(7) This section is without prejudice to section 3 of the said Act of 1986.

(8) In this section—

"community care services" has the same meaning as in section 5A of this Act;

"disabled person" has the same meaning as in the said Act of 1986;

"medical practitioner" means a fully registered person within the meaning of section 55 (interpretation) of the Medical Act 1983; and

"person" means a natural person.

Direct payments in respect of community care services

12B.—(1) Where, as respects a person in need—

(a) a local authority have decided under section 12A of this Act that his needs call for the provision of any service which is a community care service within the meaning of section 5A of this act, and

(b) the person is of a description which is specified for the purposes of this subsection by regulations,

the authority may, if the person consents, make to him, in respect of his securing the provision of the service, a payment of such amount as, subject to subsection (2) below, they think fit.

(2) If—

(a) an authority pay under subsection (1) above at a rate below their estimate of the reasonable cost of securing the provision of the service concerned, and

(b) the person to whom the payment is made satisfies the authority that his means are insufficient for it to be reasonably practicable for him to make up the difference,

the authority shall so adjust the payment to him under that subsection as to avoid there being a greater difference than that which appears to them to be reasonable practicable for him to make up.

(3) A payment under subsection (1) above shall be subject to the condition that the person to whom it is made shall not secure the provision of the service to which it relates by a person who is of a description specified for the purposes of this subsection by regulations.

(4) Regulations may provide that the power conferred by subsection (1) above shall not be exercisable in relation to the provision of residential accommodation for any person for a period in excess of such period as may be specified in the regulations.

(5) If the authority by whom a payment under subsection (1) above is made are not satisfied, in relation to the whole or any part of the payment—

(a) that it has been used to secure the provision of the service to which it relates, or

(b) that the condition imposed by subsection (3) above, or any condition properly imposed by them, has been met in relation to its use,

they may require the payment or, as the case may be, the part of the payment to be repaid.

(6) Regulations under this section shall be made by the Secretary of State and may—

(a) make different provision for different cases; and

(b) include such supplementary, incidental, consequential and transitional provisions and savings as the Secretary of State thinks fit.

Further provisions relating to direct payments

12C.—(1) Except as provided by subsection (2) below, the fact that a local authority make a payment under section 12B(1) of this Act shall not affect their functions with respect to the provision of the service to which the payment relates.

(2) Subject to subsection (3) below, where an authority make a payment under section 12B(1) of this Act they shall not be under any obligation to the person to whom it is made with respect to the provision of the service to which it relates as long as they are satisfied that the need which calls for the provision of that service will be met by virtue of the person's own arrangements.

(3) The fact that an authority make a payment under section 12B(1) of this Act shall not affect their functions under section 12 of this Act in relation to the provision, to the person to whom the payment is made, of assistance, in exceptional circumstances constituting an emergency, in cash in respect of the service to which the payment under section 12B(1) relates.

Power of local authorities to assist persons in need in disposal of produce of their work

13. Where, by virtue of section 12 of this Act, a local authority make arrangements or provide or secure the provision of facilities for the engagement of persons in need (whether under a contract of service or otherwise) in suitable work, that local authority may assist such persons in disposing of the produce of their work.

Residential accommodation with nursing

13A.—(1) Without prejudice to section 12 of this Act, a local authority shall make such arrangements as they consider appropriate and adequate for the provision of suitable residential accommodation where nursing is provided for persons who appear to them to be in need of such accommodation by reason of infirmity, age, illness or mental disorder, dependency on drugs or alcohol or being substantially handicapped by any deformity or disability.

(2) The arrangements made by virtue of subsection (1) above shall be made with a voluntary or other organisation or other person, being an organisation or person managing premises which are—

(a) a nursing home within the meaning of section 10(2)(a) of the Nursing Homes Registration (Scotland) Act 1938 in respect of which that organisation or person is registered or exempt from registration under that Act; or

(b) a private hospital registered under section 12 of the Mental Health (Scotland) Act 1984,

for the provision of accommodation in those premises.

(3) The provisions of section 6 of this Act apply in relation to premises where accommodation is provided for the purposes of this section as they apply in relation to establishments provided for the purposes of this Act.

Provision of care and after-care

Provision of care and after-care

13B.—(1) Subject to subsection (2) below, a local authority may with the approval of the Secretary of State, and shall, if and to the extent that the Secretary of State so directs, make arrangements for the purpose of the prevention of illness, the care of persons suffering from illness, and the after-care of such persons.

(2) The arrangements which may be made under subsection (1) above do not include arrangements in respect of medical, dental or nursing care, or health visiting.

Home help

Home help and laundry facilities

14.—(1) It shall be the duty of every local authority to provide on such scale as is adequate for the needs of their area, or to arrange for the provision on such a scale as is so adequate of, domiciliary services for households where such services are required owing to the presence, or the proposed presence, of a person in need or a person who is an expectant mother or lying-in, and every such authority shall have power to provide or arrange for the provision of laundry facilities for households for which domiciliary services are being, or can be, provided under this subsection.

(2) [*repealed*]

(3) [*repealed*]

(4) On the coming into operation of the provisions of this and the last two foregoing sections, the provisions of sections 13, 44 and 45 of the Health Services and Public Health Act 1968 shall cease to have effect.

Adjustments between authority providing accommodation etc., and authority of area of residence

86.—(1) Any expenditure which apart from this section would fall to be borne by a local authority—

(a) in the provision under this Act. . .of accommodation for a person ordinarily resident in the area of another local authority, or

(b) . . .

(c) for the conveyance of a person ordinarily resident as aforesaid, or

(d) in administering a supervision requirement in respect of a person ordinarily resident as aforesaid, or

(e) in the provision of accommodation, services or facilities for persons ordinarily so resident under section 7 (functions of local authorities) or 8 (provision of after-care services) of the Mental Health (Scotland) Act 1984,

shall be recoverable from the other local authority, and in this subsection any reference to another local authority includes a reference to a local authority in England and Wales.

(2) Any question arising under this section as to the ordinary residence of a person shall be determined by the Secretary of State, and the Secretary of State may determine that a person has no ordinary residence.

(3) In determining for the purposes of subsection (1) of this section the ordinary residence of any person. . ., any period during which he was a patient in a hospital provided under Part II of the National Health Service Act 1946 or Part II of the National Health Service (Scotland) Act 1978 or in a hospital managed by a National Health Service trust established under Part I of the National Health Service and Community Care Act 1990 or section 12A of the National Health Service (Scotland) Act 1978. . . .

Exclusion of powers to provide accommodation in certain cases

86A.—(1) Subject to subsection (3) below, no accommodation may be provided under this Act for any person who, immediately before the date on which this section comes into force, was ordinarily resident in relevant premises.

(2) In subsection (1) above "relevant premises" means—

(a) any establishment in respect of which a person is registered under section 62 of this Act;

(b) any nursing home within the meaning of the Nursing Homes Registration (Scotland) Act 1938 in respect of which a person is registered or exempt from registration under that Act;

(c) any private hospital registered under section 12 of the Mental Health (Scotland) Act 1984; and

(d) such other premises as the Secretary of State may by regulations prescribe.

(3) The Secretary of State may by regulations provided that in such cases and subject to such conditions as my be prescribed subsection (1) above shall not apply in relation to such classes of persons as may be prescribed in the regulations.

(4) The Secretary of State shall by regulations prescribe the circumstances in which persons are to be treated as being ordinarily resident in any premises for the purposes of subsection (1) above.

(5) This section does not affect the validity of any contract made before the date on which this section comes into force for the provision of

accommodation on or after that date or anything done in pursuance of such as contract.

Charges that may be made for services and accommodation

87.—(1) Subject to. . .the following provisions of this section, a local authority providing a service under this Act or section 7 (functions of local authorities) or 8 (provision of after-care services) of the Mental Health (Scotland) Act 1984. . .may recover such charge (if any) for it as they consider reasonable.

(1A) If a person—

(a) avails himself of a service provided under this Act or section 7 or 8 of the said Act of 1984. . .; and

(b) satisfies the authority providing the service that his means are insufficient for it to be reasonably practicable for him to pay for the service the amount which he would otherwise be obliged to pay for it,

the authority shall not require him to pay more for it than it appears to them that it is reasonably practicable for him to pay.

(2) Persons. . ., for whom accommodation is provided under this Act or section 7 of the said Act of 1984, shall be required to pay for that accommodation in accordance with the subsequent provisions of this section.

(3) Subject to the following provisions of this section, accommodation provided under this Act or section 7 of the said Act of 1984 shall be regarded as accommodation provided under Part III of the National Assistance Act 1948, and sections 22(2) to (8) and 26(2) to (4). . .and sections 42. . .and 43 of the said Act of 1948 (which make provision for the mutual maintenance of wives and husbands and the maintenance of their children by recovery of assistance from persons liable for maintenance and for affiliation orders, etc.) shall apply accordingly.

(4) In the application of the said section 22, for any reference to the Minister there shall be substituted a reference to the Secretary of State, and in the application of the said section 26, any references to arrangements under a scheme for the provision of accommodation shall be construed as references to arrangements made by a local authority with a voluntary organisation or any other person or body for the provision of accommodation under this Act or section 7 of the said Act of 1984.

(5) The Secretary of State may, with the consent of the Treasury, make regulations for modifying or adjusting the rates at which payments under this section are made, where such a course appears to him to be justified, and any such regulations may provide for the waiving of any such payment in whole or in part in such circumstances as may be specified in the regulations.

Mental Health (Scotland) Act 1984

Part III

Local Authority Services

7.–(1) In relation to persons who are or have been suffering from mental disorder a local authority may, with the approval of the Secretary of State and shall, to such extent as he may direct, make arrangements for any of the following purposes–

(a) the provision, equipment and maintenance of residential accommodation, and the care of persons for the time being resident in accommodation so provided;

(b) the exercise by the local authority of their functions under the following provisions of this Act in respect of persons under guardianship (whether under the guardianship of a local authority or of any other person);

(c) the provision of any ancillary or supplementary services;

(d) the supervision of persons suffering from mental handicap who are neither liable to detention in a hospital nor subject to guardianship.

(2) The reference in subsection (1)(a) of this section to the care of persons for the time being resident in accommodation provided by a local authority includes, in the case of persons so resident who are under the age of 16 years, the payment to those persons of such amounts as he local authority think fit in respect of their personal expenses where it appears to that authority that no such payment would otherwise be made.

8.–(1) A local authority shall provide after-care services for any persons who are or have been suffering from mental disorder.

(2) In providing after-care services under subsection (1) of this section a local authority shall co-operate with such health board or boards and such voluntary organisations as appear to the local authority to be concerned.

(3) The duty imposed by this section is without prejudice to any other power or duty which a local authority may have in relation to the provision of after-care services.

NHS (Scotland) Act 1978

Secretary of State

1.–(1) It shall continue to be the duty of the Secretary of State to promote in Scotland a comprehensive and integrated health service designed to secure–

(a) improvement in the physical and mental health of the people of Scotland, and

(b) the prevention, diagnosis and treatment of illness,

and for that purpose to provide or secure the effective provision of services in accordance with the provisions of this Act.

1

(2) The services so provided shall be free of charge, except in so far as the making and recovery of charges is expressly provided for by or under any enactment, whenever passed.

Part III

Other Services and Facilities

36.—(1) It shall be the duty of the Secretary of State to provide throughout Scotland, to such extent as he considers necessary to meet all reasonable requirements, accommodation and services of the following descriptions–

(a) hospital accommodation, including accommodation at state hospitals;

(b) premises other than hospitals at which facilities are available for any of the services provide under this Act;

(c) medical, nursing and other services, whether in such accommodation or premises, in the home of the patient or elsewhere.

(2) Where accommodation or premises provided under this section afford facilities for the provision of general medical, general dental or general ophthalmic services, or of pharmaceutical services, they shall be made available for those services on such terms and conditions as the Secretary of State may determine.

37. The Secretary of State shall make arrangements, to such extent as he considers necessary to meet all reasonable requirements, for the purposes of the prevention if illness, the care of persons suffering from illness or the after-care of such persons.

Scotland Act 1998

Section 117 Ministers of the Crown

So far as may be necessary for the purpose or in consequence of the exercise of a function by a member of the Scottish Executive within devolved competence, any pre-commencement enactment or prerogative instrument, and any other instrument or document, shall be read as if references to a Minster of the Crown (however described) were or included references to the Scottish Ministers.

Appendix 2

Key guidance

The key circulars issued by the Department of Health to social services departments, which set out the guidance to be followed in community care practice, are listed below.

	England	Wales	Scotland
Charges			
Includes the full guidance for charges with previous circulars annexed	LAC(99)98 CRAG	WOC 17/99	
Covers discretionary charges for adult services	Advice note for use by Social Services Inspectorate		
Other Important Circulars in date order			
Home help service			SWSG 7/71
Choice of Accommodation	LAC(92)27 & LAC(93)18	WOC 12/93	SWSG 5/93
Registered Establishments (Scotland) Act			SWSG 16/88
Assessment and care management			SWSG 11/91
LA powers for people with preserved rights	LAC(93)6	WOC 25/93	

LA powers to make arrangements for people who are in independent sector residential care and nursing homes on 31 March 1993			SWSG11/93
Ordinary residence	LAC(93)7	WOC 35/93	
Approvals and directions for arrangements made from April 1993	LAC(93)10	WOC 35/93	
Choice of accommodation – cross border placements			SWSG 6/94
Community care – the housing dimension			SWSG 7/94
Continuing care of the frail elderly			SWSG102/94
NHS responsibilities for meeting continuing health care needs (please note there will be changes to this by the end of 1999)	LAC(95)5 HSG 95/8	WOC 16/95 WHC(95)7	
Discharge from NHS inpatient care arrangements for receiving decision on eligibility for NHS continuing care	LAC(95)7 HSG 95/39	WHC(95)7	
LA complaints procedures			SWSG5/96
Carers (Recognition and Services) Act 1995: policy and practical guidance			SWSG11/96
Includes guidance on the Sefton judgement			SWSG6/98
Community care needs of frail older people			SWSG10/98

Guidance on the Community Care (Residential Accommodation) Act 1998	LAC(98)19	WOC 27/98	SWSG2/99
Promoting independence Partnership, prevention and carers' grants	LAC(99)13		
Promoting independence Prevention strategies and support for adults	LAC(99)14		
Follow-up action of Coughlan	LAC(99)30 HSC 1999/ 180		

Other circulars

In Scotland the charging guidance has not been issued in full since SWSG 8/96.

Circular number

SWSG 13/93

SWSG 15/93

SWSG 4/94

SWSG 5/94

SWSG 13/95

SWSG 8/96

SWSG7/97

Appendix 3

Useful addresses

Benefits Agency
Chief Executive
Mr P Mathison
Quarry House, Quarry Hill
Leeds LS2 7UA
Tel: 0113 232 4000

DSS Solicitor
New Court
48 Carey Street
London
WC2A 2LS
Tel: 020 7962 8000

Health Service Ombudsman
Millbank Tower
London
SW1P 4QP
Tel: 020 7217 4051

Local Government Ombudsman
England
21 Queens Anne's Gate
London
SW1H 9BU
Tel: 020 7915 3210

Scotland
23 Walker Street
Edinburgh
WH3 7HX
Tel: 0131 225 5300

Wales
Derwen House, Court Road
Bridgend
CF31 1BN
Tel: 01656 661 325

Northern Ireland
Progressive House
33 Wellington Place
Belfast
BT1 6HN
Tel: 01232 233 821

The Parliamentary Ombudsman
Office of the Parliamentary Com-
missioner
Millbank Tower
Millbank
London
SW1P 4QP
Tel: 020 7217 4163

Disabled Living Centres Council
Red Bank House
4 St Chads Street
Manchester
M8 8QA
Tel: 0161 834 1044

**National Centre for Independent
Living**
250 Kennington Lane
London

SE11 5RD
Tel: 020 7587 1663

Public Trust Office
Stewart House
24 Kingsway
London
WC2B 6HD
Tel: 020 7664 7300

**Government departments and
Benefits Agency**
Benefits Agency
Chief Executive's Office
Room 4CO6
Quarry House
Quarry Hill
Leeds
LS2 7UA
Tel: 0113 232 4000

Department for Education and Employment
Sanctuary Buildings
Great Smith Street
London
SW1P 3BT
Tel: 020 7925 5555

Department of Social Security
The Adelphi
1-11 John Adam Street
London
WC2N 6HT
Tel: 020 7962 8000

*Department of the Environment,
Transport and the Regions*
Mobility Unit
1/11 Great Ministers House
76 Marsham Street
London
SW1P 4DR
Voice and minicom 020 7890 6100

Disability Benefit Centres
Belfast DBC
Disability Living Allowance Branch
Castle Court
Royal Avenue
Belfast
BT1 1SL
Tel: 01232 336 556
Deals with claims for DLA and AA
from all over Northern Ireland.

Birmingham DBC
Five Ways Complex
Frederick Road
Edgbaston
Birmingham
B15 1SL
Tel: 0121 626 2000
Deals with claims from West Midlands, Shropshire, Hereford and
Worcester, Staffordshire, Leicestershire, Warwickshire, Northamptonshire, Derbyshire,
Nottnghamshire, Lincolnshire.

Bootle DBC
St Martin's House
Stanley Precinct
Bootle Merseyside
L69 9BN
Tel: 0151 934 6000
Deals with claims from Merseyside,
Central and Nort-West Lancashire,
Cumbria, North, South and West
Cheshire.

Bristol DBC
Government Buildings
Flowers Hill
Bristol
BS4 5LA
Tel: 0117 971 8311

Deals with claims from Cornwall, Devon, Avon, Gloucestershire, Wiltshire, Somerset, Dorset.

Cardiff DBC
Government Buildings
St Agnes Road
Gabalfa
Cardiff
CF4 4YJ
Tel: 01222 586 002
Deals with claims from all over Wales

Edinburgh DBC
Argyle House
3 Lady Lawson Street
Edinburgh
EH3 0XY
Tel: 0131 229 9191
Minicom: 0131 222 5494
Deals with claims from all over Scotland except Strathclyde.

Glasgow DBC
29 Cadogan Street
Glasgow
G2 7BN
Tel: 0141 249 3500
Minicom: 0141 249 3507
Deals with the claims from The West of Scotland and Outer Hebrides (postal districts G, HS, KA, ML, PA).

Leeds DBC
Government Buildings
Otley Road
Lawnswood
Leeds
LS16 5PU
Tel: 0113 230 9000

Deals with claims from Greater Manchester, East Lancashire, Derbyshire (High Peak), East Cheshire.

Newcastle DBC
Regent Centre
Arden House
Gosforth
Newcastle upon Tyne
NE3 3JN
Tel: 0191 223 3000
Deals with claims from Tyne and Wear, Durham, Northumberland, Cleveland.

Sutton DBC
Sutherland House
29-37 Brighton Road
Sutton
Surrey
SM2 5AN
Tel: 020 8652 6000
Deals with claims from London postal districts WC1 and WC2, SE1-SE28, SW1-SW20, W1, W6, W8 and W14, Hounslow, Twickenham, Berkshire, Hampshire, Surrey, Kent, East Sussex, West Sussex, Isle of Wight, Kingston, Woking.

Wembley DBC
Olympic House
Wembley
Middlesex
HA9 0DL
Tel: 020 8795 8400
Deals with claims from London postal districts EC1-EC4, E1-E18, N1-N27, NW1-NW11, W2-W5, W7, W9-W13, Buckinghamshire, Bedfordshire, Cambridgeshire, Essex, Hertfordhire, Middlesex (ex-

cept Hounslow and Twickenham), Oxfordshire, Suffolk, Norfolk.

Central Units
Disability Benefit Unit
Warbreck House
Warbreck Hill Road
Blackpool
Lancashire
FY2 0YE
Tel: 0345 123 456
Textphone: 0345 224 433
Handles all DLA and AA claims (except initial claim which is processed by Disability Benefits Centres listed above).

Independent Review Service for the Social Fund
4th Floor, Centre City Podium
5 Hill Street
Birmingham
B5 4UB
Tel: 0121 606 1200

Independent Tribunal Service
4th Floor, Whittington House
19-30 Alfred Place
London
WC1E 7LW
Tel: 020 7814 6500

Invalid Care Allowance Unit
Palatine House
Lancaster Road
Preston
Lancashire
PR1 1HB
Tel: 01253 856 123
Deals with all ICA claims.

Medical Services
Dr C Hudson
Medical Director

Government Buildings
1 Cop Lane
Penwortham
Preston
PR1 0SP
Tel: 01772 237 992
Provided by Sema Group on behalf of the Benefits Agency (formerly BAMS).

Pensions and Overseas Benefits Directorate
Tyneview Park
Whiteley Road
Benton
Newcastle upon Tyne
NE98 1BA
Tel: 0191 218 7878
Textphone: 0191 218 2160.

Social Security and Child Support Commissioners England and Wales, Office of the
5th Floor, Newspaper House
8-16 Great New Street
London
EC4A 4DH
Tel: 020 7353 5145

Social Security and Child Support Commissioners Scotland, Office of the
23 Melville Street
Edinburgh
EH3 7PW
Tel: 0131 225 2201

Phone lines
Benefit Enquiry Line (BEL)
0800 882 200
Textphone: 0800 243 355
(in Northern Ireland
0800 220 674;

Textphone: 0800 243 787) BEL specialises in benefits for disabled people, their carers and representatives. BEL has no access to personal records and so provides general advice only.

Disability Benefits Customer Care Helpline
0345 123456
Textphone: 0345 224 433
For claimants with an enquiry on their DLA or AA claim and for general enquiries on disability benefits.

Senior line
0808 800 6565
General advice for older people about benefits, community care and housing, run by Help the Aged.

England and UK-wide organisations

Action for Blind People
14-16 Verney Road
London
SE16 3DZ
Tel: 020 7732 8771
Employment, grants, information and benefits advice.

African-Caribbean Mental Health Association
Suit 37
Eurolink Business Centre
49 Effra Road
London
SW2 1BZ
Tel: 020 7737 3603

Age Concern England
Astral House
1268 London Road

London
SW16 4ER
Tel: 0800 009 966

AIDS Helpline
Tel: 0800 567 123
Minicom: 0800 521 361
Confidential advice by trained advisers.
Ethnic minority language lines
Welsh 0800 371 131
Cantonese 0800 282 446
Bengali 0800 371 132
Punjabi 0800 371 133
Hindi 0800 371136
Urdu 0800 371 135
Gujurati 0800 371 134
Arabic 0800 282 447

Al-Anon Family Groups UK and Eire
61 Great Dover Street
London
SE1 4YF
(24 hour helpline 020 7403 0888)
Self-help groups for relatives and friends of problem drinkers.

Alcohol Concern
Waterbridge House
32-36 Loman Street
London
SE1 0EE
Tel: 020 7928 7377

Alcoholics Anonymous
PO Box 1
Stonebow House
Stonebow
York
YO1 7NJ
Tel: 01904 644 026
London helpline: 020 7352 3001

Alzheimer's Disease Society
Gordon House
10 Greencoat Place
London
SW1P 1PH
Tel: 020 7306 0606
Helpline: 0845 300 0336
Advice and support for those
coping with dementia.

Asian People with Disabilities Alliance
The Disability Alliance Centre
The Old Refectory
Central Middlesex Hospital
Acton Lane
London
NE10 7NS
Tel: 020 8961 6773
Respite care, advice and advocacy,
daycare for elderly Asians and
disabled people.

Association of Blind Asians
65 Bolsover Street
London
W1P 7HL
Tel: 020 7388 2555
Organisation of blind and partially
sighted Asian people.

Care and Repair England
Castle House
Kirtley Drive
Nottingham
NG7 1LD
Tel: 0115 979 9091

Carers National Association
20-25 Glasshouse Yard
London
EC1A 4JT
Tel: 020 7490 8818

Advice Line: 0345 573 369
Informs and supports carers, brings
needs of carers to the attention of
government.

Child Poverty Action Group
94 White Lion Street
London
N1 9PF
Tel: 020 7837 7979

Chinese Mental Health Association
Terrino Chan
Oxford House
Derbyshire Street
London
E2 6HG
Tel: 020 7613 1008

Counsel and Care for the Elderly
Twyman House
16 Bonny Street
London
NW1 9PG
Tel: 0845 300 7585
Advice service on care at home,
residential care and nursing homes,
community care and financial
help.

Cruse Bereavement Care
126 Sheen Road
London
TW9 1UR
Tel: 020 8940 4818
Bereavement Line: 020 8332 7227
Counselling, support groups, practical information, advice and
publications. For details send sae.

Dial UK
St Catherine's Hospital
Park Lodge

Tickhill Road
Balby
Doncaster
DN4 8QN
Tel: 01302 310 123
Supports UK-wide disability information and advice services and details of local groups

The Disabilities Trust
1st Floor, Market Place
Burgess Hill
West Sussex
RH15 9NP
Tel: 01444 239 123
Care and accommodation for physically disabled people.

The Disabled Driver's Association
National Headquarters
Ashewellthorpe
Norwich
NR16 1EX
Tel: 01508 489 449
Self-help association aiming for independence through mobility.

Disabled Drivers' Motor Club
Cottingham Way
Thrapston
Northamptonshire
NN14 4PL
Tel: 01832 734 724
Advice for disabled motorists. Various discounts and concessions available.

Disabled Living Centres Council
The Vassil Centre
Gill Avenue
Fishponds
Bristol
BS16 2QQ

Tel: 0117 958 5130
Co-ordinates work of Disabled Living Centres UK wide. List of centres available.

Disabled Motorists Federation
National Mobility Centre
Unit 2, Atcham Estate
Shrewsbury
SY4 4UG
Tel: 01743 761 181

The Disablement Income Group
Unit 5, Archway Business Centre
19-23 Wedmore Street
London
N9 4RZ
Tel: 020 7263 3981

Equal Opportunities for People with Disabilities
1 Bank Buildings
Prince's Street
London
EC2R 8EU
Tel: 020 7726 4961
Minicom: 020 7726 4963
Employment services (17 regional centres).

Equal Opportunities Commission
Overseas House
Quay Street
Manchester M3 3HN
Voice and minicom: 0161 833 9244

The Family Fund Trust
PO Box 50
York
YO1 9ZX
Tel: 01904 621 115
Textphone: 01904 658 085

Financial help and information for families with severely disabled children under 16 years old

GLAD (Greater London Action on Disability)
see London-wide organisations

Help the Aged
St James's Walk
London
EC1R 0BE
Tel: 020 7253 0253
Minicom: 0800 269 626
Seniorline: 0800 800 6565
Free advice and information for older people and their carers about benefits, housing and community care.

Independent Living Fund
PO Box 183
Nottingham
NG8 3RD
Tel: 0115 942 8191
A government funded trust set up to provide monies to severely disabled people to enable them to employ personal or domestic care.

Jewish Blind and Disabled
164 East End Road
London
N2 0RR
Tel: 020 8883 1000
Sheltered housing and welfare services.

Jewish Care
17 Highfield Road
London
NW11 9LS
Tel: 020 7922 2590

Specialist services for people with a physical or sensory disability.

Joint Council for the Welfare of Immigrants
115 Old Street
London
EC1V 9RT
Tel: 020 7251 8708
Advice line: 020 7251 9706

Law Centres Federation
Duchess House
18-19 Warren Street
London
W1P 5DB
Tel: 020 7387 8570

Law Society
114 Chancery Lane
London
WC2A 1PL
Tel: 020 7320 5793
Group for solicitors with disabilities. Contact Judith McDermott

Leonard Cheshire
30 Millbank
London
SW1P 4QG
Tel: 020 7802 8200
Provides a wide range of support services for disabled people and their carers.

Macfarlane Trust
Alliance House
12 Caxton Street
London
SW1H 0QS
Tel: 020 7233 0342
Grants to people infected with HIV through treatment for haemophilia.

Macmillan Cancer Relief
Anchor House
15-19 Britten Street
London
SW3 3TZ
Tel: 020 8222 7708
Information line: 0845 601 6161
Information on cancer support
services, grants for patients in
financial difficulties.

Marie Curie Cancer Care
28 Belgrave Square
London
SW1X 8QG
Tel: 020 7942 7419
Provides free nursing care at home
and specialist care at 11 centres
across the UK, and conducts research.

Mental After Care Association
25 Bedford Square
London WC1B 3HW
Tel: 020 7436 6194
Provides services for people de-
tained under the Mental Health
Act.

Mental Health Act Commission
Maid Marian House
56 Houndsgate
Nottingham
NG1 6BG
Tel: 0115 943 7100
Statutory body to protect the rights
of people with mental health
problems.

Mental Health Foundation (includ-
ing The Foundation for People with
Learning Difficulties)
20-21 Cornwall Terrace
London NW1 4QL
Tel: 020 7535 7400

*Mind (The National Association of
Mental Health)*
Granta House
15-19 THe Briadway
London
E15 4BQ
Tel: 020 8519 2122
London Info Line 020 8522 1728
Outside London: 0345 660163

Mobility Centre, Banstead
Damson Way
Fountain Drive
Carshalton
Surrey
SM5 4NR
Tel: 020 8770 1151

Mobility Information Service
National Mobility Centre
Unit 2, Atcham Estate
Shrewbury
SY4 4UG
Tel: 01743 761 889
Information on mobility. Driving
assessment for disabled drivers.

Motability
Goodman House
Station Approach
Harlow
Essex
CM20 2ET
Tel: 01279 635 666

National Association of Citizens Advice Bureaux
Myddelton House
115-123 Pentonville Road
London
N1 9LZ
Tel: 020 7833 2181
Will provide details of your local
Citizens Advice Bureau.

National Centre for Independent Living
250 Kennington Lane
London
SE11 5RD
Tel: 020 7587 1663
Provides information, consultancy
and training on personal assistance
and direct payments.

National Council of Voluntary Organisations
Regent's Wharf
8 All Saint's Street
London
N1 9RL
Tel: 020 7713 6161
Minicom: 020 7278 1289

Organisation of Blind African-Caribbeans
1st Floor, Gloucester House
8 Camberwell New Road
London
SE5 0RZ
Tel: 020 7735 3400

The Patient's Association
PO Box 935
Harrow
Middlesex
HA1 3YJ
Tel: 020 8423 9111

Helpline: 020 8423 8999
Help and advice for patients.
Leaflets and self-help directory
available.

Public Law Project
Room E608, Birckbeck College
University of London
Malet Street
London
WC1E 7HX
Tel: 020 7467 9807, advisors only)

Racial Equality, Commission for
Elliot House
10-12 Allington Street
London
SW1E 5EH
Tel: 020 7828 7022

RADAR (Royal Association for Disability and Rehabilitation)
12 City Forum
250 City Road
London
EC1V 8AF
Tel: 020 7250 3222
Minicom: 020 7250 4119
National disability campaigning
and information service.

Royal Air Forces Association
43 Grove Park Road
London
W4 3RX
Tel: 020 8994 8504
Providing welfare support to serving and former RAF personnel and
their dependants.

Royal National Institute for Deaf People
19-23 Featherstone Street
London

EC1Y 8SL
Helpline: 0870 605 0123; Text:
0870 603 3007
Tinnitus Helpline: 0345 090 210
Campaigns for a better quality of
life for people with hearing impairment, provides services and under-
takes research. See also - Typetalk.

Royal National Institute for the Blind
224 Great Portland Street
London
W1N 6AA
Helpline 0345 669 999
Advice, assistance and information
on benefits, equipment, employ-
ment and support.

SANE
1st Floor, Cityside House
40 Adler Street
London
E1 1EE
Tel: 020 7375 1002
Saneline 0345 678 000
Provides information and support
for anyone affected by mental
illness.

SSAFA Forces Help
Special Needs and Disability Advi-
sor
18 Queen Elizabeth Street
London
SE1 2LP
Tel: 020 7403 8783
Tel: 020 7463 9234

Turning Point
New Loom House
101 Blackchurch Lane
London
E1 1LU

Tel: 020 7702 2300
Help with drinks, drugs, mental
health and learning disabilities.

Typetalks
John Wood House
Glacier Building
Harrington Road
Brunswick Business Park
Liverpool
L3 4DF
Tel: 0151 709 9494
Text: 0800 500 888
Text user's help scheme, Typetalk
national telephone relay service,
text rebate scheme.

Women's Royal Voluntary Service
Milton Hill House
Milton Hill
Oxfordshire OX13 6AF
Tel: 01235 442 900
Provides care and practical help for
disabled people through referral
from social services, etc.

Scotland
Age Concern Scotland
113 Rose Street
Edinburgh
EH2 3DT
Tel: 0131 220 3345

*Alzheimer Scotland - Action on
Dementia*
22 Drumsheugh Gardens
Edinburgh
EH3 7RN
Tel: 0131 243 1353
Advice: 0131 220 6155
24 hour Freephone 0800 217 817
Information and support for peo-
ple with dementia and their carers.

British Red Cross Society
(Headquarters, Scotland)
Alexander House
204 Bath Street
Glasgow
G2 4HL
Tel: 0141 332 9591
Limited medical equipment loan,
escort and transport services.

ENABLE (formerly The Scottish Soci-
ety for the Mentally Handicapped)
6th Floor, 7 Buchanan Street
Glasgow
G1 3HL
Tel: 0141 226 4541

Energy Action, Scotland
Suite 4a
Ingram House
227 Ingram Street
Glasgow
G1 1DA
Tel: 0141 226 3064
Promotes affordable warmth and
investment in practical energy
efficiency initiatives.

Law Society of Scotland
26 Drumsheugh Gardens
Edinburgh
EH3 7YR
Tel: 0131 226 7411
Provides details of Scottish solici-
tors.

**Mental Welfare Commission for Scot-
land**
K Floor, Argyle House
3 Lady Lawson Street
Edinburgh
EH3 9SH
Tel: 0131 222 6111

Statutory body to protect the right
of people with mental health
problems.

Royal British Legion Scotland
New Haig House
Logie Green Road
Edinburgh
EH7 4HR
Tel: 0131 557 2782

Scottish Association for Mental Health
Cumbrae House
15 Carnton Court
Glasgow
G5 9JP
Tel: 0141 568 7000

Scottish Association for the Deaf
Clerwood House
96 Clemiston Road
Edinburgh
EH12 6UT
Tel: 0131 312 6075

**Scottish National Institution for the
War Blinded**
Gillespie Crescent
Edinburgh
EH10 4HZ
Tel: 0131 229 1456

**Scottish Trust for the Physically
Disabled**
Craigievar House
77 Craigmount Brae
Edinburgh
EH12 8YL
Tel: 0131 317 7227
Grant applications considered in
relation to housing and transport
only.

Turning Point Scotland
The West Street Centre
121 West Street
Glasgow
G5 8BA
Tel: 0141 418 0882
Help with drinks, drugs, mental
health and learning disabilities.

Women's Royal Voluntary Service
44 Albany Street
Edinburgh
EH1 3QR
Tel: 0131 558 8028

Wales
Cardiff Law Centre
15 Splott Road
Splott
Cardiff
CF2 2BU
Tel: 01222 498 117
Provides a free legal and commu-
nity service in housing, welfare
rights, immigration and discrimi-
nation in employment.

Disablement Welfare Rights
Canolfan Lafan
2 Glanrafon
Bangor
Gwynedd
LL57 1LH
Tel: 01248 352 227

*Mind, Cymru/Wales (National Asso-
ciation for Mental Health)*
Infoline: 0345 660 163
A national mental health information line, translators available upon
request.

Wales Council for the Blind
Shand House
20 Newport Road
Cardiff
CF2 1DB

Wales Council for the Deaf
Glenview House
Courthouse Street
Pontypridd
CF37 1JW
Tel: 01443 485 687
Text: 01443 485 686

Appendix 4

··

Getting information and advice

Independent advice and representation

It is sometimes difficult for unsupported individuals to get a positive response from the Benefits Agency or social services or other local authority departments or the health authorities. You may be taken more seriously if it is clear you have taken advice about your entitlement or have an adviser assisting you.

If you want advice or help with a benefit problem, the following agencies may be able to assist. (If you cannot fund any of these agencies in the telephone book, your local library should have details.)

- Citizens Advice Bureaux (CABx) and other local advice centres provide information and advice on most matters and may be able to represent you.
- Law Centres can often help in a similar way to CABx/advice centres.
- Local authority welfare rights workers provide a service in many areas particularly on benefits, and some arrange advice sessions and take-up campaigns locally.
- National organisations for particular groups have national free (or local rate) helplines. They can put you in touch with the local group of their organisation or give you the information you need. Many produce a range of factsheets either on the particular condition or about getting community care services.
- Local organisations for particular groups of claimants may offer help. For instance, there are pensioners groups and centres for people with disabilities.
- Some voluntary agencies provide information advice and advocacy services. For details of your nearest group contact your local Council for Voluntary Services (CVS).
- Some social workers (but not all) help with benefit problems, especially if they are already working with you on another problem,

- Solicitors can give free legal advice under the green form scheme (pink form in Scotland). This does not cover the cost of representation certain appeal hearings but can cover the cost of preparing written submissions and obtaining evidence such as medical reports. However, solicitors do not always have a good working knowledge of the community care or benefit rules and you may need to shop around until you find one who does.
- Some of the larger national organisation have lists of solicitors who have expressed an interest in community work.
- Community Health Councils can give advice and information about health services.
- Refugee Council, 3 Bondway, London, SW8 1SJ tel: 020 7820 3038.
- Joint Council for the Welfare of Immigrants (JCWI), 115 Old Street, London, EC1V 9JR tel: 020 7251 8706.

Unfortunately, CPAG is unable to deal with enquiries about benefits directly from members of the public, but if you are an adviser you can phone the advice line from 2-4pm, Monday to Friday on 020 7833 4627. This is a special phone line; do not ring the main CPAG number. Alternatively, you can write to us at the Citizen's Rights Office, CPAG, 94 White Lion Street, London, N1 9PF. We can take up a limited number of test cases including appeals to the Social Security Commissioners or courts.

Advice from the Benefits Agency

You can obtain free telephone advice on benefits on the following number which is for general advice and not specific queries on individual claims:

Enquiry line for people with disabilities 0800 882 200 (in Northern Ireland 0800 220 674), (minicom: 0800 243 355)

If Englsih is not your first language, ask your local Benefits Agency office to arrange for advice in your own language.

Finding help on the Internet

Some information about benefits and a selection of leaflets is available on the Benefits Agency website at www.dss.gov.uk

The RightsNet website at www.rightsnet.org.uk carries details of new legislation and policies affecting social security benefits. It also has links to other useful sites.

Most Acts and Regulations can be found on the central government information website at www.open.gov.uk.

Appendix 5

....

Books, leaflets and periodicals

Many of the books listed here will be in your local public library. Stationary Office books are available from Stationary Office bookshops and also from many others. They may be ordered by post, telephone or fax from The Publications Centre, PO Box 276, London SW8 5DT (tel: 020 7873 9090 fax: 020 7873 8200; general enquiries tel: 020 7873 0011 fax: 020 7873 8247). They also have a website for further information at www.hmso.gov.uk

1. Textbooks

From poor law to community care, Means and Smith 1998 (second edition) (Policy Press). A history of the development of welfare services for older people.
Community Care and the Law, Luke Clements 1997 (Legal Action Group). An overview of the legislation up to and including the Court of Appeal *R v Gloucestershire ex parte Barry*.
Community Care Practice and the Law, Second edition. 1999 Michael Mandelstam (Jessica Kingsley Publishers). A comprehensive guide to both law and practice containing digests of over three hundred legal judgements and ombudsman investigations.
Managing Other People's Money, Second edition 1998 by Penny Letts (Age Concern). A guide to the power available to take over arrangements.
Home from Home: your guide to choosing a care home 1998 (Kings Fund). Suggests questions to ask when choosing a home.

2. Case law and legislation

Welfare Benefits Handbook, (2 vols) (CPAG). Comprehensive interpretation of all social security law.

Encyclopaedia of Social Services and Child Care Law (4 Vols) (Sweet & Maxwell). The legislation affecting social services with some commentary. Loose leaf with regular updates.

Community Care Law Reports (LAG). Quarterly update of legal cases and guidance.

The Law Relating to Social Security, (Stationary Office, looseleaf, 11 vols). All the legislation but without any comment. Known as the 'Blue Book'. Vols 6,7,8, and 22 deal with means-tested benefits.

CPAG's Income Related Benefits: The Legislation, (Mesher) updated by P Wood (Sweet & Maxwell). The most useful legislation with a detailed commentary.

Non-means Tested Benefits: The Legislation, by D Bonner *et al* (Sweet & Maxwell). The legislation with a detailed commentary.

CPAG's Housing Benefit and Council Tax Benefit Legislation, by L Findlay, R Poynter, P Stagg, and M Ward (CPAG). Contains legislation with a detailed commentary.

Medical and Disability Appeal Tribunals: The Legislation, by M Rowland (Sweet & Maxwell). The 3rd edition main volume (1998) of legislation with commentary is available from CPAG, priced £36 incl p&p – if you are a CPAG member. A Supplement to the 3rd edition is published in autumn, priced £17.

The Social Fund: Law and Practice, By T Buck (Sweet & Maxwell). Includes legislation, guidance and commentary. The 2nd edition is available from CPAG from December 1999 priced £46 (prov) incl p&p if you are a CPAG member. Reduced to £42 if ordered from CPAG before 30 July 1999.

Social Fund Directions, are available on the IRS website at www.irssf.demon.co.uk/ssdir.htm.

3. **Official guidance**

Adjudication Officer's Guide (Stationary Office, looseleaf, 13 vols). Vols 4-8 deal with means-tested benefits. Supplementary guidance notes are issued internally – eg, Memo AOG Vol 3/77. Also available on the CAS website at www.cas.gov.uk. (The Central Adjudication Service will be wound down from November 1999 as the decision making and appeal changes are phased in, Therefore, *Adjudication Officers' Guidance* will no longer be in this format.)

Charging for Residential Accommodation Guide, (Department of Health, one vol).

Housing Benefit and Council Tax Benefit Guidance Manual, (Stationery Office, looseleaf).

The Social Fund Guide, (Stationery Office, looseleaf, 2 vols.)

The Social Fund Cold Weather Payments Handbook, (Stationery Office, looseleaf).

4. **Leaflets and booklets**

The Benefits Agency and DSS publish many leaflets which cover particular benefits or particular groups of claimants or contributors, They are free from your local Benefits Agency office, or on Freephone 0800 666 555, or from your local DSS office. If you want to order large numbers of leaflets, you can join the Benefits Agency Publicity Register by contacting the Benefits Agency, 3rd Floor South, 1 Trevelyan Square, Leeds LS1 6EB, tel. 0645 540 000 (local rate). The DSS also has a leaflets Unit at Block 4, Government Buildings, Honeypot Lane, Stanmore, Middlesex HA7 1AY. Free leaflets on HB/CTB are available from the relevant department of your local council.

A selection of leaflets is available on the Benefits Agency Website at www.dss.gov.uk

A Guide to receiving Direct Payments (Department of Health).

A Practical Guide for Disabled People (Department of Health).

Most local authorities also produce a range of leaflets on the services they provide.

5. **Periodicals**

CPAG's *Welfare Rights Bulletin* is published every two months by CPAG. It covers developments in social security law and updates this *Handbook* between editions. The annual subscription is £23 but is sent automatically to CPAG Rights and Comprehensive Members, For subscription and membership details contact CPAG.

Articles on social security and social welfare can also be found in *Legal Action* (Legal Action Group, monthly magazine), the *Journal of Social Security Law* (Sweet & Maxwell, quarterly), and the *Adviser* (NACAB, bimonthly).

Journal of Social Welfare and Family Law, quarterly (Routledge).

Community Care Magazine, weekly.

Appendix 6

Abbreviations used in the notes

References are to statutes and regulations as amended up to 30 November 1999. All regulations are (General) Regulations unless otherwise stated.

reg(s)	regulation(s)	para	paragraph
Sch(s)	Schedule(s)	s(s)	section(s)

Acts of Parliament

B(S)A 1985	Bankruptcy (Scotland) Act 1985
CC(RA)A 1998	Community Care (Residential Accommodation) Act 1998
CCA 1990	Community Care Act 1990
CCDPA 1996	Community Care (Direct Payments) Act 1996
CO(RA)(S)O 1993	Charging Order (Residential Accommodation) (Scotland) Order 1993
CSDPA 1970	Chronically Sick and Disabled Persons Act 1970
DPSCRA 1986	Disabled Persons (Services, Consultation and Representation) Act 1986
H(S)A 1987	Housing (Scotland) Act 1987
HA 1985	Housing Act 1985
HA 1999	Health Act 1999
HASSASSA 1983	The Health and Social Services and Social Security Adjudication Act 1983
HCPA 1995	Hospital Complaints Procedure Act 1995
HGCRA 1996	Housing Grants, Construction and Regeneration Act 1996
HSCA 1993	Health Service Commissioners Act 1993
HSPHA 1948	Health Services and Public Health Act 1948
IA 1986	Insolvency Act 1986
LASSA 1970	Local Authority Social Services Act 1970
LG(S)A 1975	Local Government (Scotland) Act 1975
LGA 1970	Local Government Act 1970

LGA 1974	Local Government Act 1974
MH(S)A 1984	Mental Health Scotland Act 1984
NAA 1948	National Assistance Act 1948
NHS&CCA 1990	National Health Services Act and Community Care Act 1990
NHSA 1977	National Health Services Act 1997
RHA 1984	Registered Homes Act 1984
RHA(Amdt)1991	Registered Homes (Amendment) Act 1991
SSA 1998	Social Security Act 1998
SSAA 1992	Social Security Administration Act 1992
SSCBA 1992	Social Security Contributions and Benefits Act 1992
SW(RP)(S)D 1996	Social Work (Representation Procedure) (Scotland) Directions 1996
SW(S)A 1968	Social Work (Scotland) Act 1968

Regulations

AR Regs	Assessment of Resources Regulations 1992
CB Regs	The Child Benefit (General) Regulations 1976 No. 965
CCDP Regs	Community Care (Direct Payments) Regulations 1997 No. 734
CTB Regs	The Council Tax Benefit (General) Regulations 1992 No. 1814
DP (BMV) Regs	The Disabled Persons (Badges for Motor Vehicles) Regulations 1982
HB Regs	The Housing Benefit (General) Regulations 1987 No. 1971
HB(Amdt) Regs	The Housing Benefit (General) Amendment Regulations 1995 No. 1644
HRA Regs	The Home Repair Assistance Regulations 1996
HRG Reg	The Housing Renewal Grants Regulations 1996
HRG(PF&P) Regs	The Housing Renewal Grants (Prescribed Form and Particulars) Regulations 1996
IRBS(Amdt2) Regs	The Income-related Benefits Schemes (Miscellaneous Amendments) (No.2) Regulations 1995 No. 1339
ISG Regs	The Income Support (General) Regulations 1987 No. 1967
JSA Regs	The Jobseeker's Allowance Regulations 1996 No. 207
NA(AR) Regs	The National Assistance (Assessment and Resources) Regulations 1992 No. 2977

NA(AR)(Amdt 2) Regs	The National Assistance (Assessment and Resources) (Amendment No.2) Regulations 1998 No. 1730
NA(SPR) Regs	The National Assistance (Sums for Personal Requirements) Regulations
NHS(CDA) Regs	The National Health Service (Charges for Drugs and Appliances) Regulations 1980 No. 1503
NHS(DC) Regs	The National Health Service (Dental Charges) Regulations 1989 No. 394
NHS(GOS) Regs	The National Health Service (General Opthalmic Services) Regulations 1986 No. 975
NHS(OCP) Regs	The National Health Service (Optical Charges and Payments) Regulations 1997 No. 818
NHS(TERC) Regs	The National Health Service (Travelling Expenses and Remission of Charges) Regulations 1988 No. 551
RA(RPORE) Regs	The Residential Accommodation (Relevant Premises, Ordinary Residence and Exemptions) Regulations 1993 No. 477
RCH Regs	Residential Care Homes Regulations 1984 No. 1345
SF Regs	The Social Fund Regulations
SFCWP Regs	The Social Fund Cold Weather Payments (General) Regulations 1988 No. 1724
SFM&FE Regs	The Social Fund Maternity and Funeral Expenses (General) Regulations 1987 No. 481
SFWFP	The Social Fund Winter Fuel Payments Regulations 1998 No. 19
SS&CS Regs	The Social Security and Child Support Regulations
SS&CS(D&A) Regs	The Social Security and Child Support (Decisions and Appeals) Regulations 1999 No. 991
SS(AA) Regs	The Social Security (Attendance Allowance) Regulations 1991 No. 2740
SS(C&P) Regs	The Social Security (Claims and Payments) Regulations 1987 No. 1968
SS(CE) Regs	The Social Security (Computation of Earnings) Regulations 1996 No. 2745
SS(DLA) Regs	The Social Security (Disability Living Allowance) Regulations 1992 No. 2890
SS(GB) Regs	The Social Security (General Benefits) Regulations 1982 No. 1408

SS(HIP) Regs	The Social Security (Hospital In-Patients) Regulations 1975 No. 555
SS(IB) Regs	The Social Security (Incapacity Benefit) Regulations 1994 No. 2946
SS(IB)T Regs	The Social Security (Incapacity Benefit) Transitional Regulations 1995 No.310
SS(IB-ID) Regs	The Social Security (Incapacity Benefit – Increases for Dependants) Regulations 1994 No. 2945
SS(ICA) Regs	The Social Security (Invalid Care Allowance) Regulations 1976 No. 409
SS(IFW) Regs	The Social Security (Incapacity for Work) (General) Regulations 1995 No. 311
SS(IIPD) Regs	The Social Security (Industrial Injuries) (Prescribed Diseases) Regulations 1985 No. 967
SS(ME) Regs	The Social Security (Medical Evidence) Regulations 1976 No. 615
SS(OB) Regs	The Social Security (Overlapping Benefits) Regulations 1979 No. 597
SS(PAOR) Regs	The Social Security (Payments on account, Overpayments and Recovery) Regulations 1988 No. 664
SS(SDA) Regs	The Social Security (Severe Disablement Allowance) Regulations 1984 No. 1303
SS(WB&RP) Regs	The Social Security (Widow's Benefit and Retirement Pensions) Regulations 1979 No. 642
SSB(Dep) Regs	The Social Security Benefit (Dependency) Regulations 1977 No. 343

Other information

AA	Attendance allowance
CA	Court of Appeal
CAO	Chief Adjudication Officer
DLA	Disability living allowance
HBRB	Housing Benefit Review Board
HSG	Health Service Guidance
LGOR	Local Government Ombudsman Report
MEL	Management Executive Letter
SBAT	Supplementary Benefit Appeal Tribunal
SBC	Supplementary Benefits Commission
SW(S)G	Social Work Services Group
WOC	Welsh Office Circular

Index

. . . .

How to use this Index

Because the Handbook is divided into separate sections covering the different benefits, many entries in the index have several references, each to a different section. Where this occurs, we use the following abbreviations to show which benefit each reference relates to:

(AA)	Attendance allowance	(C-JSA)	Contribution-based jobseeker's allowance
(CTB)	Council tax benefit	(I-JSA)	Income-based jobseeker's allowance
(DLA)	Disability living allowance		
(DPTC)	Disabled person's tax credit	(JSA)	Jobseeker's allowance
(DWA)	Disability working allowance	(MA)	Maternity allowance
(ETU)	Earnings top-up	(SDA)	Severe disablement alllowance
(FC)	Family credit		
(HB)	Housing benefit	(SF)	Social fund
(IB)	Incapacity benefit	(SMP)	Statutory maternity pay
(ICA)	Invalid care allowance	(SSP)	Statutory sick pay
(IS)	Income support	(WFTC)	Working families' tax credit

Entries against the bold headings direct you to the general information on the subject, or where the subject is covered most fully. Sub-entries are listed alphabetically and direct you to specific aspects of the subject.

Paying for Care Handbook

....

1st edition

Geoff Tait
Pauline Thompson
Helen Winfield
David Simmons

Child Poverty Action Group

Published by CPAG
94 White Lion Street, London N1 9PF

Charity no 294841

© CPAG 2000

A CIP record for this book is available from the British Library.

ISBN 1 901698 24 6

Design by Devious Designs 0114 275 5634
Typeset and printed by Clowes, Beccles, Suffolk